A Life Course Approach to Mental Disorders

A Life Course Approach to Adult Health series

A Life Course Approach to Chronic Disease Epidemiology, Second Edition
Edited by Diana Kuh and Yoav Ben Shlomo
ISBN 9780198578154

A Life Course Approach to Women's Health
Edited by Diana Kuh and Rebecca Hardy
ISBN 9780192632890

Epidemiological Methods in Life Course Research
Edited by Andrew Pickles, Barbara Maughan, and Michael Wadsworth
ISBN 9780198528487

Designing, Analysing and Understanding Family Based Studies in Life Course Epidemiology
Edited by Deborah A. Lawlor and Gita D. Mishra
ISBN 9780199231034

A Life Course Approach to Mental Disorders
Edited by Karestan C. Koenen, Sasha Rudenstine, Ezra Susser, and Sandro Galea
ISBN 9780199657018

A Life Course Approach to Healthy Ageing
Edited by Diana Kuh, Rachel Cooper, Rebecca Hardy, Marcus Richards, and Yoav Ben-Shlomo
ISBN 9780199656516

A Life Course Approach to Mental Disorders

Edited by

Karestan C. Koenen

Sasha Rudenstine

Ezra Susser

Sandro Galea

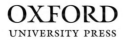

OXFORD
UNIVERSITY PRESS

OXFORD

UNIVERSITY PRESS

Great Clarendon Street, Oxford, OX2 6DP,
United Kingdom

Oxford University Press is a department of the University of Oxford.
It furthers the University's objective of excellence in research, scholarship,
and education by publishing worldwide. Oxford is a registered trade mark of
Oxford University Press in the UK and in certain other countries

Published in the United States of America by Oxford University Press
198 Madison Avenue, New York, NY 10016, United States of America

British Library Cataloguing in Publication Data
Data available

Library of Congress Control Number: 2013940566

ISBN 978-0-19-965701-8

Printed and bound by
CPI Group (UK) Ltd, Croydon, CR0 4YY

Oxford University Press makes no representation, express or implied, that the
drug dosages in this book are correct. Readers must therefore always check
the product information and clinical procedures with the most up-to-date
published product information and data sheets provided by the manufacturers
and the most recent codes of conduct and safety regulations. The authors and
the publishers do not accept responsibility or legal liability for any errors in the
text or for the misuse or misapplication of material in this work. Except where
otherwise stated, drug dosages and recommendations are for the non-pregnant
adult who is not breast-feeding

Links to third party websites are provided by Oxford in good faith and
for information only. Oxford disclaims any responsibility for the materials
contained in any third party website referenced in this work.

Foreword

We coined the term 'life course epidemiology' in the first book in this series (*A life course approach to chronic disease epidemiology*, 1997) to encourage epidemiologists with allegiances to three different models of disease causation (adult lifestyle, fetal origins, and social determinants) to work together to study the long term effects on adult chronic disease risk of physical or social exposures across the whole of life, and across generations. The first book focused on chronic physical disease, although we noted that a life course perspective was applicable to many health and social outcomes. The second and third books in the series (*A life course approach to women's health*, 2002, and the second edition of *A life course approach to chronic disease epidemiology*, 2004) had a greater emphasis on understanding lifetime functional trajectories. Methodological challenges raised were tackled by the fourth book on *Epidemiological methods in life course research* (2007), and extended by the fifth book (*Family matters*, 2009), which showed how family-based studies could help in determining causal associations in life course epidemiology. Most recently, in the latest book *A life course approach to healthy ageing* (2014) we have reviewed the factors across life that optimize well-being and function at the individual, body system and cellular levels; and we highlighted the importance of studying variations in physiological reserve, and social and behavioural adaptability.

From the start, we acknowledged that some of the concepts in life course epidemiology (e.g. trajectories, transitions and turning points) and models (e.g. critical period and chain of risk models) were borrowed from other research fields which had a stronger life course tradition. These included developmental psychopathology and the life span developmental perspective which form the foundations for this book in the series—*A life course approach to mental disorders*. A short historical excursion into these research fields sheds light on today's research priorities in life course epidemiology.

At the beginning of the twentieth century, the 'critical' effects of early life experiences were central to psychoanalysis and behaviourist research (exemplified by the work of Sigmund Freud and John B. Watson), as well as to developmental biology. Interdisciplinary studies of child growth and development emphasized continuity, homogeneity and universality of developmental processes. In the UK, John Bowlby, with his treatise on the effects of maternal care on mental health, continued the psychoanalytical tradition into the post-war era, and influenced the shift from institutional to foster care and the growth of preventive work with families. In the USA, behavioural scientists had a particular impact on social policy in the 1960s when they joined forces with policy-makers to create project Head Start. The central question in the programme's evaluation was whether any long-term benefits were due to the early intervention inoculating the children against failure, as initially expected, or being the start of a chain of positive events.

During the 1960s and 1970s the dominant early life paradigm began to be challenged by reviews of the available evidence suggesting that the timing and nature of the critical stimulus and the critical system affected were poorly defined and, in almost every example, there was also evidence of recovery or resilience. Out of this controversy, the life span developmental perspective in psychology emerged. Its aim was to study constancy and change in human development from birth to death. A role of early life experiences was not denied but the research imbalance was to be redressed by studies that focused on adolescent and adult plasticity, and on the gains as well as the losses of later life. In developmental psychopathology, there was a move away from a simple correlation between child and adult behaviours, with the implicit assumption of some underlying structure that could be irreparably damaged, towards a 'chain of risk' model (exemplified by the research led by Michael Rutter) where one adverse event would make another more likely, and so on. Attention was paid to the heterogeneity of outcomes, factors influencing resilience in the face of adversity, and triggers for discontinuity when chains of risk were broken.

This book brings together the latest conceptual and empirical developments linking back to these two traditions in psychology, while at the same time considering the population causes and consequences of mental disorders within a life course epidemiological perspective. Life course patterns of mental and physical functions and risk of mental disorders differ. However, both physical and mental outcomes in later life are shaped by biological and social factors operating across life, and some risk factors are shared. They also share an exciting research agenda that exploits technological developments to characterize better longitudinal phenotypes and environmental exposures, and attempts to understand why some population subgroups function well, despite an increased lifetime risk factor burden. In designing, implementing and evaluating interventions at key life transitions, both mental and physical health outcomes should be considered together, given the potential bidirectional relationships, and placed within the wider social context to promote an integrated approach to health and social care.

Diana Kuh
Yoav Ben-Shlomo
May 2013

Contents

Contributors

Jessica Agnew-Blais
School of Public Health,
Harvard University,
Boston, MA, USA

Jennifer Ahern
Division of Epidemiology,
School of Public Health,
University of California, Berkeley,
California, USA

Ananda B. Amstadter
Department of Psychiatry,
Virginia Commonwealth University,
Virginia Institute for Psychiatric and
Behavioral Genetics,
Richmond, USA

Katja Beesdo-Baum
Institute of Clinical Psychology and
Psychotherapy,
Technische Universität Dresden,
Dresden, Germany

Elisabeth B. Binder
Max-Planck Institute of Psychiatry,
Munich, Germany and
Department of Psychiatry and Behavioral
Sciences,
Emory University School of Medicine,
Atlanta, Georgia, USA

Bekh Bradley
Atlanta VA Medical Center, and
Department of Psychiatry and Behavioral
Sciences,
Emory University School of Medicine,
Atlanta, Georgia, USA

Michaeline Bresnahan
Mailman School of Public Health,
Columbia University, and
New York State Psychiatric Institute,
New York, USA

Ruth Brown
Department of Psychiatry,
Virginia Commonwealth University,
Virginia Institute for Psychiatric and
Behavioral Genetics,
Richmond, USA

Traolach Brugha
Department of Health Sciences,
University of Leicester, UK

Stephen L. Buka
Department of Epidemiology,
Brown University,
Providence, Rhode Island, USA

Cynthia M. Bulik
Departments of Psychiatry and Nutrition,
University of North Carolina,
Chapel Hill, USA

Mary Cannon
Department of Psychiatry,
Royal College of Surgeons in Ireland, and
Beaumont Hospital,
Dublin, Ireland

Mary Clarke
Departments of Psychiatry and Psychology,
Royal College of Surgeons in Ireland,
Dublin, Ireland

Patricia Cohen
Mailman School of Public Health,
Columbia University,
New York, USA

Ian Colman
Department of Epidemiology and Community
Medicine,
University of Ottawa,
Ottawa, Ontario, Canada

Pam Factor-Litvak
Department of Epidemiology,
Mailman School of Public Health,

Columbia University,
New York, USA

Sandro Galea
Department of Epidemiology,
Mailman School of Public Health,
Columbia University,
New York, USA

Stephen E. Gilman
Department of Social and Behavioral Sciences
and Department of Epidemiology,
Harvard School of Public Health, and
Department of Psychiatry
Massachusetts General Hospital,
Boston, Massachusetts, USA

Renee D. Goodwin
Department of Psychology,
Queens College and The Graduate Center,
City University of New York (CUNY), and
Department of Epidemiology,
Mailman School of Public Health,
Columbia University,
New York, USA

Clyde Hertzman
University of British Columbia,
Vancouver, Canada

Leslie Hulvershorn
Department of Psychiatry,
Indiana University School of Medicine,
Indianapolis, USA

Sara R. Jaffee
University of Pennsylvania, USA, and
King's College London, UK

Peter B. Jones
Department of Psychiatry,
University of Cambridge,
Cambridge, UK

Katherine M. Keyes
Department of Epidemiology,
Mailman School of Public Health,
Columbia University,
New York, USA

Golam M. Khandaker
Department of Psychiatry,

University of Cambridge,
Cambridge, UK

Susanne Knappe
Institute of Clinical Psychology and
Psychotherapy Technische Universität
Dresden,
Dresden, Germany

Karestan C. Koenen
Department of Epidemiology,
Mailman School of Public Health,
Columbia University,
New York, USA

Laura D. Kubzansky
Department of Social and Behavioral
Sciences,
Harvard School of Public Health,
Harvard University,
Boston, USA

Mary E. Lacy
Department of Epidemiology,
Brown University,
Providence, Rhode Island, USA

Hannah H. Leslie
Division of Epidemiology,
School of Public Health,
University of California Berkeley,
California, USA

Leah Li
MRC Centre of Epidemiology for
Child Health,
Institute of Child Health,
University College London,
London, UK

Charley Liu
Department of Epidemiology,
Columbia University,
New York, USA

Jessica R. Marden
Department of Social and Behavioral
Sciences,
Harvard School of Public Health,
Boston, Massachusetts, USA

Lauren M. McGrath
Psychiatric and Neurodevelopmental
Genetics Unit,
Center for Human Genetic Research,
Massachusetts General Hospital,
Boston, Massachusetts, USA

Katie A. McLaughlin
Boston Children's Hospital,
Harvard Medical School,
Harvard Center on the Developing Child,
Boston, USA

Karen S. Mitchell
Women's Health Sciences Division,
National Center for PTSD,
VA Boston Healthcare System, and
Department of Psychiatry,
Boston University,
Massachusetts, USA

Kiyuri Naicker
Department of Epidemiology and
Community Medicine,
University of Ottawa,
Ontario, Canada

Arijit Nandi
Institute for Health and Social Policy and
Department of Epidemiology, Biostatistics,
and Occupational Health,
McGill University,
Montreal, Quebec, Canada

Charles A. Nelson, III
Boston Children's Hospital,
Harvard Medical School,
Harvard Center on the Developing Child,
Boston, USA

Nicole R. Nugent
Department of Psychiatry and Human
Behavior,
Brown Medical School, and
Department of Psychiatry
Rhode Island Hospital,
Providence, USA

John Nurnberger, Jr.
Institute of Psychiatric Research,
Departments of Psychiatry and Medical and

Molecular Genetics,
Indiana University School of
Medicine,
Indianapolis, USA

Candice L. Odgers
Center for Child and Family Policy,
Sanford School of Public Policy,
Duke University,
North Carolina, USA

Demetris Pillas
National Perinatal Epidemiology Unit,
University of Oxford,
Oxford, UK

Kerry Ressler
Department of Psychiatry and Behavioral
Sciences,
Emory University School of Medicine, and
Howard Hughes Medical Institute,
Maryland, USA

Marcus Richards
MRC Unit for Lifelong Health and Ageing,
London, UK

Elise B. Robinson
Department of Epidemiology,
Harvard School of Public Health,
Boston, Massachusetts, USA

Sasha Rudenstine
Department of Epidemiology,
Mailman School of Public Health,
Columbia University,
New York, USA

Susan L. Santangelo
Department of Epidemiology,
Harvard School of Public Health,
Boston, Massachusetts, USA

Larry J. Seidman
Commonwealth Research Center,
Massachusetts Mental Health Center Public
Psychiatry Division
of the Beth Israel Deaconess
Medical Center, and
Department of Psychiatry,
Harvard Medical School,
Boston, Massachusetts, USA

Margaret A. Sheridan
Boston Children's Hospital,
Harvard Medical School,
Harvard Center on the Developing Child,
Boston, USA

Levent Sipahi
Center for Molecular Medicine and Genetics,
Wayne State University,
Detroit, Michigan, USA

Kelly Skelton
Atlanta VA Medical Center, and
Department of Psychiatry and Behavioral
Sciences,
Emory University School of Medicine,
Atlanta, Georgia, USA

Andrew E. Skodol
Department of Psychiatry,
Columbia University College of Physicians
and Surgeons, and
Department of Psychiatry,
University of Arizona College of Medicine,
Tucson, Arizona, USA

Dan J. Stein
Department of Psychiatry,
University of Cape Town,
Cape Town, South Africa

Kelcey Stratton
Hunter Holmes McGuire VA Medical Center,
and Department of Psychology,
Virginia Commonwealth University,
Richmond, USA

Ezra Susser
Departments of Epidemiology and Psychiatry,
Mailman School of Public Health,
Columbia University, and
New York State Psychiatric Institute,
New York, USA

Monica Uddin
Center for Molecular Medicine and Genetics,
Department of Psychiatry and Behavioral
Neurosciences,
Wayne State University,
Detroit, Michigan, USA

Virginia Warner
New York State Psychiatric Institute,
New York, USA

Myrna M. Weissman
Department of Psychiatry,
Columbia University College of Physician and
Surgeons and
Department of Epidemiology,
Mailman School of Public Health,
New York State Psychiatric Institute,
New York, USA

Lauren Welsh
McGill University,
Montreal, Quebec, Canada

Ashley Winning
Department of Social and Behavioral
Sciences,
Harvard School of Public Health,
Harvard University,
Boston, USA

Part 1

Introduction

Chapter 1

Life course approaches to mental illness: the emergence of a concept

Karestan C. Koenen, Sasha Rudenstine, Ezra Susser, and Sandro Galea

A life course approach to mental disorders is concerned with the interplay of social and biological factors in the production and consequences of mental illness over the life span—from the prenatal period to death and across generations. As described by Drs Kuh and Ben-Shlomo in the Preface, the life course approach to mental disorders draws on two foundations: the psychological life span perspective and the developmental psychopathology perspective. A life course epidemiological approach applies these perspectives to understand the distribution, causes, and consequences of mental disorders in human populations. Life course epidemiology is inherently interdisciplinary, drawing on expertise from fields ranging from basic neuroscience to sociology. However, the focus on populations and implications for public health and prevention distinguishes the life course epidemiology of mental disorders from other fields interested in similar questions, such as developmental psychology and child psychiatry.

Research on the life course epidemiology of mental disorders has long historical roots, exemplified by the study of the Dutch Hunger Winter published in the 1970s.[1] In the past twenty years, however, we have seen an explosion in research on the life course epidemiology of mental disorders motivated by three factors. The first is the ageing into adulthood of numerous birth cohorts.[2] Research grounded in these cohorts has provided increasing evidence that mental disorders previously perceived to emerge in adulthood have their origins early in life. For example, periconceptional exposure to famine has been strongly linked to schizophrenia (see Chapter 6), and reports also suggest that prenatal famine may be linked to mood disorder (see Chapter 8) and antisocial personality disorder (see Chapter 15).[1,3–8] Early childhood factors, such as childhood adversity, have been linked to new onsets of mental disorders throughout the life course.[9] Data from prospective birth cohorts have documented that new onsets of mental disorders in adulthood are, in fact, the exception. When careful prospective assessments are available, it appears that the majority of adults with mental disorders will have had a mental disorder by age 15 years.[10]

The second factor involves the integration of biological measures into extant cohorts made possible by rapid advances in technology that make the collection and analysis of biological samples feasible and inexpensive. Although the importance of gene–environment interplay in the production of mental disorders has been recognized for more than a century, researchers have not, until relatively recently, had the tools to be able to study that interplay. Inspired largely by the highly original work of Caspi et al.,[11] research on the examination of gene–environment interaction over the life course has mushroomed over the past decade. A search on PubMed using the terms 'gene environment interaction mental disorder' produced almost 600 papers since 2002 versus only 40 prior to that year. Until recently, such research focused on a limited number of candidate genes, but robust findings from large scale genomics studies has also begun to open further opportunities for research on gene–environment interplay over the life course (see Chapters 18 and 24).

The third factor that has motivated research on the life course epidemiology of mental disorders is the revolution in our understanding of the mechanisms through which external environmental exposures get 'under the skin' and cause disease. Groundbreaking work by Nelson and colleagues on Romanian orphans documented the effects of extreme childhood adversity on brain development early in life and the relation between these effects and the emergence of psychopathology (see Chapter 23). This research has motivated work examining the impact of more common adverse exposures, such as poverty in US children, on brain development and the emergence of mental disorders. Such work has been critical in providing a neurobiological basis for findings from cohort studies documenting the relation between early childhood adversity and increased risk of mental disorders. No less important has been the growth in research on epigenetic mechanisms and mental disorders (Chapter 22). Broadly epigenetic mechanisms regulate gene function without the alteration of underlying DNA sequence[11] and are known to change in response to individuals' physical, biological, and social exposures in a manner that influences the long-term regulation of gene expression.[12] The field of epigenetics has made the study of gene–environment interplay truly possible by enabling researchers to examine a mechanism via which environmental exposures change gene expression.

As the body of research in the field grows, our foundational texts on life course approaches to mental disorders have not kept pace. We have been struck by how the profound transformation in our understanding of the origins of mental disorders through research is not yet reflected in our training, policy or practice in population health. There currently exists no single source that has brought this research together with the goal of forging a consensus on the current state and the important next steps for the field. This book therefore aims to be first comprehensive articulation of a life course perspective on mental disorders. The book brings together researchers across disparate disciplines—epidemiology, developmental psychopathology, psychiatric genetics, sociology, developmental cognitive neuroscience—to review the methods and synthesize the existing knowledge about the life course epidemiology of mental disorders in populations. This book also considers research on mechanisms driving the production of mental disorders and emerging areas of research. The goal of this book is to bring together the state of the science of life course epidemiology to inform training, research, practice, and policy with regard to mental disorders.

The book is divided into six parts. Part One is this introduction, which gives an overview of the book. Part Two provides a current, state-of-the-science review of the methods used in the life course epidemiology of mental disorders. Although the prospective cohort study, and particularly the birth cohort study, is the design that lends itself most easily to life course questions, Chapter 2 also discusses case–control studies, including nested case–control studies within larger cohorts, cross-sectional studies, quasi-experimental designs, and randomized controlled trials in relation to how such designs may be applied to life course research using examples of well-known studies. An important methodological area in life course research is measurement, which is the focus of Chapter 3. The author gives an overview of the broad areas that may be measured including environmental risks, biological assays and archival data, discusses the challenge of assessment of mental disorders in the face of developmental change, and reviews the practical issues of training good interviewers. Chapter 4 focuses on the analysis of longitudinal data within subjects and the specific issues raised by such data including missingness due to attrition and non-normal distributions. The author describes some of the different models, including growth curve and random effects models, that can be used for study designs with repeated measures of risk and protective factors, as well as mental disorders in the same participants over time. Chapter 5 provides a clear explanation of the distinction between age, period, and cohort effects and why they are important for life course studies of mental disorders using the examples of major depression, substance use disorders, and autism spectrum disorders to illustrate age, period, and cohort effects.

Part Three is divided into eleven individual chapters that review the scientific literature on the life course epidemiology for either a major mental disorder or class of disorders. Chapter 6 focuses on schizophrenia, reviewing the literature regarding putative mechanisms and early life risk factors as manifest from conception to onset of illness. Chapter 7 discusses the phenomenology and aetiology of bipolar disorder over the life course and concludes with recommendations for future directions in the field. Chapter 8 reviews the characteristics of depression that lend themselves to a life course analytic perspective, discusses individual risk factors for both depression's onset and trajectory, and addresses the multifactorial nature of depression. Chapter 9 examines the prevalence, correlates, risk factors, trajectory, and treatment of anxiety disorders other than post-traumatic stress disorder. The chapter includes a discussion of the implications of a life course approach on the epidemiology of anxiety disorders for clinical work, public health, and future research. Chapter 10 uses a life course approach to summarize the distribution and patterns of exposure to traumatic events and associated development of post-traumatic stress disorder with particular attention to socio-cultural context. Chapter 11 reviews existing research on the life course of substance use in the areas of timing of substance use onset, early life determinants, trajectories, broader contexts, and historical periods. Chapter 12 reviews methodological issues prominent in autism research and then focuses on the actual and potential contributions of a life course approach to key areas of research in this disorder. Chapter 13 challenges the stereotype that eating disorders are only a problem among young women by reviewing the evidence on the prevalence and distribution of such disorders over the life course. Chapter 14 discusses the attention deficit hyperactivity disorder symptom profile, gender breakdown, comorbidities, and associated problems, risk factors, persistence into adolescence and adulthood, and methodological issues in studying this disorder. Chapter 15 synthesizes the literature on conduct disorder with a focus on the developmental course, attention to taxonomic issues as well as predictors and sequelae of different trajectories of conduct problems and concludes by describing implications for public health. Chapter 16 focuses on personality disorders, challenging the traditional view that such disorders are stable over time by reviewing data from studies of their naturalistic course. Part Three ends with Chapter 17 that examines lifetime risk of cognitive disorder, highlighting key influences across this trajectory, from conception into childhood, adulthood, and old age.

Part Four of the book examines potential mechanisms underlying the production of mental disorders. The genomics revolution over the past decade has driven large scale investigations of the genetic architecture of mental disorders. These efforts have determined that the genetic architecture of all major mental disorders is highly polygenic and likely overlaps across diagnosis.[12] Chapter 18 describes how the tools of genetic epidemiology may be used to address life course questions such as whether the genetic contribution to mental disorders varies over the life course. The book then turns to environmental exposures starting with pre- and postnatal exposures in Chapter 19, which focuses on summarizing the adverse associations between both pre- and postnatal exposure to environmental lead and a variety of cognitive and behavioural outcomes over the life course. Chapter 20 systematically reviews the evidence linking exposures in the individual-level social environment over the life course with the risk of psychiatric disorders. The authors discuss the specificity of the associations between environmental exposures and subsequent psychiatric disorders, the consistency of associations with disorder onset and disorder recurrence, the clustering of environmental exposures, and the implications of these findings for clinical practice. The focus on environmental exposures then moves from the individual to the macro-social level in Chapter 21 where the authors examine evidence for the role of contextual factors, such as neighbourhoods, in the production of mental disorders over the life course.

The next three chapters examine mechanisms via which external environmental factors 'get under the skin', resulting in neurobiological alterations that produce mental disorders. Chapter 22 discusses emerging developments in the field of epigenetics as applied to mental disorders. Chapter 23 examines adverse childhood experiences and brain development, with a focus on the influence of maltreatment, institutional rearing, and poverty or socio-economic status. Chapter 24 brings together, based on the previous chapters, evidence for the interplay of social and biological factors including evidence from animal models and human studies.

Part Five focuses on new directions in the life course epidemiology of mental illness. Chapter 25 describes the new developments in research from three generation cohort studies and the implications of findings from these studies for our understanding of the intergenerational transmission of mental disorder. Chapter 26 examines the role of mental disorders in physical health over the life course with a focus on cardiovascular health.

As noted in the beginning of this chapter, this book was motivated by a desire to bring together research on the life course epidemiology of mental disorders from a variety of disciplines in order to inform not only research but training, policy, and practice. The implications of a life course approach are summarized in the conclusion of the book, Part Six, Chapter 27, which highlights the implications of a life course approach for public health.

We aimed this book to be a text on the life course approaches to mental disorders that can inform our training, policy, and practice. We realize that this goal is subject to limitations, but hope that *A Life Course Approach to Mental Disorders* may nevertheless catalyse our collective discussion and contribute to the growth of the field.

References

1 **Stein AD, Pierik FH, Verrips GH, Susser ES, Lumey LH.** Maternal exposure to the Dutch famine before conception and during pregnancy: quality of life and depressive symptoms in adult offspring. *Epidemiology* 2009;**20**(6):909–915.

2 **Susser E, Terry MB, Matte T.** The birth cohorts grow up: new opportunities for epidemiology. *Paediatr Perinat Epidemiol* 2000;**14**(2):98–100.

3 **Susser E, Terry MB.** A conception-to-death cohort. *Lancet* 2003;**361**(9360):797–798.

4 **St Clair D, Xu M, Wang P, et al.** Rates of adult schizophrenia following prenatal exposure to the Chinese famine of 1959–1961. *JAMA* 2005;**294**(5):557–562.

5 **Susser E, St Clair D.** Prenatal famine and adult mental illness: interpreting concordant and discordant results from the Dutch and Chinese Famines. *Social Sci Med* 2013 Mar 7 [Epub ahead of print].

6 **Xu MQ, Sun WS, Liu BX, et al.** Prenatal malnutrition and adult schizophrenia: further evidence from the 1959–1961 Chinese famine. *Schizophr Bull* 2009;**35**(3):568–576.

7 **Brown AS, van Os J, Driessens C, Hoek HW, Susser ES.** Further evidence of relation between prenatal famine and major affective disorder. *Am J Psychiatry* 2000;**157**(2):190–195.

8 **Neugebauer R, Hoek HW, Susser E.** Prenatal exposure to wartime famine and development of antisocial personality disorder in early adulthood. *JAMA* 1999;**282**:455–462.

9 **Kessler RC, McLaughlin KA, Green JG, et al.** Childhood adversities and adult psychopathology in the WHO World Mental Health Surveys. *Br J Psychiatry* 2010;**197**(5):378–385.

10 **Kim-Cohen J, Caspi A, Moffitt TE, Harrington H, Milne BJ, Poulton R.** Prior juvenile diagnoses in adults with mental disorder: developmental follow-back of a prospective-longitudinal cohort. *Arch Gen Psychiatry* 2003;**60**(7):709–717.

11 **Caspi A, McClay J, Moffitt TE, et al.** Role of genotype in the cycle of violence in maltreated children. *Science* 2002;**297**(5582):851–854.

12 **Purcell SM, Wray NR, Stone JL, et al.** Common polygenic variation contributes to risk of schizophrenia and bipolar disorder. *Nature* 2009;**460**(7256):748–752.

Part 2

Methods in life course approaches

Chapter 2

Study designs: traditional and novel approaches to advance life course research

Stephen L. Buka and Mary E. Lacy

2.1 Introduction

2.1.1 Goals in life course studying mental illness

A life course approach provides a framework to understand the interactions of multiple determinants of health and disease across the lifespan. The theories underlying life course approaches are varied, but each emphasizes the importance of understanding the occurrence and accrual of risk over time and how these contribute to the development of psychopathology.[1-3] A number of key questions can be addressed using life course epidemiology that would otherwise be difficult to ascertain: from furthering our understanding of familial and genetic contributions to the aetiology of mental disorders (see Chapter 25), to exploring the natural course of mental disorders in varying populations (see Chapter 5), to examining the role of social and environmental factors in mental disorders (see Chapters 19–21), the use of a life course framework has greatly advanced the field of psychiatric epidemiology.

In psychiatric epidemiology, as in other disciplines, we have come to understand that few, if any, events occur in isolation.[4,5] Hence, the central focus in life course epidemiology is on the occurrence and accrual of risk conditions at multiple levels. For example, the probability that two male infants will develop major depressive disorder (MDD) may diverge due to a number of subtle environmental differences that each encounters over the course of his life. In a recent editorial, Stephen Gilman described life course and developmental epidemiology as 'shar[ing] the fundamental principles that health at any given point in time is substantially influenced by prior circumstances, and that disease processes unfold through a combination of risks operating at multiple levels—ranging from genetic inheritance and psychological vulnerability to social conditions.'[6]

Epidemiological research advances through a variety of traditional and more recently developed study designs.[7,8] Each study design represents a different approach to common research questions and has implications for the ways in which participants are selected and information is collected and analysed. The design chosen by a researcher is influenced by many factors, driven by the research question being posed along with considerations of cost, efficiency, and ethical and practical considerations.[7,9] While many epidemiological questions can be addressed through a large number of alternative designs, many of these have limited utility for issues at the core of a life course approach to the aetiology of mental disorders.

2.1.2 **Framework for this chapter**

This chapter reviews the major design options for studying psychiatric disorders across the life course. The organization is by study design and describes major features of each design approach, key instances of each design, and potential challenges and limitations associated with each design. To limit the scope of this chapter, we highlight key studies that have assessed formal psychiatric diagnoses. Study designs included are: (i) prospective cohort studies (general prospective cohort studies, perinatal/birth cohorts, and high risk prospective cohort studies); (ii) case–control studies, including nested case–control studies within larger cohorts; (iii) cross-sectional studies; (iv) quasi-experimental designs; and (v) randomized controlled trials (RCTs). Although certain design strategies, namely prospective cohort studies, lend themselves more readily to the life course approach, we have chosen to describe other study designs that can also be used to further our understanding of psychiatric epidemiology from the life course perspective. The chapter concludes with remarks on general considerations for designing life course studies, as well as recommendations for future directions of the field.

> One of the classic topics in life course epidemiology is the relationship between socioeconomic status (SES) and mental health. Over the past century, this question has been examined using a variety of different study designs in an effort to more thoroughly probe the potential causal link between social conditions and the aetiology of mental disorder. As the chapter progresses, we use this topic to illustrate the ways in which various threats to the validity of a claim for causality manifest themselves under different study designs. For the purposes of a clear illustration we focus on diagnosed depression as our outcome.

2.2 **Major design options**

In the epidemiological literature, studies are typically grouped into observational and experimental studies.[7,10]

2.2.1 **Observational**

The majority of life course studies of psychiatric disorders are observational studies.[10] As compared with experimental studies, in which exposures are randomly assigned to study participants, in observational designs the investigator observes and records data on a group of people, with no active manipulation of exposure conditions, generating information on the relationships between exposure and disease as they naturally unfold. While the causal inferences that can be derived from observational studies are typically not as strong as those in experimental studies, observational studies are free from the ethical dilemmas associated with allocating exposure in experimental designs. Observational studies typically take two forms: cohort studies or case–control studies; each form has a number of variations that are now discussed in detail.

2.2.1.1 Cohort studies

In epidemiology, a prospective cohort study is one in which participants are enrolled in a study before the outcome of interest has occurred and are then followed for a period of time. This study design is one of the preferred design options for studying mental health across the life course because it allows for direct measurement of both exposures and outcomes as they occur, providing strong evidence for temporality of exposure–disease relationships. There remain, however, many important design considerations, challenges, and limitations in the design and conduct of such studies.

In a prospective cohort study, participants are often selected to be representative of a larger population of interest—defining the relevant population of interest is central to designing a maximally informative prospective cohort study. In some instances, the population may be defined by the set of key exposures of interest—e.g. a pregnancy, school-age or midlife cohort. In others, the most informative population may be those at elevated risk of developing disease, e.g. family history of disorder, certain environmental exposures. If an investigator has multiple outcomes of interest, it can be difficult to identify specific subpopulations at risk of disease, in which case a more general population may be most appropriate.

Data are collected in order to provide information on the outcomes that are the focus for the study; the implications for this are particularly important in a prospective study because, as the cohort ages, an investigator may wish that additional data had been prospectively collected on another exposure or disease.[11] Additionally, decisions related to study design and data collection are made relative to the science of the field when the study is initiated. This phenomenon is referred to as the scientific period effect.[11,12] It has become a truism that many of the greatest discoveries of long-term prospective cohort studies were not anticipated at the time of initiation, and, as a corollary to this scientific period effect, that certain data (such as genetic material) that become relevant at a later scientific time are overlooked at the onset of earlier projects.

Another key consideration in designing a prospective cohort study is minimizing study drop-out and loss to follow-up. Given the long-term follow-up in prospective cohort studies, it is especially important to consider procedures to minimize study drop-out and loss to follow-up during the planning phase. A number of strategies have been used in previous studies to minimize study attrition: collection of detailed contact information, sending reminders of follow-up interviews, and sharing study findings with participants in the form of newsletters or bulletins.[12,13]

Prospective cohort studies: socio-economic status and depression across the life course Using data from nearly 40 years of follow-up, Gilman et al. examined the relationship between SES in childhood and the lifetime risk for major depression.[14] They found that participants who had lower SES in childhood had a nearly two-fold increase in risk of lifetime major depression compared with those from the highest SES category, after controlling for a number of potential confounders. This study exemplifies the value of prospective cohort studies to advance causal inference in the absence of experimentation: it clearly establishes temporality of exposure (childhood SES) and outcome (lifetime depression), it uses a valid measure to identify diagnoses of depression (DSM-III and -IV diagnoses), and it takes into account a number of important factors that could potentially confound the true association between SES and depression. However, despite the study's many strengths, because it is an observational study, there remain a number of potential threats to validity. Typically, selection bias is one of the greatest threats to the validity of an observational study. In this case, however, because exposure (childhood SES) is out of the control of study participants, the threat of selection bias may be less pronounced than in other instances (e.g. choice of marital partner), which is more influenced by the individual. Information bias is also reduced in this example, as diagnoses of depression were generated independent of knowledge of family socio-economic circumstances. Finally, there remains the potential that there is residual and unmeasured confounding. It would be impossible to measure every potential confounder that occurs over the more than forty years that the study spans and, further, the study was not designed solely to address this particular research question. In any study with such a wide scope and with multiple decades of follow-up, there is always the possibility that an important potential confounder was overlooked or was not adequately measured.

2.2.1.2 Examples of major prospective cohort studies of mental disorder

There are several important and well-known general prospective cohort studies examining psychiatric disorders across the life course. Due to space limitations we summarize the considerations and decisions made for two recent study designs.

The Netherlands Mental Health Survey and Incidence Studies (NEMESIS-I and -II) These studies serve as excellent examples of the unique type of question that can be answered, as well as the unique challenges that arise in conducting a nationally representative, prospective cohort study. Both studies employed a three-wave prospective cohort design and were designed to enrol a nationally representative sample of the Dutch population in terms of gender, age, ethnicity, and urbanicity. NEMESIS-I utilized a multistage, stratified random sampling framework to enroll a cohort of participants that were representative of the Dutch population; a total of 7,076 participants was enrolled in the study, with baseline data collected in 1996 and follow-up data collected at 12 months (n = 5,618) and 36 months after baseline (n = 4,796).[15] NEMESIS-II utilized a sampling framework similar to that of NEMESIS-I to enrol a nationally representative sample; 6,646 participants completed baseline interviews from 2007 to 2009.[16] Similar to NEMESIS-I, NEMESIS-II is designed to have a total of three waves of data collection; however, a longer follow-up period between the waves (three years) was chosen for NEMESIS-II. As such, data from waves 1 and 2 have not yet been publicized. For both studies, in-person interviews were conducted in the home using the Composite International Diagnostic Interview (CIDI; version 1.1 for NEMESIS-I and version 3.0 for NEMESIS-II) with diagnoses based on the *Diagnostic and Statistical Manual of Mental Disorders* (DSM-III-R for NEMESIS-I and DSM-IV for NEMESIS-II).[15–18] Both NEMESIS studies share similar aims of providing data on the prevalence, incidence, and course of mental disorders in the Dutch population, as well as providing a framework for studying financial and healthcare burden of mental disorders in The Netherlands. Further, the two cohorts are separated by the span of a decade, thus providing information on trends in mental disorders and service utilization in The Netherlands. Founded on these shared aims, the scope of the study was expanded for NEMESIS-II to enable researchers to assess a broader range of diagnoses in the Dutch population and the study was also designed to collect genetic information on participants. Being able to do a side-by-side comparison of these two studies with such similar structure and aims allows for a useful discussion of some key design considerations and potential challenges. As evidenced by the changes made from NEMESIS-I to NEMESIS-II, the investigators were able to use NEMESIS-I not only to answer proposed research questions, but also to better define the scope of their research and further perfect their study protocol. NEMESIS-II was expanded to include collection of genetic data and was designed to have a longer length of time between follow-ups. This change in study design would allow for a more in-depth understanding of the natural course and familial characteristics of mental illness in the Dutch population.

Challenges and limitations Prospective cohort studies have contributed greatly to our understanding of the prevalence and distribution of mental disorders, the course of disorders across
time and information related to utilization of mental health services. They have also been useful
in illustrating a number of the challenges and limitations associated with carrying out a long-term
prospective cohort study. Considerable human and fiscal resources are needed to enrol, track,
and retain participants, and to carry out meaningful follow-up for such a long span of time. These
challenges are especially prominent in life course studies of mental illness, due to the time and
effort needed to accurately assess psychiatric outcomes and the multiple potential contributing
risk and protective factors that operate at multiple levels of influence (from molecular to societal)
on the initiation and progression of psychopathology. In addition, as in all observational studies,
the designers of cohort studies must anticipate concerns about both imprecisely measured and
unmeasured confounding which can undermine the utility of such efforts. Faced with limited
resources, investigators must balance breadth, depth, and the size of such cohorts: breadth in
terms of the range of contributing conditions and potential confounds assessed; depth regarding
the length and intensity of assessment; and size in terms of the number of participants enrolled.
Informative cohort studies have ranged from hundreds to hundreds of thousands of participants with commensurate trade-offs between statistical power, on the one hand, and richness of
data regarding the multiple complex developmental trajectories that may eventually manifest as
mental disorder.

Finite resources demand additional trade-offs between cohort enrolment versus retention.
Successful cohort studies not only need a rich array of data regarding potential risk factors and
psychiatric outcomes, but meaningful inference also requires a high level of retention and protection against threats to validity resulting from attrition and resulting selection bias. While some
attrition is inevitable, considerable creative effort and investment in subject retention is necessary
to ensure that costly cohort studies yield data of maximal scientific utility. While this applies for
cohort studies in general, the close relationship between many forms of mental disorder and
social engagement (such as participation in a prospective cohort study) poses a particularly serious challenge for life course studies of mental illness. The extent to which attrition is also associated with risk conditions of interest may irrevocably reduce the potential of cohort studies to
generate unbiased estimates of interest.

Despite these challenges, however, cohort studies will remain at the forefront of design options
to advance understanding of mental illness and the life course.

2.2.1.3 Perinatal and birth cohorts

In addition to the general design features of a prospective cohort study, in a birth or perinatal
cohort there are additional challenges involved with recruiting and enrolling participants at
or before birth. Parents are the primary target for recruitment and, depending on the length
of follow-up, parents may serve as the primary respondent even though the cohort of interest comprises the offspring generation. In a perinatal cohort study, the emphasis is on factors
that occur in the months immediately prior to and following birth. Therefore, studies of this
design typically will recruit and enrol parents (usually mothers) who are pregnant or planning to become pregnant in the near future. Data are generally collected on mother and fetus
throughout the pregnancy, at birth and for a defined length of time following birth. In a birth
cohort, investigators typically design a sampling scheme to target births that occur in a specific
geographic region within a specified period of time. For both perinatal and birth cohorts, the
length of follow-up is determined by the research questions being posed and the resources
available for the study.

Issues related to data collection are another unique concern for perinatal and birth cohorts. While parents may serve as the primary respondent during the child's infancy and toddler years, it is possible to collect data directly on very young children. Special consideration, however, must be given to the length and appropriateness of data collection procedures, training of interviewers, and study consent and assent procedures to ensure adequate protection of human subjects.

Over the years, birth and perinatal cohorts have proved an invaluable source of information in the study of the life course of psychiatric disorders. This study design enables investigators to examine the impact of the foetal, infant and early childhood experience on mental health outcomes across the life course. We now describe two influential perinatal and birth cohorts, again limiting our scope to studies that have generated psychiatric diagnoses.

The Collaborative Perinatal Project (CPP) and New England Family Study (NEFS) The CPP was initiated more than 50 years ago to investigate prospectively the prenatal and familial antecedents of paediatric, neurological, and psychological disorders of childhood. Nationwide, 12 university–affiliated medical centres participated, including two in New England (in Boston and Providence). More than 50,000 pregnancies were enrolled between 2 January 1959 and 31 December 1965 (16,557 in the NEFS sites).[19,20] The study followed up 88% of survivors at 1 year, 75% at 4 years and 79% at 7 years.

Data from examinations and interviews were recorded by trained staff at each site beginning at the time of registration for prenatal care, using standardized protocols, forms, manuals, and codes. At the first prenatal visit, a complete reproductive and gynaecological history, recent and past medical history, socio-economic interview, and family history were recorded. A socio-economic index was assigned to each pregnancy, adapted from the Bureau of the Census and derived from education and occupation of the head of household along with household income.[21] Prenatal clinic visits were scheduled monthly during the first 7 months of pregnancy, every 2 weeks during the 8th month, and every week thereafter. Blood samples were collected for serology and for storage of frozen sera. After admission for delivery, trained observers recorded the events of labour and delivery, and the obstetrician completed labour and delivery protocols. Approximately 75% of subjects had cord blood samples drawn and stored. The neonate was observed in the delivery room, examined by a paediatrician at 24 h intervals in the newborn nursery, and received a neurological examination at 2 days. Study offspring received five subsequent assessments: at ages 4, 8, and 12 months, and 4 and 7 years. At each follow-up examination the mother was interviewed about the child's interval history, records of medical treatment obtained if appropriate, and physical measurements were taken. Paediatric–neurological examinations occurred at 4 and 12 months and at 7 years; and psychological examinations at 8 months, and at 4 and 7 years. Family and social history information was obtained from the mother at intake and at 7 years. Diagnostic summaries were prepared by study physicians following the 12-month and 7-year assessments.

The Boston and Providence CPP cohorts comprised 16,557 births. Adult follow-up of these two New England CPP cohorts began in 1983 with the Providence sample (4140 pregnancies).[22] The first major study selected about 500 infants born with moderate perinatal complications and 500 matched comparison subjects, and conducted standardized psychiatric diagnostic assessments at mean age 23 years.[23] The generally null results indicated no elevated risk for psychiatric disorder in relation to perinatal complications, with two exceptions. Infants born with conditions suggestive of chronic foetal hypoxia were at marginally elevated risk for both cognitive impairment and psychotic disorders, including schizophrenia. The roles of perinatal complications, infections during pregnancy and family history of psychosis have been investigated in multiple projects involving both the Providence and Boston sites.[24-26] This work resulted in the first uses of stored CPP maternal serum samples relative to adult outcomes, including the initial serologically based finding of elevated maternal antibodies[27] and cytokine levels[28] in relation to subsequent psychosis. These schizophrenia projects now include more than 1000 CPP cohort members with and without psychotic disorders and incorporate detailed clinical diagnostic, neuropsychological, structural and functional imaging procedures, and more.[29,30]

In recent years, this team has extended the follow-up and assessment of three-generation pedigrees (i.e. CPP mothers, their offspring who comprise the CPP cohort members, and the offspring of the CPP cohort members). These projects all seek to integrate family designs with early life risk conditions, capitalizing upon the large number of cohort members with multiple offspring. With the increased emphasis on family designs, the overall effort was renamed 'The New England Family Study' (NEFS).

2.2.1.4 High risk cohort

The high risk cohort study is a variation on the general prospective cohort study described above, with the key distinction being that subjects are recruited because they have been selected on the basis of their exposure history. Often, subjects are identified as being at high risk for developing the outcome of interest based on manifestations of psychopathology in their parents. Given the familial nature of psychiatric disorders, in psychiatric epidemiology, high risk studies often take the form of multi-generation family studies.

Studies such as these allow researchers to better examine the natural history of psychiatric disorders in relation to parental mental illness. One potential limitation of high risk studies, however, is that their results, and, ultimately, the conclusions they draw, may only be applicable for high risk populations. By contrast, high risk studies do provide an efficient means of examining relatively rare disorders.

High risk cohort studies: the example of SES and depression A landmark investigation into the relationship between SES and depression utilizing a high risk cohort was conducted by Ritsher et al.[31] These investigators drew upon the well-known cohort developed by Weissman et al.[32] which included a sizeable number of parents with major depressive disorder (MDD—recruited from a treatment centre) and a group-matched sample of parents without MDD recruited randomly from the same community. In this high risk design, the offspring cohort was selected for and classified according to presence or absence of parental depression. Analyses examined the occurrence of MDD among offspring with respect to parent SES while adjusting for parent MDD. The high risk design ensured a large number of parents with and without MDD and a powerful method to examine the influence of parental SES, independent of the potentially confounding influence of parent MDD. Analyses revealed a strong and consistent association between low parental education and subsequent onset of MDD among offspring, in support of a 'social causation' model. Neither parental depression nor the offspring's own depression predicted downward drift in educational attainment, occupational status, or income, failing to support the model of 'social drift'. Using this high risk design to control for the well-established intergenerational transmission of MDD, this investigation demonstrated that low parental SES results in a more than tripled risk of MDD among offspring and highlighted the role of the social environment in the aetiology of MDD, whether or not genetic vulnerability is present.

High risk cohorts have been developed for most major forms of psychopathology, including schizophrenia, depression, and substance use disorders. We provide one example from our work in schizophrenia.

Schizophrenia: high risk component of the New England Family Study The New England Family Study (NEFS) included the offspring of 13,464 women whose pregnancies were studied between 1959 and 1966.[33] Buka et al.[24] followed up a subsample of the NEFS cohort for a study of families at high risk for psychosis. The goal of this study was to ascertain about 200 of the original mothers and fathers who had psychoses and a comparable group of unaffected parents to examine the combined influence of parental psychosis and perinatal risk factors on the development of psychopathology in adult offspring. The details of parent ascertainment and diagnoses are described in Goldstein et al.[29] From a total pool of 26,928 parents, 859 with a history of psychiatric treatment were identified through prior record review and record linkage with private and public psychiatric treatment facilities. Unaffected parents were selected to be comparable with affected parents based on a number of factors including parent's age, ethnicity, and G2 offspring's age, sex, and history of prenatal complications. (This last factor was included to enable maximum capacity to investigate the interaction between parent diagnosis and birth complications in relation to offspring status).

2.2.1.5 Case–control

Unlike the study designs we have described up to this point in which participants are recruited into the study and followed over time to ascertain their outcome status, in a case–control study, participants are selected based on presence or absence of a disorder and exposure data are obtained after the outcome has been ascertained. Although case–control studies are not the strongest design option for conducting life course psychiatric research, this particular study design has a number of benefits.[34] Because participants are selected after the outcome of interest has occurred, case–control studies are typically extremely cost-effective, especially in studying rare diseases. As compared with cohort studies, in which the investigator may need to follow a large number of participants for years to identify the outcome of interest, in a case–control study the outcome has already occurred and the investigator seeks to determine those exposures or conditions that may have contributed to this occurrence. This, however, leads us to one of the most important potential limitations of this study design: the threat of recall bias.[34-36] Exposures, by definition, occurred in the past, and those collected through participant self-report introduce the possibility of people inaccurately recalling their exposure history. Often, those who have developed the outcome of interest are more likely to examine their past exposures more carefully in an attempt to find an explanation for why they developed the disease. In a case such as this, where cases are systematically reporting exposure differently from controls, recall bias has been introduced into the study and, because it systematically differs among exposed and unexposed, this bias may potentially skew study findings. The challenge lies in identifying a way to measure past exposures without introducing bias or inconsistencies in their assessment. In the psychiatric epidemiology literature, there have been some informative examples of novel ways to minimize or avoid the potential of recall bias being introduced into the study. For example, in a classic study, Walker et al.[37] obtained childhood home videos of 32 schizophrenic patients and their healthy siblings as a source of unbiased data on early emotional expression. Differences were found from infancy through adolescence, with fewer expressions of joy and greater expressions of negative affect among cases than controls. Thus, despite using a case–control design, the existence of informative and stable early risk indicators (in this instance, video evidence of emotional expressivity) yielded important new insight regarding the manifestation, early in the life course, of differences that later manifest as or predispose towards clinical schizophrenia.

Another important limitation is the potential for selection bias. In a case–control study, identification of cases is fairly straightforward; it is the identification of controls, however, that presents a challenge.[34,38] Cases and controls must arise from the same study base; if controls were to have developed the outcome of interest, they must have been eligible to be identified as cases. Although this sounds relatively straightforward, in practice it can be quite difficult to ensure that the controls properly represent the study base from which cases have been have drawn. This is an especially important point because, in order to estimate accurately the effect of exposure on the outcome, the controls are being used to estimate the exposure distribution in the study population; therefore, a misrepresentative selection of controls could bias study results significantly.[35]

> **Case–control studie: the example of SES and depression** In a case–control study, the primary threats to study validity lie in the selection of controls and in the ascertainment of exposure status. Returning to our research question examining the relationship between SES and depression, Jacobson et al.[39] investigated the relationship between childhood deprivation and the occurrence of, and severity of, adult depression. In this study, researchers identified 347 depressed inpatient women, 114 outpatient women, and 198 'normal' women who served as controls. Childhood deprivation was assessed using documented events in childhood; interviews with subjects were also conducted in an attempt to assess depriving childrearing experiences. The use of archival data from childhood to document significant events which could be considered deprivation (i.e. loss of a parent) lends strength to this study as it minimizes the introduction of recall bias. However, data from participant interviews are potentially biased. Further, there is the potential for selection bias insofar as the 'normal' women selected as controls may not be representative of the population from which the cases arose, for instance if these tended to include women who were atypical in terms of having especially favourable childhoods (so-called 'supernormal' controls). If so, any apparent differences in rates of childhood deprivations might result from controls who were less deprived than expected, and not cases who had relatively high levels of childhood deprivation. In a study such as this, where cases are identified from hospital inpatients and outpatients, it can be difficult to define clearly what constitutes the study base, i.e. what group of patients would have eventually been identified at that hospital had they developed major depression.

2.2.1.6 Cross-sectional studies

In life course research, cross-sectional studies provide information on both the prevalence of disease as well as associations between risk factors and disease, but typically provide little definitive information to further understanding of causal relationships. In a typical cross-sectional study, participants are sampled and interviewed at a single time-point.[7] As compared to case–control studies described above, cross-sectional studies typically place less emphasis on reconstructing past exposure; rather they provide a snapshot of prevalence of disease and associations between exposure and disease in a given sample at a given time often limiting the inference we can make regarding the temporal sequence between exposure and disease. Another difference from case–control studies is the sampling framework. In case–control studies a great deal of effort is placed on sampling an informative set of controls that are representative of the population that gave rise to the case. In cross-sectional studies, participants may include either a sample of convenience (based on their availability and willingness to participate) or they are often based on a representative sample of the general population (which allows for high generalizability). Cross-sectional studies, while not typically considered a strong design option for life course research, provide important insight into the prevalence of psychiatric disorders in a population and can provide initial evidence as to potential associations that can be investigated further using a more stringent study design.[40] Additionally, retrospective data can be collected from participants either using archival data or during the interview process in an attempt to reconstruct past exposure history.

> **Cross-sectional studies: the example of SES and depression** Returning to our examination of the relationship between SES and depression, a recent study utilized cross-sectional data from a household telephone survey in the USA and in Germany to examine the association between SES and depression.[41] Using basic demographic information, given the size and relative low cost of a single cross-sectional assessment, researchers were able to conduct stratified analyses to examine the association between SES and depression within different age groups, for example. However, cross-sectional data do not allow for causal inferences to be made about the relationship between SES and depression; given that all data are from one time-point, there is no evidence as to the temporality of the exposure–outcome relationship. Further, information bias can arise depending on how data are collected. In the example above, information on SES and depression was self-reported and collected by telephone interview, introducing the possibility of reporting bias. Cross-sectional studies also have the potential for unmeasured confounding. Given that all data are collected from one time-point, many other factors that could be influencing the association of interest are not captured by the one-time assessment.

2.2.2 Quasi-experimental designs

Unlike true experiments, where the investigator manipulates the exposures or conditions affecting research participants, quasi-experiments are characterized by investigator manipulation of observations (not treatments). Given the focus of this chapter, observations would typically be assessments of psychopathology and mental health, implemented after the occurrence of major events of relevance to life course theory—such as natural disasters (e.g. Hurricane Katrina), acts of terrorism, OR positive events resulting from policy changes and the like, such as income supplements. Such quasi- or natural experiments largely differ from traditional observational studies in that participants are largely 'selected' into exposed or unexposed groups by an event that is substantially not within their own control. As such, these often are less subject to selection bias than typical observational studies. However, at the same time, attempts to study the mental health consequences of such quasi-experiments may be hampered by the challenges of responding quickly to initiate an investigation soon after a natural occurrence of interest has taken place. Poorly implemented efforts may introduce problems related to both information bias (where respondents are typically not blind to the event of interest and may provide non-comparable information) and confounding, where the investigation may not be able to assess the full relevant set of potential confounding factors. One excellent example of the potential to advance understanding of life course theories in mental health is that of Costello et al.[42] who superimposed a unique 'natural experiment' on to an ongoing high quality cohort study, thus effectively reducing most major threats to typical observational studies.

Natural experiments: the example of SES and depression Returning to our example on depression and SES, Costello et al. found themselves in the fortuitous position to examine the impact of income supplements on mental health.[42] In 1993, the Great Smoky Mountains study enrolled a representative population sample of 1,420 rural children aged 9 to 13 years at baseline. One-quarter of study participants were American Indian; the remainder were predominately White. The study was designed as an 8-year prospective cohort study, but midway through the study, a casino was opened on the Indian reservation which increased annual income for participants living on the reservation (i.e. the quarter of participants that were American Indians). Researchers, having collected 4 years of data on the children prior to the increase in income, were now able to examine the role of income on the development of childhood psychopathology using a within-subject design. Contrary to previous study designs, which examined the impact of income on mental health, Costello et al. were able to examine this relationship in a setting in which income, a potentially strong explanatory variable for mental illness, was directly manipulated by forces outside the control of the family. The exposure (income supplements) was directly tied to the opening of the casino on the reservation; therefore, only families living on the reservation (i.e. only Native American families) were 'exposed'. Compared with an observational design, in which there are very many inter-related factors impacting a family's income level, in this study income was controlled by a force outside of the family's control (an 'exogenous' factor). It was not, however, randomly assigned; the income supplements were 100% correlated with ethnicity, raising remaining potential concerns of confounding. Therefore, any factors related to culture or ethnicity that differ between Native American families and Caucasian families were not addressed by the manipulation of income. The authors accounted for this possibility in analyses that considered several major potential confounding variables, and they observed a significant reduction in rates of childhood conduct and oppositional defiant disorders associated with income supplementation, providing important new evidence supporting the social causation of these conditions.

2.2.3 Experimental designs

In experimental studies, participants are randomly assigned to receive exposure or not with the exposure being manipulated by study investigators. The implications of this randomization and manipulation of exposure are related to the inferences that may be made about causality. When exposure is truly assigned at random to study participants, it may be assumed that, on average, all known and unknown confounders are evenly distributed across the study arms and, therefore, that the two arms of the study are exchangeable. The ability to make assumptions such as these has led RCTs to be considered the gold standard in epidemiological studies. However, in psychiatric epidemiology, investigators typically examine the impact of harmful exposures or 'risk factors' on mental disorders; obviously, the random allocation of harmful exposures to study participants is not ethically permissible. To illustrate: researchers have long wanted to understand the impact of trauma on the development of mental disorder, nevertheless it would be unethical to randomly assign participants to undergo a traumatic life event so that investigators could study their psychological response. Further, logistic considerations and the high cost associated with the long-term follow-up of subjects further limit the use of RCTs in life course research. As a result, due to the ethical considerations combined with practical constraints, experimental studies (in particular of potentially harmful conditions)— considered the gold standard in epidemiologic research—are not often used in psychiatric research. For further reading on experimental studies with incident psychiatric disorders as the outcome, please refer to the excellent reviews conducted by Cuijpers et al.[43,44]

Randomized controlled trials: the example of SES and depression These are considered the gold standard in epidemiological studies. As implied by the name, in RCTs participants are randomly assigned to receive the exposure. Given a large enough sample, it may be assumed that, on average, all known and unknown confounders are evenly distributed across the study arms (i.e. the two arms are exchangeable). In the preceding example of a natural experiment investigating the relationship between income and mental health, we saw that we could not make this assumption about exchangeability and, therefore, we had to acknowledge the potential for bias due to confounding. The Child and Family Study of the New Hope Project (New Hope) will serve as our final example examining the relationship between income and mental health in the setting of an RCT. This study was designed to examine the effectiveness of an employment-based anti-poverty project on children's development. In 1994–1995, 745 low-income adults who had at least one child between the ages of 1 and 11 were randomly assigned to treatment ($n = 366$) or control ($n = 379$). Families randomized to treatment had access to a package of benefits (income supplements, childcare assistance, and health care subsidies) which were intended to increase employment and reduce family poverty. The children were evaluated at 2- and 5-year follow-up on their academic performance, competence beliefs, values and efficacy, perceived quality of social relationships, and positive/problem behaviours (internalizing and externalizing). At the 2- and 5-year follow-up, New Hope boys were rated more positively on positive social behaviour and externalizing problem behaviours, and were performing better in respect of academic achievement and educational aspirations than children from control families. When examining the effects of the programme among girls, however, the findings were mixed; at the 2-year follow-up, New Hope girls were rated higher in terms of externalizing problem behaviours and had been subject to more disciplinary actions than girls in the control group; at 5-year follow-up, New Hope girls were rated higher for internalizing problems than control girls.[45,46] The authors suggested, however, that gender differences in programme effects resulted from the nature of the absolute differences in behavioural and academic measures among boys and girls; girls in both arms were performing better than boys, so had less room for improvement. Whereas this study does not perfectly map on to previous examples examining the relationship between income and mental health, it does illustrate the strengths of the RCT for life course research. In this study, the randomization of low income adults with young children created groups that appear to be exchangeable at baseline.[46] Exchangeability of the groups allows us to make comparisons between the groups under the assumption that the groups are identical with the exception of the New Hope programme. Further, we would expect that randomization would eliminate the potential for selection bias to occur in the allocation of treatment, thus preventing systematic differences between the two groups (i.e. all families have equal probability of receiving treatment or control).

2.3 **Conclusions**

Life course approaches to advance understanding of the causes and prevention of mental disorder are rich in both potential and challenges. Relatively rare disorders require large sample sizes; complex conditions require considerable effort and resources for accurate assessment; multiple contributing factors from the molecular to the societal level require rich exposure assessments; and the complexity of the human condition introduces a range of potential confounding factors. Each of the study designs presented in this chapter has advanced our knowledge of how mental disorders originate, progress, and may diminish over the life course.

References

1 George LK. *Life-course perspectives on mental health.* New York: Springer; 1999. p. 565–583.

2 Kuh D, Ben-Shlomo Y, Lynch J, Hallqvist J, Power C. Life course epidemiology. *J Epidemiol Community Health* 2003;**57**(10):778–783.

3 Ben-Shlomo Y, Kuh D. A life course approach to chronic disease epidemiology: conceptual models, empirical challenges and interdisciplinary perspectives. *Int J Epidemiol* 2002;**31**(2):285–293.

4 Barker DJP. The developmental origins of adult disease. *J Am Coll Nutr* 2004;**23**(Suppl 6):588S–595S.

5 Elder GH, Shanahan MJ. The life course and human development. In: *Handbook of child psychology*, 6th ed. New York: John Wiley & Sons; 2007. pp. 665–715.

6 Gilman SE. Commentary: Childhood socioeconomic status, life course pathways and adult mental health. *Int J Epidemiol* 2002;**31**(2):403–404.

7 Aschengrau A, Seage GR. *Essentials of epidemiology in public health.* 2nd ed. Sudbury, MA: Jones & Bartlett; 2008.

8 Rothman KJ, Greenland S, Lash TL. *Modern epidemiology.* 3rd ed. Philadelphia: Lippincott Willams & Wilkins; 2008.

9 Woodward M. *Epidemiology: study design and data analysis.* 2nd ed. Boca Raton, FL: Chapman & Hall/CRC Press; 2005.

10 Pickles A, Maughan B, Wadsworth M. *Epidemiological methods in life course research.* New York: Oxford University Press; 2007.

11 Susser E, Terry MB, Matte T. The birth cohorts grow up: new opportunities for epidemiology. *Paediatr Perinat Epidemiol* 2000;**14**(2):98–100.

12 Wadsworth MEJ, Butterworth SL, Hardy RJ, et al. The life course prospective design: an example of benefits and problems associated with study longevity. *Soc Sci Med* 2003;**57**(11):2193–2205.

13 Stratford R, Mulligan J, Downie B, Voss L. Threats to validity in the longitudinal study of psychological effects: the case of short stature. *Child Care Health Dev* 1999;**25**(6):401–419.

14 Gilman SE, Kawachi I, Fitzmaurice GM, Buka SL. Socioeconomic status in childhood and the lifetime risk of major depression. *Int J Epidemiol* 2002;**31**(2):359–367.

15 Bijl RV, van Zessen G, Ravelli A, de Rijk C, Langendoen Y. The Netherlands Mental Health Survey and Incidence Study (NEMESIS): objectives and design. *Soc Psychiatry Psychiatr Epidemiol* 1998;**33**(12):581–586.

16 de Graaf R, Ten Have M, van Dorsselaer S. The Netherlands Mental Health Survey and Incidence Study—2 (NEMESIS-2): design and methods. *Int J Methods Psychiatr Res* 2010;**19**(3):125–141.

17 Bijl RV, De Graaf R, Ravelli A, et al. Gender and age-specific first incidence of DSM-III-R psychiatric disorders in the general population. Results from the Netherlands Mental Health Survey and Incidence Study (NEMESIS). *Soc Psychiatry Psychiatr Epidemiol* 2002;**37**(8):372–9.

18 de Graaf R, ten Have M, van Gool C, van Dorsselaer S. Prevalence of mental disorders and trends from 1996 to 2009. Results from the Netherlands Mental Health Survey and Incidence Study—2. *Soc Psychiatry Psychiatr Epidemiol* 2012;**47**(2):203–13.

19 Broman S. *The collaborative perinatal project: an overview.* New York: Praeger; 1984.

20 Broman S, Bien E, Shaughnessy P. *Low achieving children: the first seven years.* Hillsdale, NJ: Lawrence Erlbaum Associates; 1985.

21 Myrianthopoulos NC, French KS. An application of the U.S. Bureau of the Census socioeconomic index to a large, diversified patient population. *Soc Sci Med* 1968;**2**(3):283–299.

22 Buka SL, Lipsitt LP, Tsuang MT. Birth complications and psychological deviancy: a 25-year prospective inquiry. *Acta Paediatr Jpn* 1988;**30**(5):537–546.

23 Buka SL, Tsuang MT, Lipsitt LP. Pregnancy/delivery complications and psychiatric diagnosis. A prospective study. *Arch Gen Psychiatry* 1993;**50**(2):151–156.

24 Buka SL, Goldstein JM, Seidman LJ, et al. Prenatal complications, genetic vulnerability, and schizophrenia: the New England longitudinal studies of schizophrenia. *Psychiatr Ann* 1999;**29**(3):151–156.

25 Goldstein JM, Seidman LJ, Buka SL, et al. Impact of genetic vulnerability and hypoxia on overall intelligence by age 7 in offspring at high risk for schizophrenia compared with affective psychoses. *Schizophr Bull* 2000;**26**(2):323–334.

26 Seidman LJ, Buka SL, Goldstein JM, Horton NJ, Rieder RO, Tsuang MT. The relationship of prenatal and perinatal complications to cognitive functioning at age 7 in the New England Cohorts of the National Collaborative Perinatal Project. *Schizophr Bull* 2000;**26**(2):309–321.

27 Buka SL, Tsuang MT, Torrey EF, Klebanoff MA, Bernstein D, Yolken RH. Maternal infections and subsequent psychosis among offspring. *Arch Gen Psychiatry* 2001;**58**(11):1032–1037.

28 Buka SL, Tsuang MT, Torrey EF, Klebanoff MA, Wagner RL, Yolken RH. Maternal cytokine levels during pregnancy and adult psychosis. *Brain Behav Immun* 2001;**15**(4):411–420.

29 Goldstein JM, Buka SL, Seidman LJ, Tsuang MT. Specificity of familial transmission of schizophrenia psychosis spectrum and affective psychoses in the New England family study's high-risk design. *Arch Gen Psychiatry* 2010;**67**(5):458–467.

30 Thermenos HW, Goldstein JM, Buka SL, et al. The effect of working memory performance on functional MRI in schizophrenia. *Schizophr Res* 2005;**74**(2–3):179–194.

31 Ritsher JE, Warner V, Johnson JG, Dohrenwend BP. Inter-generational longitudinal study of social class and depression: a test of social causation and social selection models. *Br J Psychiatry* Suppl 2001;**40**:s84–90.

32 Weissman MM, Kidd KK, Prusoff BA. Variability in rates of affective disorders in relatives of depressed and normal probands. *Arch Gen Psychiatry* 1982;**39**(12):1397–1403.

33 Niswander KR, Gordon M. *The women and their pregnancies: the Collaborative Perinatal Study of the National Institute of Neurological Diseases and Stroke.* Philadelphia: WB Saunders; 1972.

34 Schlesselman JJ, Schneiderman MA. Case control studies: design, conduct, analysis. *J Occup Environ Med* 1982;**24**(11):879.

35 Lee W, Bindman J, Ford T, et al. Bias in psychiatric case—control studies. *Br J Psychiatry* 2007;**190**(3):204–209.

36 Berney LR, Blane DB. Collecting retrospective data: accuracy of recall after 50 years judged against historical records. *Soc Sci Med* 1997;**45**(10):1519–1525.

37 Walker EF, Grimes KE, Davis DM, Smith AJ. Childhood precursors of schizophrenia: facial expressions of emotion. *Am J Psychiatry* 1993;**150**(11):1654–1660.

38 Wacholder S, Silverman DT, McLaughlin JK, Mandel JS. Selection of controls in case-control studies. II. Types of controls. *Am J Epidemiol* 1992;**135**(9):1029–1041.

39 Jacobson S, Fasman J, Dimascio A. Deprivation in the childhood of depressed women. *J Nerv Ment Dis* 1975;**160**(1):5–14.

40 Kraemer HC, Yesavage JA, Taylor JL, Kupfer D. How can we learn about developmental processes from cross-sectional studies, or can we? *Am J Psychiatry* 2000;**157**(2):163–171.

41 Knesebeck Ovd, Lüschen G, Cockerham WC, Siegrist J. Socioeconomic status and health among the aged in the United States and Germany: a comparative cross-sectional study. *Soc Sci Med* 2003;**57**(9):1643–1652.

42 Costello EJ, Compton SN, Keeler G, Angold A. Relationships between poverty and psychopathology—a natural experiment. *JAMA* 2003;**290**(15):2023–2029.

43 Cuijpers P, van Straten A, Smit F, Mihalopoulos C, Beekman A. Preventing the onset of depressive disorders: a meta-analytic review of psychological interventions. *Am J Psychiatry* 2008;**165**(10):1272–1280.

44 Cuijpers P, Van Straten A, Smit F. Preventing the incidence of new cases of mental disorders: a meta-analytic review. *J Nerv Ment Dis* 2005;**193**(2):119–125.

45 Huston AC, Duncan GJ, McLoyd VC, et al. Impacts on children of a policy to promote employment and reduce poverty for low-income parents: new hope after 5 years. *Dev Psychol* 2005;**41**(6):902–918.

46 Huston AC, Duncan GJ, Granger R, et al. Work-based antipoverty programs for parents can enhance the school performance and social behavior of children. *Child Dev* 2001;**72**(1):318–336.

Chapter 3

Measurement issues in epidemiology of psychiatric disorders

Patricia Cohen

3.1 Introduction

Here we review measurement issues that necessarily require thinking through the recruited population to be addressed and potential sources of information including and beyond that to be obtained from cohort members, family, friends and/or official records. Established interview assessments of psychiatric disorders cover a range of ages, inclusion of many disorders or, sometimes, only those most prevalent. Some longitudinal studies examine the extended course of a particular disorder based on clinical samples. Others, more broadly, focus on general or high risk populations. Measure planning begins by reviewing the broad areas in which data have already suggested risks related to the targeted psychiatric disorders or symptoms. Investigators then must decide which risks should be at least modestly included, any 'uncovered' risks that investigators feel should be addressed, and which risks should be included as thoroughly as possible. The potential domains of relevant measures are discussed, including measure selection, sequence, and administration issues. Measurement issues of reliability and validity are briefly introduced.

The importance of interview sites, interviewer training and selection, and consideration of respondent difficulties or limitations are discussed in relation to measurement adequacy. Included in this chapter are some of the methods employed in the 35-year longitudinal Children in the Community (CIC) study.[1]

3.2 The population to be studied

With regard to cohort recruitment, epidemiological studies may obtain study participants from a range of options that depend on the major study goals and what data may answer goal-related questions. It also matters whether the research is primarily focused on questions for which answers may be provided in a single assessment: for example, a study with the primary goal of estimating prevalence of particular problems, symptoms, or disorders in one or more subpopulations. Alternatively, given study goals involving earlier risks as predictive of later disorders, the course of disorder symptoms, life quality in persons with identified disorders, or broader changes over time in disorder-related function, repeated assessments are required. These studies are most informative when the investigators have seriously thought through what may be real—but little-investigated—risk or protective issues, as part of or distinct from already shown predictors based on earlier empirical studies.

As is well known, the highest level of psychiatric disorder is generally found in the early adulthood populations, with particularly high levels of depressive and anxiety disorders. This age requires careful consideration and measurement of variables that may be consequences of earlier mental disorder rather than a risk for such a disorder. These may include quality of relationships with family (parents, siblings), other closely involved persons, and/or peers. Physical disorders, health risks, or reports of poor social or professional well-being may be a consequence of earlier risks. Thus careful timing of potential risks and the participants' perspectives on disorder onset timing may assist assessment of the likely meaning of the connection.

Relevant participants may be recruited from residential locations, from school populations or other organizations, or from psychiatric or other health evaluation/treatment populations. Recruitment itself may be complicated. For example, will recruitment involve all available participants? A randomly selected subpopulation? Or a selection limited to those who agree to carry out required study components, such as future reassessments, or inclusion of one or more potential informants, such as mother, teacher, spouse, or close friend?

The age range of cohort members at the initial assessment is also a serious decision. Not only does inclusion of young offspring require parental agreement and usually parental information and/or interaction, but it also requires careful decisions regarding how the observed or reported behaviours or problems match the study goals. By late childhood/early adolescence, it is critical to include self-reported problems and strengths in addition to parental and, when feasible, teacher reports. Later in adolescence and into young adulthood, self-reports will be essential, although parents and/or other frequent contact persons may provide useful information.

Plans for a longitudinal sample, even starting with only two assessments, need an adjustment of recruitment size to cope with potential participant loss. Geographic moves typically vary by cohort age: whole family moves are common for offspring very early in life, much less so for offspring in middle childhood, and cohort member moving is relatively frequent as they move into full adulthood. This problem can be partly lowered when the data collection includes participant early identification of friends, relatives, or other locators who could likely provide new physical or Web-based addresses of the participant. And, of course, the Internet is another increasing source of data collection from study participants, although methods of ensuring that data are coming from consistent responders will be necessary.

3.3 **Study measures and useful sources**

3.3.1 **Cohort protocol coverage of mental disorders**

Probably the best sources of mental disorder component assessment will be found from those who have already created and employed such measures on a relevant or reasonably similar population to the anticipated one. This does not mean that changes in the *Diagnostic and Statistical Manual for Mental Disorders* (DSM) or the *International Classification of Diseases* (ICD) can be ignored, but rather that some recent disorder assessments have been developed and employed for studies of one or many of these disorders and, typically, changes are more or less easily incorporated. A disorder protocol designed for a clinical population will almost certainly need to be edited before it will be optimal for a non-clinical population. As has long been appreciated, 'the problems of a clinical instrument's validity in the general population has little to do with the instrument per se but rather with the nature of diagnoses in the general population . . . . Clinicians will have much better diagnostic agreement when dealing with severe cases . . . . This holds for both medical and psychiatric diagnosis. The general population always has proportionally more mild and borderline cases of a disorder.'[2]

Thus, in structuring a psychiatric disorder section of an interview designed for a general population, one will generally want it to be relatively easy to create scaled measures of disorder symptoms as well as (possibly 'graded') diagnostic assessments. If so, one will need some questions that can readily be scaled. For example, in the CIC assessment of paranoia in adolescents, we added specific questions including what the experienced threats or threatening behaviours were thought to be, sometimes including 'Why?' and how they reacted (with scored responses). For an initial question such as, 'Have you ever thought that people were following you or spying on you?' a 'Yes' response may be best followed by asking for description of such an experience. If the description indicates the likelihood that the respondent really had strongly believed that, next questions may cover the length of this belief and whether anyone else saw or believed it. Given a relatively strong response, follow-up questions would inquire about effects such as spending time with friends or other people more or less often, missing school or work, or having difficulty doing things s/he wants or should do.

Another assessment component is reporting sought or obtained help for psychiatric symptoms or disorders, whether from a sophistically experienced friend, a relative, or a professional adult. If professional help has been sought, questions covering treatment recommendations, behavioural changes, and the presence or absence of consequential changes in symptoms therefore follow. Again, the interviewer should be provided with response options that may be simply checked and with format locations to record responses that were not included but seem to be important and/ or distinct. For example, in the CIC study the mothers responded independently to the same set of her child's disorder items as did her child. Analyses of the disorder data in pooled parent and child assessments collected when the cohort average age was about 13 years were employed in publications. Over the next two assessments in late teens and early adulthood, it became clear that youth reports more clearly identified predictors of ongoing symptoms. Thus, cohort reports were generally employed in subsequent analyses and publications.

3.3.2 Environment and environmental risks

Regardless of age, there is a series of variables that should nearly always be at least modestly covered in addition to actual diagnostic assessment. These include physical, social, and self-evaluated quality of the respondent's environments, including dwelling/neighbourhood, education, and/or employment settings. Optimally, they also include relationship quality with persons in those settings: family members, friends, community, other students, and other employees. The CIC group found that beginning an interview with these issues works well, and usefully delays coverage of the disorders until the interview process is well established.

Research may be designed in aggregate to focus on particular environments (e.g. region or residence with a history of severe damage or violence) or population vulnerability (e.g. offspring of parents with a particular mental or physical disorder), or populations varied in already-known vulnerabilities related to certain mental disorders (e.g. maturing youth with illegal or violent behaviours who develop full antisocial personality disorder as adults). In such selections the study would be designed to identify the biological and life history differences that may influence the actual development of these disorders.

For example, given the high disorder risk associated with problematic parenting, child abuse, and/or neglect, including these measures in a cohort study may be desirable. When feasible in a study, only by asking the cohort members, such information must be carefully obtained, with efforts to avoid the risk that the disorder has produced an expanded view of personal treatment.

3.3.3 **Other measures**

3.3.3.1 Existing records

Given the increasing appreciation that risks and vulnerability-increasing experience and setting may begin very early in life, an ideal study of influences on the origin and course of mental illnesses would include birth, health, and school records. These and other records (such as disorder histories or problems of other family members) may be more readily obtained in official data in developed countries other than the USA, and study planning should consider the potential value of such data, and whether and how such data might be obtained. For example, there is a range of studies now being carried out in Quebec, Canada, where overall income and educational differences, housing quality, and other broad measures are being applied to existing data on relevant outcomes in regional subpopulations. Although it was possible for the CIC study to obtain official records of childhood abuse, such data may be difficult to obtain in other US states. Nevertheless, regional records of, for example, family income or prevalence of certain serious disorders may be available. There are also collaborative studies such as those focusing on particular disorders or symptoms to be linked to relevant measures that are available or that can be created from existing data.[3,4]

3.3.3.2 Biological measures and issues

In addition to a paper or Web-based questionnaire or verbally collected data, specific cohort member tasks may be designed to indicate relevant behavioural, emotional, intellectual, physical, or more specific brain-related activity (e.g. magnetic resonance imaging (MRI), functional MRI). DNA extracted from saliva or blood is included in many studies, with the goal of identifying genetic impacts on symptoms and disorders. There are also issues of biological and functional brain changes with age that are still to be further measured.[5] These potential sources and issues need early consideration in order to maximize the strength of the study in meeting its intended goals while 'keeping' the assessed cohort available for future assessments.

3.4 **Other measures applied to cohort members**

Disorder and disorder-risk interviews will vary across the age range of the cohort members. Nevertheless, it is not as difficult as one might expect to use very similar questions or study tasks over a substantial age range. For example, in some psychiatric assessments (often in childhood and also in late adulthood), tasks that represent measures of intellectual performance may be usefully employed, given the levels of skills and competence that strongly influence mental disorder presence and level of dysfunction. Other assessed measures will necessarily reflect hypotheses specific to the planned study. For example, included in the CIC study were ranking of life goals in adolescent assessments, on the hypothesis that high ranking of goals focusing entirely on individual well-being (e.g. wealth, health) would be predictive of the number of subsequent psychiatric disorders, as proved to be the case.[6] Childhood and adolescent traits such as irritability are another set of dimensions that have been shown to be predictive of current as well as subsequent disorders years later.[7] It is also now clear that psychiatric disorders of many kinds are seen in childhood and adolescence in rates that may often exceed those of adults.[8,9]

The number and adequacy of measured risks will also influence the time required for the assessment, whether assessed by interviewer questions or by printed or Web-based computerized questions with answer options. Therefore, careful scrutiny of the current evidence of serious influence on, or prediction of, a psychiatric disorder should be carefully examined prior to decisions on what can realistically be included and how thoroughly.

3.5 Age differences in environmental and experiential predictors of psychiatric symptoms

3.5.1 Infancy and early childhood

There is increasingly strong empirical evidence that a large component of a person's risk for many, perhaps even most, emotional, cognitive, and behavioural disorders have origins in difficult early childhood development and treatment.[10] For this reason, some longitudinal studies begin with a cohort first assessed relatively or very early in life. Neonatal children cannot tell you about their problems, but mothers generally can at least describe: (a) their own view of strengths and weaknesses of their offspring; (b) the home environment, potentially including data on who cares for the infant if they are employed or away, and what fraction of the work-day, or duration in days or weeks, describes their absences;[11] and (c) what the father, mother, or other caretakers do when they see or hear the child doing something that is forbidden, dangerous, or annoying.

Observations of interactions of infants with their mothers (e.g. Beebe et al.[12]), or evaluations of abilities of mothers to play with, read to, or comfort, their young child as observed by trained experts are often predictive of later problems in childhood. In my experience, it is possible for one or two interviewers/observers to evaluate a 2- or 3-year-old child and mother in their home, but such an effort can be both difficult and expensive. Alternatively, it may be wise to limit such observational data to an established research environment.

Not surprisingly, mothers tend to be best sources of data on pre-school offspring, although fathers or other family members, medical records, child care centre staff, or at-home employees or relatives may also provide relevant and useful information. Mothers can usually report parental attitudes about and during the pregnancy, parenting behaviour—especially disciplinary actions, and frequency of positive interactions (playing with, taking to positive active child sites, taking child along when shopping or doing other errands, quantity and nature of television shows child typically watches (and with whom)).

3.5.2 Middle childhood

As children reach pre-school/school onset ages, maternal and teacher/caretaker interviews or questionnaires and observational studies of the child with other children or with a parent are usually helpful. For example, handedness is sometimes a critical issue and readily assessed in middle childhood when 'left-handed' consequences may be problematic. Peer relationships begin to be very important, as do activities and achievement levels; often even more so as children move into later ages.

There are several variables for which assessment at an earlier age may produce strong predictors of later increase or decrease in symptoms of mental disorders. Indeed this likelihood is a strong reason for including such variables into assessments at earlier ages, even when there may be only modest evidence of their future influence magnitude. Among these are people's overall understanding of themselves early in life, including strengths and weaknesses potentially measured as traits, quality of relationship with peers, understanding of strengths and goals of close peers, and of their own life goals. When planning assessments at later ages, reassessment of these measures as well as psychiatric symptom measures may be useful.

3.5.3 Late childhood

By these ages information on activities, preferences, behaviours, environments and relationships can be elicited in interviews of the youth. Responses to simple questions covering age-relevant emotional and behavioural symptoms may produce evidence of oncoming psychiatric disorders in some children.

3.5.4 Early to mid-adolescence

Information on qualities of family interactions, school attendance and performance, peer relationships, romantic relationships, and negative and positive experiences and activities is readily elicited in these youth. In addition, they also typically respond well to the diagnostic assessments.

3.5.5 Transition to adulthood and early adulthood

This age range has the highest level of psychiatric disorders and participants can respond well in general. There are disorder-relevant life and behaviour issues including romantic relationships and commitments, parenting, education level and goals, employment/income/home responsibilities, and environment. Again, issue selection requires careful consideration of what is already known, what are dominant issues for the disorders to be studied, and what potentially important issues have been absent in the literature.

3.5.6 Middle adulthood

The issues noted for the younger adults often remain but may require restating questions to make them more relevant and informative to the symptoms and disorders that may have increased or declined. For example, relationship quality with older offspring may become more important for parental well-being. The gradual course of ageing itself may feel more threatening to some people, especially in the older age range, and may be predictive of disorders or symptoms.

3.5.7 Later adulthood

In these interviews, the focus is bound to include ageing issues, including changes in tasks and responsibilities, relationships, and activities, and their connections to psychiatric disorders, symptoms, and distress.

3.6 Assessment of statistical quality of measures

The usual statistical method employed to assess the measurement quality of the question responses is the assessment of 'reliability' of responses to a set of scaled response questions (r_{xx}). This method is a relatively simple consideration of the correlation between responses to these questions across a set of persons (such as everyone assessed by sets of items covering particular disorders, settings, or traits). The construct of this method focuses on the view that if a variable measure is adequate, a significant level of correlations among the responses to the individual questions will be found across the cohort studied. Such correlations will also reflect correlations with the 'total score' represented by the sum of the scaled responses. Reliability as a measurement quality indicator is quite appropriate to many multiple-item measures of traits, relationships, activities, and environmental settings. The primary solutions to a relatively 'low' reliability (<0.60, for example) is production of either more or better questions.

This method is somewhat problematic in the assessment of psychiatric disorders in a general population. Disorders are essentially defined by the presence and level of symptoms that are not 'normally' present, and therefore not necessarily highly connected in the population as a whole. In a person with a diagnosed psychiatric disorder, we would anticipate a relatively high relationship between symptoms because that is what 'produced' the disorder 'assignment' (and, of course, there are 'subsidiary' questions on the duration and intensity of a symptom that are not relevant to those who indicate no such symptom). One of the methods of creating 'scaled disorder' measures that have good reliabilities is to ensure that the symptom response options cover a range of levels, rather than only the minimum levels that would define full 'disorders'. Epidemiological studies may find it useful to identify the cohort members with summed scaled symptom responses in some analyses, enabling ready examination of that 'kind of problem' in the study sample or subsamples.

3.7 Selecting and training interviewers

Training, selecting, and recruiting interviewers is one of the most critical tasks for creating high quality data. Here we focus on interviewers who are not necessarily familiar with the field. Nevertheless, there is a substantial literature showing that some professionals may not accept cohort member responses to some questions, based on their own opinions or experiences.[12] This does not mean that persons with a relevant professional background are to be avoided as interviewers, but only that they also need to be carefully trained and evaluated. If they identify protocol questions that may be misunderstood, those items should be carefully reviewed and revised if necessary. But ultimately the quality of the data will depend on the quality of the interviewers.

In this respect I refer substantially to what I learned from my colleague Claudia Hartmark as we collaborated in training and selecting interviewers. Once persons potentially interested in this role are identified, interviewer candidates are invited to an initial general meeting in which the meaning and goals of the study are described. Elements of the protocol are distributed and briefly examined together. The overall issue of separation of one's personal reactions from one's administration of the study questions is described as central and discussed. Strong training focuses on conveyed 'attitude absence' or at least minimization—for example, absence of early expression to participants of gratitude for participation (including smiling expression of agreement if respondent indicates that the answers to questions are hard), and especially no reaction to identified symptoms except as required by follow-up questions in the protocol.

Interviewers who have had experience with other studies are a potential source, nevertheless study staff need to establish evidence that well-performing interviewers will thoroughly understand basic principles, including respect for the respondent regardless of respondent's attitude, behaviour, or history, and no presenting of interviewer's own opinion regarding any issue on which the respondent may have expressed a different opinion.

Interviewer candidates are then linked to non-cohort volunteers whom they will interview, all interviews being tape-recorded. These recorded interviews are then turned in and evaluated along with the scored interviews. Candidate recruitment as a study interviewer is done only following a positive evaluation. We have found that female interviewers tend to be better than males in interviews of general population samples (possibly with the exception of those psychiatric professionals with useful knowledge of the field and willingness to follow the protocol).

We have prepared a substantial manual for interviewers in our longitudinal study (available on request). Following the neutral and impartial attitudes that the interviewer should convey throughout the interview (see 'Interviewer presentation'), each section of the adult and child interviews is reviewed and the parts of these that the interviewer is expected to read are identified. Difficult or sensitive questions are noted and interviewers are advised to be as matter-of-fact as possible including pre-interview rehearsals if they find a section likely to be difficult. We remind them that they should not be acting like clinicians: they are to gather data as given by the respondent, not to evaluate it, except where we have explicitly instructed them to do so (in general only when the study member's response is not clear). As in other aspects of the protocol, in general, interviewers are not to add questions to those included in the prepared protocol. This does not mean that sometimes a clarifying question may not be relevant, but that such additions are only (rarely) communicated under strong evidence that the respondent did not understand the question. In such a case, the interviewer needs to be clear. (Such a risk suggests less-than-adequate question or question response options, which should have been picked up and changed during protocol development and testing.)

These assume that the interviewer is entering the response to read-aloud questions. For assessments of children as young as 8–10 years, the response options to some questions may be placed on a coloured cardboard placard such as NEVER, SOMETIMES, OFTEN, and ALWAYS, with the numbers 1, 2, 3, and 4 under these options representing the coding. (Note that an even number of options makes it impossible for respondents to overselect the middle option.) The interviewer reads the item and points to these options for the child to choose. If there is concern about reading ability of an older child or cohort adult, the interviewer who reads the items may employ either a placard with response options or state the options such as, 'Would you say that happens Never, Sometimes, Often, or Always?'

For later ages (and respondent agreement), and particularly after the respondent has participated in at least one earlier interview, a printed or on-computer version of the interview is an option. Computer versions easily carry the advantage of, for instance, add-on questions covering intensity, duration, associated problems, following a positive response to an initial question such as the presence of a symptom (such a program may be 'spoken' by the computer). Alternatively, an interviewer may carry a computer to the interview site, reading questions aloud as well as response options for a participant who prefers such a method or who may be a poor reader. If the cohort member prefers to complete the response options without involvement of the nominal interviewer, such a method may be carried out, given adequate programming of the questions and alternative response options. The interviewer should take a quick look at the responded protocol in order to ensure that there are selected responses to all the asked questions.

Similarly, when a study participant has moved to a location to which, for distance or funding reasons, interviewers cannot travel, options include telephone interviews following a mailing of the protocol to the participant, or an Internet-based interview of a participant who has agreed to respond. Some earlier recruited participants may also be more willing to respond via the Internet than by physical connection to an interviewer, and, given the current mobility of populations—particularly of young adults—such a connection may be the most feasible option in an ongoing study. Given substantially increasing Internet activities of both youth and adults, responding to questions presented (ideally vocally as well as visually) via the Internet may be preferred by many. If so, verbal 'interaction' with the 'game' may be necessary and workable.

In such a method, as in all others, it remains necessary for the respondents to understand fully the questions and response options, and to understand the importance of complete local privacy for their responses.

In such cases, the investigator may need to develop a method to produce reasonable evidence (such as particular earlier questions about preferred activities or other relatively unique issues) that responses are returning from the requested source.

3.8 **Summary**

In general, epidemiological studies, and especially longitudinal ones, consume a large amount of effort by a group of experts. Obtaining the strongest information regarding origins and/or course of psychiatric disorders requires several considerations. First, the professionals planning the study need to know the research and literature that are relevant to the disorders to be covered, as well as those potential risks that may not have been adequately examined. Second, these strengths may include selection and recruitment of information sources in addition to the persons who are the primary focus of the study. Data from family members, a close friend, physician, caretaker, or teacher may be very informative and within the possibilities of funding, when usefully considered. Third, quality of the data collected by interviewers is a critical issue. If interviewers are to collect the responses from cohort members they should be trained and tested before being included in the full data collection. Fourth, if methods such as Web-based questionnaires are to be employed, there need to be ways to gather information regarding the independence of cohort responses or the kind of assistance provided to the cohort respondent. Fifth, when genetic data and/or biological reactions to particular exposures via brain component responses can be linked to specific disorders or disorder symptom development, we are—or will be developing—additional understanding of the sources and consequences of these disorders.

Given these strengths, longitudinal studies can produce substantial evidence that improves understanding of these disorders, and the potential utility of efforts to maximize prevention and/or treatment success.

References

1 Cohen P, Crawford TN, Johnson JG, Kasen S. The Children in the Community Study of developmental course of personality disorder. *J Personality Disord* 2005;**19**(5):566–486.

2 Pfohl, B. Discussion following B. Dorenwend, 'The problem of validity revisited'. In: Robins LN, Barrett JE, editors. *The validity of psychiatric diagnosis*. New York: Raven Press; 1989. p. 53.

3 Lampi KM, Bannerjee PN, Gissler M, et al. Finnish prenatal study of autism and autism spectrum disorders: overview and design. *J Autism Dev Disord* 2010;**41**:1090–1096.

4 Harper KN, Hibbeln JR, Deckelbaum R, Quesenberry Jr CP, Schaefer CA, Brown AS. Maternal serum docosahexaenoic acid and schizophrenia spectrum disorders in adult offspring. *Schizophr Res* 2011;**128**:30–36.

5 Nelson E, Leibenluft E, McClure E, Pine DS. The social re-orientation of adolescence: a neuroscience perspective on the process and its relation to psychopathology. *Psychol Med* 2005;**35**:163–174.

6 Cohen P, Cohen J. *Life values and adolescent mental health*. Mahwah, NJ: Lawrence Erlbaum; 1996.

7 Leibenluft E, Cohen P, Gorrindo T, Brook JS, Pine DS. Chronic versus episodic irritability in youth: a community-based, longitudinal study of clinical and diagnostic associations. *J Child Adolesc Psychopharmacol* 2006;**16**(4):456–466.

8 Jaffee SR, Jarrington H, Cohen P, Moffitt TE. Cumulative prevalence of psychiatric disorder in youths. *J Am Acad Child Adolesc Psychiatry* 2005;**44**(5):406–407.

9 Kim-Cohen J, Caspi A, Moffitt TE, Harrington H, Milne BJ, Poulton, R. Prior juvenile diagnoses in adults with mental disorder. *Arch Gen Psychiatry* 2003;**60**:709–717.

10 Shonkoff JP, Phillips DA editors. *From neurons to neighborhoods: the science of early childhood development*. Washington DC: National Academy Press; 2000.

11 Crawford TN, Cohen PR, Chen H, Anglin DM, Ehrensaft M. Early maternal separation and the trajectory of borderline personality disorder symptoms. *Dev Psychopathol* 2009;**21**:1013–1030.

12 Robins LN, Barrett JE. *The validity of psychiatric diagnosis*. New York: Raven Press; 1989. p. 53.

Chapter 4

Analytic considerations in a life course perspective

Leah Li

4.1 Introduction

There has been growing interest in using a life course approach to study mental health outcomes.[1] Although some psychiatric disorders (e.g. autism) tend to have early onset, for more common disorders such as depression, the onset may occur in childhood, but their prevalence rises during adolescence and is much higher in adulthood.[2]

Children with behaviour problems are more likely to grow up to have mental disorder, compared to children without.[3] For example, childhood internalizing and externalizing disorders are associated with mid-life affective and anxiety disorder.[4] The trajectories of some mental health outcomes may be set early in life and childhood experiences are thought to be important in development of mental health across the life course. Part of the association between early life factors and poor adult mental health is due to the increased risk of early first onset of mental disorder, which may lead to recurrent episodes.

Early origins of mental health problems are well established, predating life course epidemiology. Adverse experiences in early life, such as socio-economic disadvantage,[5] parental divorce,[6] and sexual[7] and physical abuse,[8] are associated with poor mental health. The influence of these experiences persists into adult life.[9]

While childhood experiences are important for determining the lifetime trajectories of mental health, there are several widely accepted hypothetical models for assessing the influence of exposures during different life stages on subsequent mental health outcome. For example, we may hypothesize that childhood is a 'critical period' when adverse experiences affect adult mental well-being.[1] For example, adverse experiences during sensitive periods in childhood may have an effect on biological systems (i.e. hypothalamic–pituitary–adrenal axis) and the effect remains latent until adulthood, independent of adult exposure to adversity.[10]

We may also hypothesize that early life factors influence adult outcome through multiple developmental pathways, including cognitive, social, emotional, or neuropsychiatric development.[10] Moreover, early exposure may lead to further disadvantage which increases the risk of psychiatric disorder. In the cumulative risk models, we assume that the cumulative time with a certain exposure is associated with the outcome. It has been shown that the accumulation of socio-economic disadvantages across childhood and adulthood (though the latter may be more important) are associated with increased risk of mid-life disorder.[11]

The association between some time-dependent exposures and mental health may be bidirectional. For example, social economic status (SES) is associated with depression over the life course;[12] low childhood SES is related to increased risk of subsequent mental disorder but mental health in childhood may also influence adult SES,[11] a reverse causality argument. The life course relationship between underweight or obesity and psychological distress is also complicated by the direction of their association.[13] These time-dependent measures (psychological distress, SES, and weight status) can be both exposures and outcomes on these pathways, and thus are subject to measurement errors. Unravelling the direction of the relationship raises methodological issues.

Recent studies suggest that developmental trajectories of mental health may be associated with other outcomes. For example, psychological health throughout the life course is found to be associated with cortisol secretion in mid-adulthood.[14] Life course study also extends to the next generation. Trajectories of maternal depression have been linked to offspring psychological outcomes.[15]

4.2 Analytic considerations for longitudinal data in life course study

The application of life course perspective to mental health research poses methodological challenges associated with the complexity of the life course hypotheses and longitudinal data. In this section we discuss a number of analytic issues and provide an overview of methods for some research questions in life course study, with a focus on mental health.

4.2.1 Longitudinal data for the life course study of mental health

4.2.1.1 Longitudinal life course data

Investigating life course influences on mental health requires data collected at the relevant life stages, and ideally from before birth to adult life, and across generations. Life course study often involves repeated exposure and outcome measures. While there has been marked development in analytic methods for longitudinal outcome variables in recent decades, analysing repeated measures on exposures and mental health remains a challenge.[16]

4.2.1.2 Missing data

In longitudinal studies, missing data due to sample attrition (i.e. permanent drop-out due to death, refusal, etc.), sweep missingness, or item missingness (missing some information at a sweep) may lead to bias and loss of efficiency of the sample estimates. The complete case approach may produce biased estimates when individuals with all variables of interest are not representative of the original (or target) sample. This is particularly an issue when examining life course influence on adult mental health. For example, poor behaviour and mental illness are known predictors for the probability of dropping out of longitudinal studies.[17]

Exposures for mental disorder are also related to sample attrition. In a British birth cohort study, where individuals were followed up to mid-adulthood, measures of childhood maltreatment (known predictors for adult psychological distress) are underestimated among participants who remained in the study until adulthood.[18] This selective missingness results in biased estimates for the exposures and outcome, and may also affect their associations.

Several statistical approaches can be applied to reduce the bias and improve the efficiency of the estimates, such as multiple imputation (MI) and inverse probability weighting (IPW),[19] and a combination of MI and IPW (using MI to address missing data for exposures and confounders, and IPW for the sample attrition).[20] These methods assume that data are missing at random (MAR), i.e. that the probability of missingness of a particular variable depends on the observed values and not on the missing value itself.

4.2.1.3 Measurements for mental health

Instruments used to measure mental well-being have to be designed for particular life stages. For example, the Rutter Home Behaviour Scale[21] and Bristol Social Adjustment Guide[22] have been used to assess emotion and behaviour problems in children. In adults, the Malaise Inventory[23] and General Health Questionnaire[24] are adopted in many large studies to assess psychological symptoms. These measures include many items, each of which identifies a psychological or somatic symptom. They are often used as a cumulative score, derived as a total of many items, to reflect an aspect of mental disorder. The score is usually a count (or an ordinal) variable, although it is also treated by many as a continuous variable. The score sometimes has a skewed distribution or clusters at a specific value (i.e. zero for no symptoms) and these distributions should be taken into consideration when choosing the analytic method.

4.2.2 Choice of statistical method

The choice of statistical methods depends on the life course hypotheses and types of measures being considered. A simple model selection approach has been used to compare the distinct hypotheses of the cumulation, critical period, or mobility model for the effect of a binary exposure over the life course on a late outcome.[25] The approach is not practicable for a large number of continuous exposures.

Many life course studies of mental health are concerned with its changes over time. Repeated mental health assessments are used to establish how the trajectories vary between individuals or between groups. A key aspect of longitudinal data is that repeated measurements from the same participant are correlated. For example, data from the 1958 British Birth Cohort show that the correlation coefficient for malaise scores at ages 23, 33, 42, and 50 years ranges from 0.5 to 0.6; this within-individual correlation needed to be taken into account in the analysis of these longitudinal data.

A range of random effects models for analysing longitudinal response variables such as growth curve models and growth mixture models have provided promising tools for analysing longitudinal life course data. Sections 4.2.2.1–7 discuss several analytic approaches to address research questions in life course and intergenerational studies of mental health.

4.2.2.1 Growth curve models

Growth curve models may be used to describe longitudinal changes of a continuous variable with increasing age for individuals or groups.[26] The models assume that the response variable follows a normal distribution. As mental health measures often follow a non-normal distribution (e.g. positively skewed non-zero values), a non-linear transformation (e.g. log transformation) is commonly used to normalize the measures.

We assume that y_{ij} is a response variable (e.g. a mental health score on a continuous scale) at the occasion j for the individual i ($j = 1, 2, \ldots, n_i$; $i = 1, 2, \ldots, n$) and that x_i is an individual-specific covariate (e.g. an exposure such as childhood adversity). As individuals may differ in age at each occasion, t_{ij} is the exact age of the measurement. Supposing the response variable Y is a linear function of age (t) and the covariate (X), a growth curve model with random effects is written as

$$y_{ij} = \beta_{0i} + \beta_{1i} t_{ij} + \alpha\, x_i + e_{ij}$$

$$\beta_{0i} = \beta_0 + \mu_{0i}$$

$$\beta_{1i} = \beta_1 + \mu_{1i}.$$

(A)

The model (A) assumes that each individual has its own initial value β_{0i} (mean β_0 and variance σ_0^2) and slope β_{1i} (mean β_1 and variance σ_1^2). It assumes that random coefficients (μ_{0i}, μ_{1i}) follow a bivariate normal distribution, that e_{ij} is an independent and identically distributed random variable which follows a normal distribution, and that $\text{cov}(e_{ij}, \mu_{0i}) = \text{cov}(e_{ij}, \mu_{1i}) = 0$. The model also assumes that repeated response measures assess the same property at each occasion, and all individuals have the same shape of trajectory, characterized by the linear function of age. Individual trajectories may differ with respect to model parameters $(\beta_{0j}$ and $\beta_{1i})$.

The growth curve model is flexible in specifying the trajectory using a range of linear or nonlinear functions of age (e.g. polynomial, spline, fractional polynomial), to capture the patterns of development during different periods. Further covariates, time-invariant (x_i) or time-varying exposures (x_{ij}), can be added to the model. The growth curve models can be applied to assess the general pattern of changes over time, and whether the exposures are associated with the changes (adding an interaction term with age). The growth curve model is also flexible for the number of measurements, which may not be spaced equally over time. Individuals with a missing response variable at some occasions can be included under a MAR assumption.[19]

4.2.2.2 Longitudinal data with a non-normal distribution

In a growth curve model we assume the repeated response variable to be normally distributed. However, measures for mental health are often skewed. A simple transformation to a normally distributed variable may not always be feasible. For example, when a large proportion of data cluster at zero (i.e. with no symptoms of mental illness), a transformation will not change the fact that many scores have the same value. Figure 4.1 illustrates the distribution of the Malaise Inventory which assessed 24 psychological and somatic symptoms in the 1958 British Birth Cohort when they were aged 33 years. The distribution of the malaise score is positively skewed, with a substantial number of participants having a low score and only a few having high scores; a measure like this is unsuitable for analysis as a continuous variable.

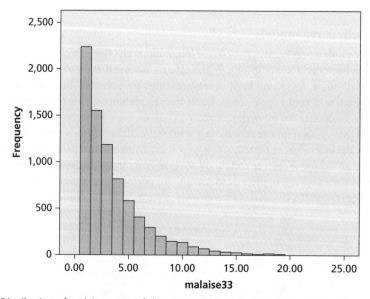

Figure 4.1 Distribution of malaise score of the 1958 British Birth Cohort (age 33 years).

One approach for dealing with the highly skewed and clustered data is to recode such measures into categories. For example, we may convert a mental health score (z) to a binary response (y) via a threshold (c).[27] The score is classified as presence ($y = 1$) if $z > c$, or otherwise absence ($y = 0$) of psychological disorder for analysis with logistic regression. For example, a malaise score (24 items) of ≥ 7 has previously been shown to identify clinically diagnosed depression with 73% sensitivity and 81% specificity.[28]

4.2.2.3 Random effects logistic models for binary outcomes

We assume that y_{ij} is a binary response variable, t_{ij} is the exact age, and x_i is an individual specific exposure, a random effects logistic model[26] is written as

$$\text{logit}(P(y_{ij} = 1)) = \beta_{0i} + \beta_{1i}\, t_{ij} + \alpha\, x_i + \theta\, x_i t_{ij} \tag{B}$$

$$\beta_{0i} = \beta_0 + \mu_{0i}$$

$$\beta_{1i} = \beta_1 + \mu_{1i}.$$

We assume that random coefficients (μ_{0i}, μ_{1i}) follow a bivariate normal distribution. Each individual has its own 'propensity' for the response (μ_{0i} and μ_{1i}). The covariance structure is explicitly modelled.

Assume that y is a repeated binary measure representing depression at multiple ages during adulthood, and that x is a binary variable of behaviour problems in childhood. The fixed effect θ represents the difference in age trends in log odds for depression between two groups (children with and without behaviour problems). A significant positive value of θ indicates that the association between childhood behaviour and adult depression strengthens with increasing adult age. The model (B) accounts for the intra-subject variability and allows the varying numbers of measures for each individual due to missing data.

4.2.2.4 Random effects logistic models for ordinal outcomes

Classifying a mental health score into a binary variable relies on a suitable threshold, which ideally should have clinical significance. An alternative method for analysing longitudinal measures with a skewed and censored distribution is to divide the score into ordered categories, and to model the ordered categories using random effects ordinal logistic models.[26] Assuming that y_{ij} is a response variable (e.g. percentiles) at the occasion j for the individual i, t_{ij} is the exact age, and x_i is an individual specific exposure, a proportional odds model is written as

$$\text{logit}(P(y_{ij} \leq c)) = \gamma_c - [\beta_{0i} + \beta_{1i}\, t_{ij} + \alpha\, x_i + \theta\, x_i t_{ij}] \tag{C}$$

where β_{0i} and β_{1i} have the same assumptions as in model (B). The fixed effect θ represents the difference in age trends between two groups (i.e. children with and without behaviour problems).

The model assumes an underlying multinomial distribution for the response variable and the effect of covariates is the same across all $C - 1$ cumulative logits (i.e. proportional odds; C is the number of categories). A significant positive value of θ indicates that the effect of the covariate on adult depression strengthens over time. The fixed effect θ represents the difference in age trends in log odds of having a higher percentile compared with a lower percentile (i.e. adult mental health score at 90th versus 80th, 80th versus 70th, and so on) between children with behaviour problems and those without. The model can be extended so that the effect of exposures may vary across cumulative logits.[27]

4.2.2.5 Other approaches for analysing skewed mental health data

The non-parametric methods such as the Mann–Whitney–Wilcoxon test can be applied to study the association between exposures and non-normally distributed mental health outcomes. These methods are based on the ranks rather than the actual values of the measures. However, they may lose power when there is a large number of observations that are tied at particular values. Most of the non-parametric methods were developed originally for cross-sectional studies. Although some extensions have been made for the longitudinal data,[29,30] they are not readily available in statistical packages.

For longitudinal data with a cluster of zero values, we might want to assess how the exposures are associated with the risk of a non-zero score and the severity among those with a non-zero score. In this case, for example, a two-stage analysis is possible; we may use a logistic regression model to discriminate zeros from non-zeros and a linear or Poisson regression model to the non-zero values (depending on the distribution of the non-zero values), fitting the two models simultaneously.[31] The estimated effects from two models, one for the proportion of zeros and one for the non-zero data, are assumed to be inter-correlated. The two models are linked by adding random effects to both the discrete and continuous parts of the model and allowing those random effects to be correlated with each other. This method is based on the assumption that non-zero values have a log–normal or a Poisson distribution. It allows the use of different sets of covariates for the zero and non-zero parts[31] and thus is flexible. The generalized linear models for log–normal, gamma, and Weibull distributions are also useful for analysing the right-skewed mental health data, for example alcohol consumption and mental health.[32]

For highly skewed data, we may want to use the median as a measure of centrality instead of the mean. Standard software is readily available to fit median or quantile regression to cross-sectional data. There has been some recent development in quantile regression models with random effects.[33] However, the approaches for longitudinal data are not available in standard software.

4.2.2.6 Growth mixture models for identifying distinct patterns of trajectories

Random effects models discussed so far (e.g. growth curve models or random effects logistic models) all assume that developmental trajectories across individuals have the same marginal shape defined by a function of age. Any heterogeneity in this is captured by random parameters of the model such as the intercept and slope. In mental health research, we are sometimes interested in specific patterns of trajectories for psychological and behavioural development, for example, the homogeneous subsets of individuals within the heterogeneous population, whose trajectories represent chronic, early onset, or late onset of mental disorders, compared with individuals with no mental health problems.

In the 1946 British Birth Cohort, using five repeated measures of anxious and depressive symptoms, Colman et al.[34] identified six distinct classes from age 13 to 53 years. These are 'absence of symptoms', 'repeated moderate symptoms', 'adult-onset moderate symptoms', 'adolescent symptoms with good adult outcome', 'adult-onset severe symptoms', and 'repeated severe symptoms over the life course'.[34] The results confirm that heterogeneity of growth trajectories exists within a large population sample.

Growth mixture modelling is an important tool[35] which allows different classes (or subpopulations) of trajectories for mental health development in the sample.[36] Within each class, growth

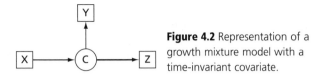

Figure 4.2 Representation of a growth mixture model with a time-invariant covariate.

trajectories are homogeneous[37] or vary around the mean trajectory.[38] Growth mixture modelling is based on the assumption that the observed data are subject to measurement error and the study population includes a mixture of individuals from a limited number of latent classes, each with their own trajectory type.

The growth mixture model illustrated in Figure 4.2 consists of the following components: (1) a latent growth curve of observed variable Y (i.e. mental health measure); (2) a categorical variable for unobserved class C (k); (3) a time-invariant covariate X; (4) a distal outcome Z. The marginal density for the data y can be expressed as

$$f(y_i \,|\, x_i) = \sum_k P(C_i = k \,|\, X_i = x_i) P(Y_i = y_i \,|\, C_i = k).$$

The first part is a logistic model for multinomial variable C, and the second part is the model for the trajectory, given the class membership. The growth mixture models can be applied to variables from a range of distributions, such as normal, categorical, and zero-inflated Poisson distributions.

The model assessment and selection of optimal number of classes are based on several statistical criteria and tests; for instance, the model with small values of the Akaike's Information Criterion (AIC) and Bayesian Information Criterion (BIC).[39] These tests include the Lo–Mendell–Rubin likelihood ratio test, the bootstrap likelihood ratio test, and Vuong–Lo–Mendell–Rubin likelihood ratio test for k versus $k-1$ classes. A low P-value (traditionally $P < 0.05$) indicates that the $k-1$ classes model needs to be rejected in favour of a model with at least k classes.

We used the 1958 British Birth Cohort to illustrate the application of a growth mixture model to study the association between behavioural difficulties in early childhood and trajectories of depression in adulthood. The Cohort included all children born in one week in March 1958 in Great Britain. Approximately 17,000 live births were followed up at ages 7, 11, 16, 23, 33, 42, 45, and 50 years.

Psychological distress at age 7 years was measured using the Bristol Social Adjustment Guide.[22] An internalizing behaviour scale was obtained by summing four syndromes (depression, unforthcomingness, withdrawal, and miscellaneous). An externalizing behaviour scale was formed by summing four syndromes (anxiety for acceptance, hostility, restlessness, and inconsequential behaviour). In adulthood, common symptoms of anxiety and depression were recorded with the Malaise Inventory.[23] A 24-item self-reported questionnaire indicating depression and anxiety tendencies (nine somatic and 15 depressive symptoms) was obtained at ages 23, 33, and 42 years.[28] A shorter version (eight psychological items) was administered at age 50 years. Only psychological items across age were used. As different ranges of malaise score were used (15 items at ages 23–42 years and eight items at age 50 years), we rescaled the scores to obtain the same total of 120 for all ages (multiplied by eight for malaise score at ages 23, 33, and 42 years, multiplied by 15 for score at age 50 years). The aim was to establish: (i) the number of classes of trajectories for adult depressive symptoms; (ii) whether there is a gender difference in profiles of adult depression; and (iii) whether childhood behaviour is associated with trajectories of depression.

We applied a growth mixture model to malaise score at all ages. As malaise scores were highly skewed with a large proportion of individuals having a score zero, we adopted a zero-inflated Poisson model for the trajectories. Sex and internalizing and externalizing behaviour at age 7 years were included as time-invariant covariates in the model. The analysis included all individuals with at least one of the four ages at which malaise scores were obtained ($n = 14,741$). Individuals with incomplete data were assigned to their most likely class on the basis of the available information and parameter estimates obtained from maximum likelihood estimation of the model under the MAR assumption.[19]

The best-fitting model (based on the AIC, BIC and statistical tests) identified five trajectory groups: individuals with: (i) 'an absence of symptoms'; (ii) 'low level symptoms'; (iii) 'a moderate stable level of symptoms'; (iv) 'mid-adulthood onset of a moderate level of symptoms'; and (v) 'high, deteriorating level of symptoms'. For each individual, the probability of belonging to each of the five groups (class membership) was estimated and the individual classified into the group of the highest probability. The association between the covariates and patterns of trajectory can be estimated, i.e. the relative risk ratio (RRR) for each trajectory group (against 'an absence of symptoms') for females and individuals with internalizing or externalizing behaviour problems, compared to males and those without behaviour problems, respectively.

As was expected, females were more likely than males to have depressive symptoms at all adult ages. In particular, females had an increased risk of a moderate, stable (RRR = 3.21) or high, deteriorating (RRR = 4.79) early onset of depressive symptoms over the life course. They were also more likely to have minor symptoms from their early 20s, and some deterioration from early 30s. Individuals with internalizing and externalizing behaviour problems in early childhood were more likely to have a persisting (RRR = 1.11) or deteriorating (RRR = 1.25) onset of depression in their early 20s over the life course (Table 4.1).

4.2.2.7 Association between trajectories of mental health and other outcomes

One important area in life course research is to establish how longitudinal development of mental health is associated with other outcomes of childhood exposure. Emotional development in childhood has been shown to be associated with affective and anxiety disorders in mid-adulthood.[4]

Table 4.1 Multinomial logistic regression model assessing the association of gender and childhood behaviour with four trajectory groups of adult mental health in the 1958 British Birth Cohort

	Relative risk ratio[a] (95% CI)			
	Group 2: Low level (25.9%)	Group 3: Moderate, stable (21.6%)	Group 4: Mid-adult onset, moderate (18.8%)	Group 5: High, deteriorating (16.7%)
Females	1.59 (1.42, 1.79)	3.21 (2.85, 3.62)	1.67 (1.47, 1.89)	4.79 (4.20, 5.45)
Internalizing behaviour	0.98 (0.93, 1.03)	1.14 (1.08, 1.20)	1.01 (0.95, 1.07)	1.24 (1.17, 1.31)
Externalizing behaviour	1.02 (0.97, 1.07)	1.11 (1.05, 1.17)	1.01 (0.95, 1.07)	1.25 (1.18, 1.32)

[a] For each trajectory group (baseline: Group 1, 'absence of symptoms') for females and individuals with behaviour problems, compared with males and those without problems, respectively.

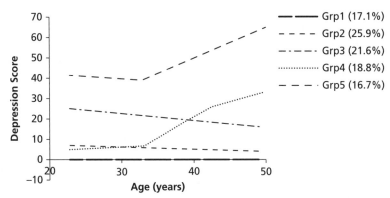

Figure 4.3 Five trajectory groups for depressive symptoms (23–50 years) in the 1958 British Birth Cohort.

Distinct trajectories of depressive symptoms are associated with changes in body size from adolescence to adulthood.[22] Trajectories of maternal pre- and postnatal depression are associated with offspring behaviour.[15]

Growth mixture models can be applied to link the distinct patterns of trajectories to other outcome(s) (Figure 4.2). Based on the growth mixture model, each individual is assigned to the trajectory group based on the highest estimated posterior probability. The class membership C can be used in subsequent analyses as an exposure and related to a single outcome. Thus the association between patterns of trajectories and the outcome Z can be estimated by regressing Z onto C. This approach can be useful when there is an a-priori reason for believing that subgroups exist within a population and that classes identified reflect the hypotheses of interest. It has been used in several studies, for example, to investigate the association between distinct maternal mental health trajectories in the pre- and postnatal periods and in child development.[40] In Figure 4.3, the trajectory groups identified could be used as an exposure measure and linked to a late outcome. This association would shed some light on the 'accumulative risk' hypothesis; for instance, that the duration (from early or mid-adulthood) and severity (mild, moderate, or high level of symptoms).

4.3 **Summary**

Life course study of mental health presents methodological challenges due to its complex research questions and the fact that these longitudinal data can have a non-normal skewed distribution, missing values and be correlated within subjects. In this chapter we have discussed some statistical methods which may be applied to this type of data to answer important questions in the life course study of mental health.

References

1 Colman I, Ataullahjan A. Life course perspectives on the epidemiology of depression. *Can J Psychiatry* 2010;**55**(10):622–632.

2 Wadsworth M, Maughan B, Pickles A. Introduction: development and progression of life course ideas in epidemiology. In: Wadsworth M, Maughan, B, Pickles A, editors. *Epidemiological methods in life course research*. Oxford: Oxford University Press; 2007.

3 **Rodgers B.** Behaviour and personality in childhood as predictors of adult psychiatric disorder. *J Child Psychol Psychiatry* 1990;**31**(3):393–414.

4 **Clark C, Rodgers B, Caldwell T, Power C, Stansfeld S.** Childhood and adulthood psychological ill health as predictors of midlife affective and anxiety disorders: the 1958 British Birth Cohort. *Arch Gen Psychiatry* 2007;**64**(6):668–678.

5 **Ritsher JE, Warner V, Johnson JG, Dohrenwend BP.** Inter-generational longitudinal study of social class and depression: a test of social causation and social selection models. *Br J Psychiatry* 2001;**40**(Suppl):s84–s90.

6 **Rodgers B, Power C, Hope S.** Parental divorce and adult psychological distress: evidence from a national birth cohort: a research note. *J Child Psychol Psychiatry* 1997;**38**(7):867–872.

7 **Fergusson DM, Horwood LJ, Lynskey MT.** Childhood sexual abuse and psychiatric disorder in young adulthood: II. Psychiatric outcomes of childhood sexual abuse. *J Am Acad Child Adolesc Psychiatry* 1996;**35**(10):1365–1374.

8 **Widom CS, DuMont K, Czaja SJ.** A prospective investigation of major depressive disorder and comorbidity in abused and neglected children grown up. *Arch Gen Psychiatry* 2007;**64**(1):49–56.

9 **Benjet C, Borges G, Medina-Mora ME.** Chronic childhood adversity and onset of psychopathology during three life stages: childhood, adolescence and adulthood. *J Psychiatr Res* 2010;**44**(11):732–740.

10 **Hertzman C, Power C.** Child development as a determinant of health across the life course. *Curr Paediatrics* 2004;**14**(5):438–443.

11 **Stansfeld SA, Clark C, Rodgers B, Caldwell T, Power C.** Repeated exposure to socioeconomic disadvantage and health selection as life course pathways to mid-life depressive and anxiety disorders. *Soc Psychiatry Psychiatr Epidemiol* 2011;**46**(7):549–558.

12 **Miech RA, Shanahan MJ.** Socioeconomic status and depression over the life course. *J Health Social Behav* 2000;**41**:162–176.

13 **Kivimaki M, Batty GD, Singh-Manoux A, et al.** Association between common mental disorder and obesity over the adult life course. *Br J Psychiatry* 2009;**195**(2):149–155.

14 **Power C, Li L, Atherton K, Hertzman C.** Psychological health throughout life and adult cortisol patterns at age 45 y. *Psychoneuroendocrinology* 2011;**36**(1):87–97.

15 **Vanska M, Punamaki RL, Tolvanen A, et al.** Maternal pre- and postnatal mental health trajectories and child mental health and development: prospective study in a normative and formerly intertile sample. *Int J Behav Dev* 2011;**35**:517–531.

16 **De Stavola BL, Nitsch D, dos Santos Silva I, et al.** Statistical issues in life course epidemiology. *Am J Epidemiol* 2006;**163**(1):84–96.

17 **Atherton K, Fuller E, Shepherd P, Strachan DP, Power C.** Loss and representativeness in a biomedical survey at age 45 years: 1958 British birth cohort. *J Epidemiol Community Health* 2008;**62**(3):216–223.

18 **Denholm R, Power C, Thomas C, Li L.** Child maltreatment and household dysfunction in a British birth cohort. *Child Abuse Review* 2013 Feb 27 [Epub ahead of print].

19 **Little RJ, Rubin DB.** *Statistical analysis with missing data.* 2nd ed. New York: John Wiley & Sons; 2002.

20 **Seaman SR, White IR, Copas AJ, Li L.** Combining multiple imputation and inverse-probability weighting. *Biometrics* 2012;**68**(1):129–137.

21 **Rutter M.** A children's behaviour questionnaire for completion by teachers: preliminary findings. *J Child Psychol Psychiatry* 1967;**8**:1–11.

22 **Stott DH.** *The social adjustment of children.* London: University of London Press; 1969.

23 **Rutter ML.** Psycho-social disorders in childhood, and their outcome in adult life. *J R Coll Physicians Lond* 1970;**4**(3):211–218.

24 **Goldberg DP, Hillier VF.** A scaled version of the General Health Questionnaire. *Psychol Med* 1979;**9**(1):139–145.

25 **Mishra G, Nitsch D, Black S, De SB, Kuh D, Hardy R.** A structured approach to modelling the effects of binary exposure variables over the life course. *Int J Epidemiol* 2009;**38**(2):528–537.

26 **Goldstein H.** *Multilevel statistical models.* 3rd ed. New York: John Wiley & Sons; 2003.

27 **Hedeker D, Mermelstein J.** A multilevel thresholds of change model for analysis of stage of change data. *Multivariate Behav Res* 1998;**33**(4):427–455.

28 **Rodgers B, Pickles A, Power C, Collishaw S, Maughan B.** Validity of the Malaise Inventory in general population samples. *Soc Psychiatry Psychiatr Epidemiol* 1999;**34**(6):333–341.

29 **Lachin JM.** Distribution-free marginal analysis of repeated measures. *Drug Info J* 1996;**30**:1017–1028.

30 **Davis CS.** Semi-parametric and non-parametric methods for the analysis of repeated measurements with applications to clinical trials. *Stat Med* 1991;**10**(12):1959–1980.

31 **Tooze JA, Grunwald GK, Jones RH.** Analysis of repeated measures data with clumping at zero. *Stat Methods Med Res* 2002;**11**(4):341–355.

32 **Azuero A, Pisu M, McNees P, Burkhardt J, Benz R, Meneses K.** An application of longitudinal analysis with skewed outcomes. *Nurs Res* 2010;**59**(4):301–307.

33 **Koenker R.** Quantile regression for longitudinal data. *J Multivariate Data Analysis* 2004;**91**:74–89.

34 **Colman I, Ploubidis GB, Wadsworth ME, Jones PB, Croudace TJ.** A longitudinal typology of symptoms of depression and anxiety over the life course. *Biol Psychiatry* 2007;**62**(11):1265–1271.

35 **Pickles A, Croudace T.** Latent mixture models for multivariate and longitudinal outcomes. *Stat Methods Med Res* 2010;**19**(3):271–289.

36 **Mora PA, Bennett IM, Elo IT, Mathew L, Coyne JC, Culhane JF.** Distinct trajectories of perinatal depressive symptomatology: evidence from growth mixture modeling. *Am J Epidemiol* 2009;**169**(1): 24–32.

37 **Nagin DS.** Analyzing developmental trajectories: a semiparametric, group-based approach. *Psychological Methods* 1999;**4**(2):139–157.

38 **Muthen B, Muthen LK.** Integrating person-centered and variable-centered analyses: growth mixture modeling with latent trajectory classes. *Alcohol Clin Exp Res* 2000;**24**(6):882–891.

39 **Schwarz GE.** Estimating the dimension of a model. *Ann Stat* 1978;**6**(2):461–464.

40 **Weaver IC, Champagne FA, Brown SE, et al.** Reversal of maternal programming of stress responses in adult offspring through methyl supplementation: altering epigenetic marking later in life. *J Neurosci* 2005;**25**(47):11045–11054.

Chapter 5

Age, birth cohort, and period effects in psychiatric disorders in the USA

Katherine M. Keyes and Charley Liu

5.1 Introduction

Risk for psychiatric disorders varies across the life course, with incidence most likely to occur during specific critical periods of development.[1] As the life course perspective increases in utility to understand disease aetiology, analysis of period and cohort effects in historical data over time has become imperative for understanding the role of biological and environmental factors in disease distribution at the population level. Temporal variation in rates of disease may reflect changes in the nature and magnitude of the effect of aetiologically important exposures, and identification of particular cohorts with higher than expected rates of psychiatric disorders is vital for public health planning and intervention efforts.

In the present chapter we review three disorders with sufficient research bases in age, period, and cohort effects such that conclusions can be generated: major depression, alcohol use disorders, and autism spectrum disorders. We focus our review on studies conducted in the USA, as trends in psychiatric disorders and related mortality vary across countries and cultures; thus a cohesive framework for investigation of age–period–cohort effects is best suited in defined geographic areas. We begin by defining and describing age, period, and cohort effects and statistical considerations in estimating and interpreting models.

5.2 What are age, period, and cohort effects?

Age effects can be conceptualized at both the individual and the ecological level. Individual-level age effects are developmentally linked pathways to health outcomes; for example, individuals are most likely to initiate cigarette use between the ages of 13 and 15 years,[2] and alcohol use between the ages of 15 and 17 years.[3] Ecological-level age effects refer to the age structure of the population (i.e. the distribution of older and younger individuals over time). For example, the prevalence of Alzheimer's disease is expected to increase as the proportion of individuals aged ≥80 years in the USA increases.[4] Period effects describe changes in the prevalence of health outcomes associated with certain years, and these affect all age groups simultaneously. Common sources of period effects are changes in law or policy, introduction of an environmental pollutant in the population, or other factors that could affect all age groups simultaneously. Cohort effects describe changes in the prevalence of an outcome associated with certain age groups in certain years. That is, cohorts share exposure to certain environmental conditions at critical developmental ages, they compete for positions in labour and educational markets, and they experience historical events such as war and recession at the same age. Cohort effects in a health outcome indicate that the shared experience of early childhood, coming of age, and growing older with others of the same age can shape health.

5.3 **Design and analysis considerations in age–period–cohort modelling**

5.3.1 **Study design: cross-sectional**

Evaluation of birth cohort effects began as a life table method dating as far back as Farr.[5] and graphical approaches were further developed throughout the first half of the 20th century.

Whereas many studies use repeated cross-sections of data taken over time for age–period–cohort research, such data are often unavailable especially for psychiatric disorders, as criteria for diagnoses have shifted over time. Thus, single cross-sectional studies comparing retrospectively reported lifetime prevalence of disorder across individuals in different cohort groups are commonly used. Assessment of age, period, and cohort effects in the cross-sectional design is limited, however, because the effects of one can confound the effects of the others. For instance, in a cross-sectional dataset in which the prevalence of an outcome is observed to be increasing across age, we cannot tell whether this increase is a true age effect or a pure cohort effect (since, in a cross-sectional study, those of different ages are also in different cohorts). Further, recall may be poorer among older individuals, especially for disorders with young age of onset, creating the appearance of a cohort effect. For example, Simon et al.[6] demonstrated that people with major depression are most likely to report onset within the last five years regardless of their age at the time of the interview. Finally, there may be survivor effects, with those surviving to older ages being healthier and less likely to have a history of substance abuse or other psychiatric problems. Thus, while retrospective cross-sectional studies provide important information on cohort effects, they should be interpreted with caution.

5.3.2 **Study design: surveillance data**

Data collection of multiple age groups observed in many periods is preferable for teasing apart age, period, and cohort effects, but even in this situation, the independent effects of age, period, and cohort cannot be uniquely estimated in standard modelling procedures. This inability to uniquely estimate effects is due to the co-linearity among the three variables; in fact, they are perfectly co-linear. Given an age X and a period Y, the birth cohort Z is fully determined by Y–X. Thus, attempts to model simultaneously all three as additive covariates renders an unidentifiable model without additional assumptions. An array of methods has been developed with varying underlying assumptions in order to achieve model identification.[7–9] Most models place some type of constraint on the age, period, and cohort covariates in order to induce a non-linear relation with the outcome. Other methods focus entirely on the second order functions of the underlying linear relations, interpreting only the direction of changes over time without specifically ascribing the underlying slope to period or cohort effects.[7] Still other methods define cohort effects as the interaction between age and period and assess systematic variation by cohort that is non-additive across age–period categories.[9] circumventing identification issues and providing a reinterpretation of common assumptions about how cohort effects arise. We recommend that researchers interested in analysing data use an age–period–cohort model: (a) develop a comprehensive set of hypotheses about how age, period, and cohort effects could arise for a particular psychiatric disorder; (b) how age, period, and cohort effects operate together (e.g. whether effects are hypothesized to be additive or interactive); (c) conduct extensive graphical analysis of the data to understand the descriptive patterns; and (d) choose the best statistical strategy that corresponds to both hypotheses and graphical data patterns.

5.4 **Major depression**

Evidence indicates that treatment for depression has become more widespread.[10,11] Whether this is an effect of increased awareness and attention, or of an increase in prevalence, remains to be determined.

We identified 18 population-based studies in the USA that have examined whether individuals in more recently born cohorts have higher prevalence rates of depression compared with older cohorts. Studies published in the 1980s and 1990s using population-based data sources unanimously reported that younger birth cohorts (the youngest birth cohorts of these studies were typically born in the late 1950s and early 1960s) had a higher lifetime prevalence of major depression compared with older birth cohorts (see Table 5.1). Whereas most of these studies were descriptive, three studies attempted formal age–period–cohort modelling in which cohort effects were estimated independently from age and period effects. Results indicated that younger birth cohorts indeed exhibited higher risk, and that there was also a strong period effect in which the risk of major depression was elevated across the whole population. However, virtually all of these studies were cross-sectional analyses relying on respondent report of lifetime depressive episodes. This approach has been widely criticized,[6,12–14] as differential mortality and recall create bias in examining lifetime rates of depression among older individuals.

Five studies of birth cohort effects in major depression have been published since 2000, and findings are not as consistent as the earlier studies.

Perhaps the most rigorous examination of the issue has been by Costello et al.'s, meta-analysis of data from more than 60,000 children and adolescents from successive birth cohorts.[15] No changes in the prevalence of depression or depressive symptoms across birth cohorts were documented, leading the authors to conclude that previous investigations based on retrospective reporting were subject to recall bias. Data from the Sterling County study, a longitudinal study across 40 years of data collection, also documented no change in incident depression across two birth cohorts.[16]

In summary, whereas early population-based studies in the 1980s and 1990s suggested an increase in the prevalence of depression among younger birth cohorts, more recent investigations have revealed little increase in incidence or prevalence, suggesting that: (a) previous studies may have been subject to recall effects, and (b) the perceived increases in depression may well be a function of increased awareness and ascertainment of cases.

5.5 **Alcohol use and alcohol use disorders**

Substantial evidence indicates that the prevalence of alcohol use, alcohol disorder, and alcohol-related mortality is sensitive to environmental changes such as increases in taxes, changes in policies and laws governing opening and closing hours, happy hours, and threshold for intoxicated driving.[17] Furthermore, surveillance data indicate substantial trends over time in use of, and mortality due to, alcohol.

Considerable research has been conducted to assess cohort effects in alcohol use disorders, although few studies have been able to formally model age, period, and cohort effects simultaneously. A recent review synthesized evidence from 12 studies that have examined birth cohort effects on alcohol use disorders.[18] Most studies have been conducted in the USA, with retrospective assessment from cross-sectional surveys used to assess differences in lifetime alcohol use disorder prevalence by birth cohort. A broad selection of birth cohorts across the 20th century has been included in studies of cohort effects on alcohol use disorders. Of these 12 studies, 10 found evidence of cohort effects in alcohol use disorder prevalence, and nine of those 10 found that the youngest cohorts were at the highest risk. These studies have by and large shown consistent

Table 5.1 Population-based studies of birth cohort effects in depression in the USA

Study	Population/design	Cohort range	Depression diagnosis	Findings	Limitations	Strengths
Weissman et al.[41]	Cross-sectional survey of community sample in New Haven	1881–1963	DSM-III MDE	Increasing 6-month and lifetime prevalence and earlier age of onset in more recently born cohorts	Retrospective report	
Gershon et al.[42]	Cross-sectional survey of relatives of US individuals with psychiatric disorders	<1910–1959	RDC unipolar depression	Increasing lifetime prevalence in more recently born cohorts	Retrospective report	
Lavori et al.[43]	Cross-sectional survey of relatives of US individuals with psychiatric disorders	1930–1959	RDC unipolar depression	Increasing lifetime prevalence and younger age of onset in more recently born cohorts; strong period effects bserved	Retrospective report	Formal age–period–cohort model
Wickramaratne et al.[44]	Cross-sectional survey of five US community samples (ECA)	1905–1965	DSM-III MDE	Increasing lifetime prevalence and younger age of onset in more recently born cohorts; period effects also observed for men	Retrospective report	Formal age–period–cohort model
Klerman et al.[45]	Cross-sectional survey of relatives of US individuals with psychiatric disorders	<1915–1955 or later	RDC unipolar depression	Increasing lifetime prevalence in more recently born cohorts	Retrospective report	
Joyce et al.[46]	Cross-sectional survey of New Zealand community adults	1921–1968	DSM-III MDE	Increasing lifetime prevalence in more recently born cohorts (increasing 12-month prevalence for more recently born cohorts in men only)	Retrospective report	
Warshaw et al.[47]	Cross-sectional survey of relatives of US individuals with psychiatric disorders	1906–1965	RDC unipolar depression	Increasing lifetime prevalence and younger age of onset in more recently born cohorts; strong period effects observed	Retrospective report	Formal age–period–cohort model

Table 5.1 (continued) Population-based studies of birth cohort effects in depression in the USA

Study	Population/design	Cohort range	Depression diagnosis	Findings	Limitations	Strengths
Ryan et al.[48]	Cross-sectional survey of siblings of children with MDD	(Range not given; mean: 1970; SD: 6)	RDC unipolar depression	Increasing lifetime prevalence in more recently born cohorts	Retrospective report	
Burke et al.[49]	Cross-sectional survey of five US community samples (ECA)	<1917–1966	DSM-III MDE	Increasing lifetime prevalence and younger age of onset in more recently born cohorts	Retrospective report	
Cross-National Collaborative Group[50]	Pooled analysis of nine cross-sectional North American general population and family studies (~39,000 subjects)	<1905–1995 or later	DSM-III MDE	Increasing lifetime prevalence in more recently born cohorts, with variation by country	Retrospective report	
Lewinsohn et al.[51]	Three cross-sectional surveys of adults and one of adolescents	1900–1972	DSM-III-R MDD	Increasing lifetime prevalence in more recently born cohorts	Retrospective report	Convergent findings across different populations
Leon et al.[52]	Cross-sectional survey of relatives of US individuals with psychiatric disorders	1915–1954 and later	RDC unipolar depression	Increasing lifetime prevalence in more recently born cohorts for men; peak in prevalence for 1945–1954 cohort for women	Retrospective report	
Kessler et al.[53]	Cross-sectional survey of US general population (NCS)	1936–1975	DSM-III-R MDE	Increasing lifetime prevalence in more recently born cohorts	Retrospective report	
Murphy et al.[16]	40-year longitudinal community study	1952 and 1970	Not specified	No difference in incidence between two cohorts; current prevalence higher among younger women		Longitudinal

Table 5.1 (continued) Population-based studies of birth cohort effects in depression in the USA

Study	Population/design	Cohort range	Depression diagnosis	Findings	Limitations	Strengths
Kessler et al.[54]	Cross-sectional survey of US general population (NCS-R)	<1941–1984	DSM-IV MDD	Increasing lifetime prevalence in more recently born cohorts	Retrospective report	
Kasen et al.[55]	20-year longitudinal study	1928–1945 vs 1945–	Depression index	Overall increases in depression in younger birth cohorts, but more declines with age compared with older birth cohorts		Longitudinal
Costello et al.[15]	Meta-analysis of epidemiological studies comprising 60,000 children (up to age 18 years)	1965–1996	ICD-9, -10, or DSM-III, III-R, or IV MDD or MDE in the past week, month or year	No effect of year of birth on depression		Large pooled sample; current diagnoses
Hasin et al.[56]	Cross-sectional survey of US general population (NESARC)	1906–1984	DSM-IV MDE	Highest lifetime prevalence in 'baby boom' cohort	Retrospective report	

DSM, *Diagnostic and Statistical Manual*; MDE, major depressive episode; RDC, Research Diagnostic Criteria; MDD, major depressive disorder; ECA, epidemiological catchment area; NCS (-R) National Comorbidity Survey (Replication); NESARC, National Epidemiologic Survey on Alcohol and Related Conditions.

and monotonic increases in the prevalence of alcohol use disorders by birth cohort, with cohorts born in the latter half of the 20th century at higher risk than those born in the early decades of the 1900s.

Interestingly, age–period–cohort modelling of alcohol consumption and high risk drinking patterns, independently of alcohol use disorders, do not show similar trends. Kerr et al.[19] documented in sequentially conducted cross-sectional samples over 26 years that two simultaneous processes are operative in alcohol consumption trends. Whereas cohorts born in the late 1970s and early 1980s consume alcohol less frequently and have a lower overall consumption mean compared with previously born cohorts, heavy episodic drinking is more prevalent. If true, this suggests that increases in risky patterns of alcohol consumption may portend greater drinking consequences for these cohorts later in life. However, other national studies have not found similar results, and instead have documented that heavy episodic drinking is either decreasing in cohorts born in the 1980s[20,21] or that period effects explain trends over time in heavy episodic drinking rather than cohort effects.[22]

The underlying mechanisms through which age, period, and cohort effects arise in alcohol use and related disorders is unclear, although studies are beginning to test specific hypotheses about the role of various environmental factors. Keyes et al.[23] recently documented the alcohol-related social norms of birth cohorts in the 1960s through the 1990s using nationally representative yearly surveys of adolescents. Investigators found that these cohort-specific social norms are strongly associated with individual risk of binge drinking and increases in alcohol-using occasions, independently of time-period-specific social norms as well as the adolescents' personal attitude toward use. This suggests that one driver of birth cohort effects in alcohol use is the amount of social sanctioning against behaviour from peers, which changes across time. Evidence also indicates that women in more recently born cohorts are increasing drinking at a faster rate than men.[18] Given that social norms for women have changed enormously over the past several decades, this accumulating research underscores the notion that social norms play an important role in shaping alcohol use at the population level.

5.6 **Autism spectrum disorders**

Diagnoses of autism and autism spectrum disorders have increased in the past two decades in the USA as well as in many other western countries.[24–28] The reasons for these increases remain controversial, and are thought to derive from some combination of increased awareness, changes in diagnoses and diagnostic practices, and an increase in the population prevalence of individual-level risk.

Autism diagnosis is strongly related to child age.[29] with diagnoses most likely to occur between the ages of 3 and 5 years, although the average age of diagnosis has been decreasing as early markers of autism symptoms are increasingly recognized.[30,31] Age effects, however, are unlikely to be driving the increased incidence of autism diagnosis as age-adjusted rates still show a marked increase over time.[32] This leaves the possibility of some combination of period and cohort effects as driving the increase in autism diagnoses.

Observations of period and cohort effects have different implications for the aetiology of the increases, with period effects suggesting that widespread environmental factors that influence all age groups at a particular time are responsible for the increase, whereas cohort effects indicate that environmental influences that affect specific age groups at a particular time should be considered. Given the relatively constrained age range over which autism diagnoses typically occur, however, period effects are unlikely drivers of diagnostic increases. Environmental factors would need to have the same effect on autism diagnoses among children of all ages in order for a period effect to explain the increases in autism incidence, which is unlikely based on the developmental epidemiology of autism.

Indeed, evidence to date is strongly suggestive of powerful cohort effects in the incidence and prevalence of autism.[33–35] For example, data from the Centers for Disease Control and Prevention funded Autism and Developmental Disabilities Monitoring Network indicate a more than two-fold increase in the prevalence of autism spectrum disorders among eight-year-olds in the USA born in 1998 compared to 1994.[36] (with substantial variation in the size of the increase across states.[34] and more recent data indicate that the prevalence continues to increase.26 Population-based data from the California Department of Developmental Services (DDS) and Denmark indicate consistent increases in the incidence of autism diagnoses across age for each successively younger birth cohort from approximately 1990 onward.[32,33]

California DDS data also indicate that cohort effects in autism diagnosis incidence are stronger in children who exhibit higher functioning on social interaction, language, and communication compared to those with lower functioning (Figure 5.1).[37] Although the odds of an autism diagnosis among those exhibiting low functioning were four times higher in the 2002 cohort than in the 1992 cohort, the odds of an autism diagnosis among those exhibiting high functioning were almost 15 times higher.

Cohort effects could arise in autism diagnoses through a number of potential mechanisms. For example, if the prevalence of a risk factor acting at conception exhibits change over time (e.g. paternal age[38]), then each successively younger cohort will be differentially exposed, manifesting as a cohort effect (e.g. each successively younger cohort has older fathers). Alternatively, an exposure introduced into the population as a whole could differentially affect autism incidence depending on age of exposure. This would also manifest as a cohort effect. As the prevalence of autism diagnoses is continuing to increase, continued surveillance of period and cohort effects in autism spectrum disorders will continue to be an important public health activity.

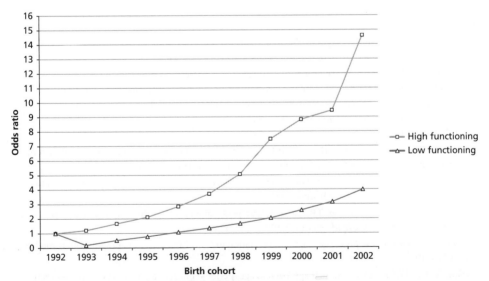

Figure 5.1 Cohort effects in autism diagnosis in California from 1994 to 2005 by child's functioning at the time of diagnosis.

5.7 **Other disorders**

This chapter discusses evidence for age, period, and cohort effects for psychiatric disorders with a well-documented evidence base regarding these effects. Bipolar disorder and attention deficit/hyperactivity disorder (ADHD) have also demonstrated increases in childhood diagnoses.[39,40] but limited investigations have been made into possible age, period, and cohort effects. The rapid changes in trends over time suggest the need for continued surveillance and age–period–cohort modelling.

5.8 **Summary**

Assessment of age, period, and cohort effects is vital for a life course approach to psychiatric epidemiology. Variation in the incidence and prevalence of psychiatric disorders by birth cohort, independent of age and period, suggests that the social structures in which individuals are embedded during important developmental time-periods can influence the risk of psychiatric disorder onset for groups of individuals exposed to those structures. Published research supports a role for birth cohort effects in the incidence and prevalence of alcohol use disorders. Whereas cohort effects in major depression have been found, the existence of cohort effects remains controversial due to data suggesting that a retrospective reporting bias may explain a large part of these results. Autism diagnoses have robust evidence for cohort effect. The increase in the prevalence of many psychiatric disorders during childhood, adolescence, and young adulthood my portend greater consequences in numerous domains of social, medical, and psychiatric morbidity throughout the next several decades as these young cohorts reach middle and old age.

Acknowledgements

This research was supported in part by support from New York State Psychiatric Institute and the Department of Epidemiology at the Mailman School of Public Health (K. Keyes).

References

1 Kessler RC, Amminger GP, Aguilar-Gaxiola S, Alonso J, Lee S, Ustun TB. Age of onset of mental disorders: a review of recent literature. *Curr Opin Psychiatry* 2007;**20**(4):359–364.

2 Everett SA, Warren CW, Sharp D, Kann L, Husten CG, Crossett LS. Initiation of cigarette smoking and subsequent smoking behavior among U.S. high school students. *Prev Med* 1999;**29**(5):327–333.

3 Grant BF. Prevalence and correlates of alcohol use and DSM-IV alcohol dependence in the United States: results of the National Longitudinal Alcohol Epidemiologic Survey. *J Stud Alcohol* 1997;**58**(5):464–473.

4 Hebert LE, Scherr PA, Bienias JL, Bennett DA, Evans DA. Alzheimer disease in the US population: prevalence estimates using the 2000 census. *Arch Neurol* 2003;**60**(8):1119–1122.

5 Farr W. *Vital statistics: memorial volume of selections from the reports and writings of William Farr.* London: Offices of the Sanitary Institute; 1885.

6 Simon GE, VonKorff M, Ustun TB, Gater R, Gureje O, Sartorius N. Is the lifetime risk of depression actually increasing? *J Clin Epidemiol* 1995;**48**(9):1109–1118.

7 Clayton D, Schifflers E. Models for temporal variation in cancer rates. II: Age–period–cohort models. *Stat Med* 1987;**6**(4):469–481.

8 Yang Y, Land KC. A mixed models approach to age–period–cohort analysis of repeated cross-section surveys: trends in verbal test scores. In: **Stolzenberg RM** editor. *Sociological methodology.* Boston: Blackwell; 2006.

9   Keyes KM, Li G. A multi-phase method for estimating cohort effects in age-period contingency table data. *Ann Epidemiol* 2010;**20**(10):779–785.

10 Olfson M, Marcus SC. National patterns in antidepressant medication treatment. *Arch Gen Psychiatry* 2009;**66**(8):848–856.

11 Olfson M, Marcus SC, Druss B, Elinson L, Tanielian T, Pincus HA. National trends in the outpatient treatment of depression. *JAMA* 2002;**287**(2):203–9.

12 Simon GE, VonKorff M. Reevaluation of secular trends in depression rates. *Am J Epidemiol* 1992;**135**(12):1411–1422.

13 Giuffra LA, Risch N. Diminished recall and the cohort effect of major depression: a simulation study. *Psychol Med* 1994;**24**(2):375–83.

14 Patten SB. Recall bias and major depression lifetime prevalence. *Soc Psychiatry Psychiatr Epidemiol* 2003;**38**(6):290–296.

15 Costello EJ, Erkanli A, Angold A. Is there an epidemic of child or adolescent depression? *J Child Psychol Psychiatry* 2006;**47**(12):1263–1271.

16 Murphy JM, Laird NM, Monson RR, Sobol AM, Leighton AH. Incidence of depression in the Stirling County Study: historical and comparative perspectives. *Psychol Med* 2000;**30**(3):505–514.

17 Anderson P, Chisholm D, Fuhr DC. Effectiveness and cost-effectiveness of policies and programmes to reduce the harm caused by alcohol. *Lancet* 2009;**373**(9682):2234–2246.

18 Keyes KM, Li G, Hasin DS. Birth cohort effects and gender differences in alcohol epidemiology: a review and synthesis. *Alcoholism: Clin Exp Res* 2011;**35**(12):2101–2112.

19 Kerr WC, Greenfield TK, Bond J, Ye Y, Rehm J. Age-period-cohort modelling of alcohol volume and heavy drinking days in the US National Alcohol Surveys: divergence in younger and older adult trends. *Addiction* 2009;**104**(1):27–37.

20 Bachman JG, Freedman-Doan P, O'Malley PM, Johnston LD, Segal DR. Changing patterns of drug use among US military recruits before and after enlistment. *Am J Public Health* 1999;**89**(5):672–677.

21 Keyes KM, Grant BF, Hasin DS. Evidence for a closing gender gap in alcohol use, abuse, and dependence in the United States population. *Drug Alcohol Depend* 2008;**93**(1–2):21–29.

22 Karlamangla A, Zhou K, Reuben D, Greendale G, Moore A. Longitudinal trajectories of heavy drinking in adults in the United States of America. *Addiction* 2006;**101**(1):91–99.

23 Keyes KM, Schulenberg JE, O'Malley PM, et al. Birth cohort effects on adolescent alcohol use: the influence of social norms from 1976 to 2007. *Arch Gen Psychiatry* 2012;**69**(12):1304–1313.

24 Blaxill MF. Any changes in prevalence of autism must be determined. *BMJ* 2002;**324**(7332):296.

25 Schechter R, Grether JK. Continuing increases in autism reported to California's developmental services system: mercury in retrograde. *Arch Gen Psychiatry* 2008;**65**(1):19–24.

26 Centers for Disease Control and Prevention. *Autism and Developmental Disabilities Monitoring (ADDM) Network*. 2010. <http://wwwcdcgov/ncbddd/autism/addmhtml>

27 Senecky Y, Chodick G, Diamond G, Lobel D, Drachman R, Inbar D. Time trends in reported autistic spectrum disorders in Israel, 1972–2004. *Isr Med Assoc J* 2009;**11**(1):30–33.

28 Honda H, Shimizu Y, Imai M, Nitto Y. Cumulative incidence of childhood autism: a total population study of better accuracy and precision. *Dev Med Child Neurol* 2005;**47**(1):10–18.

29 Fountain C, King MD, Bearman PS. Age of diagnosis for autism: individual and community factors across 10 birth cohorts. *J Epidemiol Community Health* 2011;**65**(6):503–510.

30 Mandell DS, Novak MM, Zubritsky CD. Factors associated with age of diagnosis among children with autism spectrum disorders. *Pediatrics* 2005;**116**(6):1480–1486.

31 Liu K, King M, Bearman P. Social influence and the autism epidemic. *Am J Sociol* 2010;**115**(5):1387–1434.

32 Hertz-Picciotto I, Delwiche L. The rise in autism and the role of age at diagnosis. *Epidemiology* 2009;**20**(1):84–90.

33 **Parner ET, Schendel DE, Thorsen P.** Autism prevalence trends over time in Denmark: changes in prevalence and age at diagnosis. *Arch Pediatr Adolesc Med* 2008;**162**(12):1150–1156.

34 **Rice C, Nicholas J, Baio J, et al.** Changes in autism spectrum disorder prevalence in 4 areas of the United States. *Disabil Health J* 2010;**3**(3):186–201.

35 **Gurney JG, Fritz MS, Ness KK, Sievers P, Newschaffer CJ, Shapiro EG.** Analysis of prevalence trends of autism spectrum disorder in Minnesota. *Arch Pediatr Adolesc Med* 2003;**157**(7):622–627.

36 **Centers for Disease Control and Prevention.** Prevalence of autism spectrum disorders—Autism and Developmental Disabilities Monitoring Network, United States, 2006. *Morb Mortal Wkly Rep* 2009;**58**(SS10):1–20.

37 **Keyes KM, Susser E, Cheslack-Postava K, Fountain C, Liu K, Bearman PS.** Cohort effects explain the increase in autism diagnosis among children born from 1992 to 2003 in California. *Int J Epidemiol* 2012;**41**(2):495–503.

38 **Reichenberg A, Gross R, Weiser M, et al.** Advancing paternal age and autism. *Arch Gen Psychiatry* 2006;**63**(9):1026–1032.

39 **Moreno C, Laje G, Blanco C, Jiang H, Schmidt AB, Olfson M.** National trends in the outpatient diagnosis and treatment of bipolar disorder in youth. *Arch Gen Psychiatry* 2007;**64**(9):1032–1039.

40 **Centers for Disease Control and Prevention.** Increasing prevalence of parent-reported attention-deficit/hyperactivity disorder among children—United States, 2003 and 2007. *Morb Mortal Wkly Rep* 2010;**59**(44):1439–1443.

41 **Weissman MM, Leaf PJ, Holzer CE, 3rd, Myers JK, Tischler GL.** The epidemiology of depression. An update on sex differences in rates. *J Affective Disorders* 1984;**7**(3–4):179–188.

42 **Gershon ES, Hamovit JH, Guroff JJ, Nurnberger JI.** Birth-cohort changes in manic and depressive disorders in relatives of bipolar and schizoaffective patients. *Arch Gen Psychiatry* 1987;**44**(4):314–319.

43 **Lavori PW, Klerman GL, Keller MB, Reich T, Rice J, Endicott J.** Age–period–cohort analysis of secular trends in onset of major depression: findings in siblings of patients with major affective disorder. *J Psychiatr Res* 1987;**21**(1):23–35.

44 **Wickramaratne PJ, Weissman MM, Leaf PJ, Holford TR.** Age, period and cohort effects on the risk of major depression: results from five United States communities. *J Clin Epidemiol* 1989;**42**(4):333–343.

45 **Klerman GL, Weissman MM.** Increasing Rates of Depression. *JAMA* 1989;**261**(15):2229–2235.

46 **Joyce PR, Oakley-Browne MA, Wells JE, Bushnell JA, Hornblow AR.** Birth cohort trends in major depression: increasing rates and earlier onset in New Zealand. *J Affective Disorders* 1990;**18**(2): 83–89.

47 **Warshaw MG, Klerman GL, Lavori PW.** The use of conditional probabilities to examine age-period-cohort data: further evidence for a period effect in major depressive disorder. *J Affective Disorders* 1991;**23**(3):119–129.

48 **Ryan ND, Williamson DE, Iyengar S, et al.** A secular increase in child and adolescent onset affective disorder. *J Am Acad Child Adolesc Psychiatry* 1992;**31**(4):600–605.

49 **Burke KC, Burke JD, Jr, Rae DS, Regier DA.** Comparing age at onset of major depression and other psychiatric disorders by birth cohorts in five US community populations. *Arch Gen Psychiatry* 1991;**48**(9):789–795.

50 **Cross-National Collaborative Group.** The changing rate of major depression. Cross-national comparisons. Cross-National Collaborative Group. *JAMA* 1992;**268**(21):3098–3105.

51 **Lewinsohn PM, Rohde P, Seeley JR, Fischer SA.** Age-cohort changes in the lifetime occurrence of depression and other mental disorders. *J Abnormal Psychol* 1993;**102**(1):110–120.

52 **Leon AC, Klerman GL, Wickramaratne P.** Continuing female predominance in depressive illness. *Am J Public Health* 1993;**83**(5):754–7.

53 **Kessler RC, McGonagle KA, Nelson CB, Hughes M, Swartz M, Blazer DG.** Sex and depression in the national comorbidity survey. II: Cohort effects. *J Affective Disorders* 1994;**30**(1):15–26.

54 **Kessler RC, Berglund P, Demler O, et al.** The epidemiology of major depressive disorder: results from the National Comorbidity Survey Replication (NCS-R). *JAMA* 2003;**289**(23):3095–3105.

55 **Kasen S, Cohen P, Chen H, Castille D.** Depression in adult women: age changes and cohort effects. *Am J Public Health* 2003;**93**(12):2061–2066.

56 **Hasin DS, Goodwin RD, Stinson FS, Grant BF.** Epidemiology of major depressive disorder: results from the National Epidemiologic Survey on Alcoholism and Related Conditions. *Arch Gen Psychiatry* 2005;**62**(10):1097–1106.

Part 3

Life course approach to specific mental disorders

Chapter 6

Schizophrenia and related psychosis

Golam M. Khandaker, Mary Clarke, Mary Cannon, and Peter B. Jones

6.1 Introduction

The characteristic age-at-onset function for schizophrenia and related psychoses provides prima facie evidence for a life course dimension to these disorders. The incidence of the clinical syndrome is vanishingly rare before puberty, accelerates during the epoch of post-pubertal brain development over the following decade and a half before declining into middle-age. Understanding the biology of this close association between psychotic illness and development undoubtedly holds keys to the epigenetic puzzle that is schizophrenia.[1] Here, we take a life course approach to schizophrenia by reviewing the literature regarding putative mechanisms and early life risk factors as manifest from conception to onset of illness. We include environmental, developmental, and cognitive domains, and emphasize evidence from population-based studies that has accrued rapidly over the past quarter century.

6.2 Prenatal risk factors for schizophrenia

6.2.1 Maternal infection

Recent studies have used serological assays or clinical examination to determine exposure to prenatal infection at the individual level, implicating a range of prenatal infections and inflammatory responses as being associated with risk of schizophrenia in offspring.[2] Based on representative, general population cohorts, the evidence from these studies has good internal and external validity.

6.2.1.1 Herpes simplex virus

One Danish nested case–control study reported 50% increased risk of schizophrenia for prenatal exposure to herpes simplex virus type 2 (HSV-2)-2, which remained significant after adjustment for family history of mental illness and other confounders.[3] This risk estimate is in line with a previous report from the National Collaborative Perinatal Project (NCPP) birth cohort.[4] However, not all studies have found an association between HSV-2 and schizophrenia.[5] So far, no studies have reported an association between prenatal HSV-1 and schizophrenia.

6.2.1.2 Toxoplasma gondii

Around two-fold increased risk of schizophrenia has been reported for elevated level of maternal IgG antibody to *Toxoplasma gondii* in the Prenatal Determinants of Schizophrenia (PDS) and a Danish cohort.[6,7] In the latter, *T. gondii* was specifically associated with 'narrowly defined' schizophrenia (*International Classification of Diseases*, 10th revision: F20), out of all outcomes studied.[7]

One study from the NCPP cohort suggests exposure to *T. gondii* serotype I may be associated with five-fold increased risk of affective psychosis.[8]

6.2.1.3 Influenza

In the PDS cohort, a seven-fold increased risk of schizophrenia spectrum disorder for exposure to influenza during first trimester and a three-fold increased risk for exposure during first half of pregnancy was observed.[9] There was no increase in risk for exposure during late pregnancy. Due to relatively small sample size, none of the risk estimates reached statistical significance.

6.2.1.4 Other prenatal infections

As well as specific infections, risk of schizophrenia in offspring has been examined in relation to maternal non-specific bacterial, viral, respiratory, genital, reproductive, and other infection during pregnancy.[2] A recent Danish study found that serious maternal infection during pregnancy was not significantly different from that before or after pregnancy in terms of offspring's risk of schizophrenia.[10]

6.2.1.5 Inflammatory cytokines

Cytokines are mediators of host response to infection and act as markers of inflammation and immune activation.[11] Elevated level of inflammatory cytokines, such as tumour necrosis factor-α or interleukin-8 (IL-8) have been reported, during pregnancy, in mothers of individuals who developed schizophrenia as adults compared with control mothers.[12,13] It has been suggested that inflammatory cytokines may mediate the risk of psychosis in offspring related to prenatal infection.[13]

6.2.1.6 Prenatal maternal infection and neurodevelopment

Studies from NCPP and PDS cohorts suggest that exposure to various infections (influenza, respiratory, genital, or reproductive, etc.) or increased IL-8 during pregnancy is associated with increased ventricular volume,[14] and length of cavum septum pallucidum,[15] deficits in childhood verbal IQ,[16] and adult executive function,[17] in schizophrenia. However, some of these associations were only present in schizophrenic individuals who were exposed to prenatal maternal infection compared with unexposed cases, but not in controls.[14,16] This suggests that prenatal maternal infection operates in combination with genetic and/or other risk factors (discussed in Section 6.5.2).

6.2.1.7 Timing of exposure

The issue of 'sensitive period' has not been adequately addressed in most studies, primarily due to limited sample size. However, in general there is a trend for greater risk of psychotic illness in offspring for exposure to infection during early stages of gestation.[2]

6.2.2 Maternal nutritional status

Historical cohort studies based on populations exposed to severe famine have demonstrated an increased risk of schizophrenia in adult offspring of mothers exposed to famine during pregnancy.[18] These findings, along with observations such as increased congenital central nervous system (CNS) defects due to famine exposure during pregnancy,[19] increased risk of schizophrenia in offspring for low maternal pre-pregnant body mass index (BMI), and low placental weight,[20] implicate severe malnutrition during pregnancy in the aetiology of schziophrenia. Specific micronutrient deficiencies have also been implicated, including vitamin D, iron, and folic acid among others.[21]

Recently, maternal obesity, as determined by pre-pregnancy BMI, has been associated with two- to three-fold increased risk of schizophrenia in offspring in two birth cohorts.[22] High pre-pregnancy and pregnancy BMI increases the risk of a range of adverse neurodevelopmental outcomes in offspring including neural tube defect.[23] However, increased risk of infection, gestational diabetes, obstetric complications, etc., among obese mothers may also underlie the association between maternal obesity and schizophrenia in offspring.[22]

6.3 **Obstetric complications**

The broad category of 'obstetric complications' (OCs) is a well-replicated risk factor for schizophrenia. The association between obstetric complications and schizophrenia is in the region of a 1.5–2.0-fold increase in the odds of developing schizophrenia among those exposed to OCs compared with those unexposed.[24]

6.3.3 **Mechanisms of action**

The mechanism through which OCs exert their effect on risk for schizophrenia is unclear. There is evidence that perinatal hypoxia may have direct lasting effects on dopaminergic function.[25] There is also evidence to suggest that birth insults have an indirect effect through altering the manner in which dopamine function is regulated by stress in adulthood.[26] Additionally, Cannon et al.[27] found that, among schizophrenia patients, birth hypoxia was associated with a 20% decrease in brain-derived neurotrophic factor (BDNF) whereas, among the matched healthy controls, birth hypoxia was associated with a 10% increase in BDNF.

There is evidence that hypoxia itself may mediate the effects of other OCs. Cannon et al.[28] found a linear relationship between the number of hypoxia-causing OCs and risk of schizophrenia, suggesting that any association between these specific OCs and schizophrenia is accounted for by the effect of hypoxia on risk for schizophrenia. These data also suggest that hypoxia interacts with genetic susceptibility to further increase risk.

6.4 **Motor development**

Longitudinal studies of childhood development in individuals who later go on to develop schizophrenia[29-33] show motor, language, and cognitive developmental impairments evident from middle childhood and possibly earlier.

6.4.1 **Motor developmental abnormalities during infancy and childhood in schizophrenia**

6.4.1.1 High risk studies

High risk research in schizophrenia has almost exclusively concentrated on offspring of schizophrenic parents gathered from treatment samples. The most consistent finding from recent high risk studies is that offsprings of schizophrenic parents display motor co-ordination problems in middle childhood.[34]

6.4.1.2 General population birth cohort studies

A study from the 1946 British Birth Cohort by Jones et al. showed that individuals who developed schizoiphrenia as adults had delayed acquisition of motor and language milestones by age 2 years compared with healthy controls.[35] Further work using population-based data from the 1966 Finnish Birth Cohort has confirmed that delayed attainment of milestones in infancy significantly increases the risk of later schizophrenia in a dose–response manner.[36] Additionally, delayed attainment of developmental milestones and exposure to obstetric complications combined may significantly increase the risk of schizophrenia beyond that associated with each factor independently.[37] Neuoimaging data from the 1966 Finnish birth cohort suggest that disconnectivity between brain frontal cortical and posterior regions may underlie both delayed infant motor milestones and adult cognitve function in schizophrenia.[38]

6.5 Childhood infection as a risk factor for adult schizophrenia

6.5.1 Central nervous system infection

A recent meta-analysis of three population-based cohorts by Khandaker et al. suggests that childhood CNS viral infection, as a group, is associated with nearly two-fold increased risk of adult non-affective psychosis (risk ratio: 1.7).[39] Increased risk of adult schizophrenia for exposure to meningococcal meningitis in childhood has been reported in another study.[40]

6.5.2 Mechanisms for early life infections and schizophrenia

6.5.2.1 Gene–environment interaction

Infection during pregnancy is widespread in the general population, yet only a fraction of the exposed offspring develops schizophrenia. Clarke et al. found an additive effect of family history of psychosis and prenatal infection in the causation of schizophrenia.[41] Possible exposure to several infections in the same group of case mothers (PDS and NCPP cohorts) might indicate confounding by other factors, such as social class. Alternatively or in addition, clusters of infections in a few mothers might suggest some overlap of genetic liability between schizophrenia and infection, in general.[2,42] Recent genome-wide association studies have reported a significant association between schizophrenia and markers close to the major histocompatibility complex region on chromosome 6, which includes several immunity-related genes.[42,43] Thus, it is possible that early life infection, by affecting gene expression or in the presence of pre-existing genetic liability, leads to a distinct or pathological immune response, which in turn increases the risk of schziophrenia.

6.5.2.2 Inflammatory response

Since a range of prenatal infections has been linked with schizophrenia in offspring, it has been suggested that a common pathway may be involved, such as the inflammatory response arising from activation of the innate immune system following infection. Simulated viral or bacterial infection or direct injection with a proinflammatory cytokine (IL-6) in pregnant mice has been reported to produce intermediate phenotypes related to schizophrenia in the adult offspring.[44] Some of these phenotypes such as deficits in sensory gating or altered latent inhibition are reversible with treatment with the anti-psychotic clozapine.[45]

6.5.2.3 Fetal programming

Programming of the fetal hypothalamic–pituitary–adrenal (HPA) axis as a result of exposure to excess maternal glucocorticoids following infection may be another common pathway.[46,47] Such a model suggests that early life programming would lead to an exaggerated or otherwise abnormal

HPA response to stress in adult life. The abnormal response during the period of risk for schizo-phrenia may contribute to onset through neurotoxic or other mechanisms.

6.5.2.4 Direct interference

None of the studies of HSV-2 or *T. gondii* reported an increase in specific IgM antibodies, sug-gesting that acute infections with these agents during pregnancy were unlikely.[48] However, direct interference with brain development is possible as these organisms are neurotropic. The observed association between childhood viral (but not bacterial) CNS infection and adult psychosis is in line with this suggestion.[39]

6.5.2.5 Microglial 'priming'

In a series of experiments, Dantzer et al. demonstrated that systemic infection may lead to changes in cognition, mood, and behaviour by activating immune system cells (microglia) in the brain.[49] It has been suggested that areas containing previously activated microglia tend to respond more strongly to a new stimulus.[50] Thus, childhood infection may have a priming effect on the CNS microglial cells.[50] This is consistent with the 'two hit' model of schizophrenia,[51] whereby exposure to various risk factors during early life is thought to prime the CNS for a pathological response to a 'second hit' via the same signalling pathway.[52]

6.6 Childhood cognitive development in schizophrenia

Identification of premorbid IQ deficit in people who will later develop schizophrenia is one of the most consistent findings in schizophrenia.[35,53] This is a key piece of evidence underpinning a developmental aspect to the disorder.[54,55] Recently, in a systematic review and meta-analysis of the population-based studies Khandaker et al. showed a significant deficit in premorbid IQ in schizophrenia[53] and confirmed that this deficit is due to a decrement in premorbid IQ in the majority of future cases (a left-shift of this population)[35,56], rather than due to a minority effect driven by a subgroup with conspicuously low IQ.

6.6.1 Magnitude of premorbid IQ deficit

The mean childhood IQ of people who develop schizophrenia as adults is around 93.[53] Compared with a mean IQ of 100 in the general population, this is a large deficit at the population level of around half a standard deviation. Premorbid verbal and performance IQ are significantly lower in schizophrenia; both measures are equally affected.

6.6.2 Dose–response relationship between IQ and risk of schizophrenia

Premorbid IQ is associated with the risk of schizophrenia in a dose–response manner (i.e. linear association), which equates to a 3.7% increase in risk for every one-point decrease in premorbid IQ.[53] It has been shown that compared with the group of people with IQ 100–115, the risk of developing schizophrenia is double among people with IQ 70–85 (odds ratio: 2.36), while the risk is nearly five-fold for those with IQ <70 (odds ratio: 4.78) (Figure 6.1). Conversely, risk of schizophrenia is reduced by half in people with higher premorbid intelli-gence (IQ >115), suggesting that higher IQ may be protective.[53] Moreover, in the meta-analysis by Khandaker et al. greater premorbid IQ deficits were strongly associated with an earlier illness onset.[53]

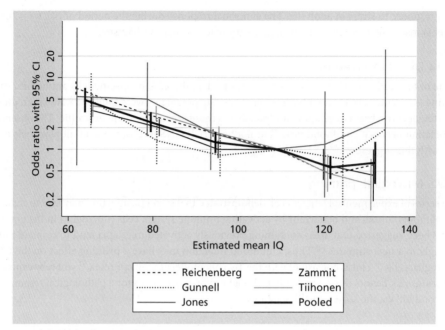

Figure 6.1 Odds ratio for risk of schizophrenia across six IQ categories. Estimated mean IQ refers to mean IQ of each category calculated according to proportion of people in the category. IQ category 100–115 is used as reference. CI, confidence interval.

Reproduced from *Schizophrenia Research*, Volume 2–3, Khandaker GM et al., A quantitative meta-analysis of population-based studies of premorbid intelligence and schizophrenia, pp. 220–7, Copyright © 2011, with permission from Elsevier, http://www.sciencedirect.com/science/journal/09209964.

6.6.4 **Is the IQ deficit progressive?**

It has been hypothesized that neurodevelopmental impairment in schizophrenia is progressive over the premorbid period, which would be reflected by deterioration in IQ. Birth cohort studies of schizophrenia have measured IQ relatively early, at ages 6–12 years, whereas military conscript cohort studies have measured IQ at ages 16–18 years. However, there is no significant difference in the magnitude of IQ deficit between these two groups of studies.[53] This suggests no appreciable change in IQ during the premorbid period. However, this question can only be settled by repeated assessment within the same individuals. Currently, such data are available for few schizophrenia cases.[53]

6.6.5 **Premorbid IQ and functional outcome**

It has been shown that general cognitive ability, as measured by IQ, is a more sensitive and reliable predictor of functional outcome in schizophrenia than measures of specific ability.[57] Studies of first-episode psychosis have found that premorbid IQ is a significant predictor of outcome up to 10 years of follow-up,[58–60] even after controlling for duration of untreated psychosis and previous functional status.[60]

6.6.7 Interpretation and implication of findings

The existence of two approximately linear relationships, where lower premorbid IQ is associated with both increased risk and earlier illness onset,[53] argues for a widespread neurodevelopmental contribution to schizophrenia. This is not to suggest that other factors, alone or in combinations, are not important causes of schizophrenia; discrete combinations of genetic and environmental factors are likely to be involved. The majority of causal constellations are either manifest as, or mediated by, a cognitive or IQ-related factor. Such an effect may involve either risk or protection.

6.7 Childhood social and behavioural development in schizophrenia

6.7.1 Social and behavioural impairment preceding illness onset in schizophrenia

Deficits in social functioning have been shown to precede the onset of schizophrenia.[33,61–64] In the 1946 British Birth Cohort Jones et al. showed that children who went on to develop schizophrenia preferred solitary play and had self-reported anxiety in social situations.[35] In another population cohort, Bearden et al.[65] found that social maladjustment at age 7 years increased the risk of adult schizophrenia, and that unusual behaviour at ages 4 and 7 years was present to a greater extent among those who would later develop schizophrenia and their siblings compared with those who did not later develop schizophrenia. Social deficits appear to deteriorate from childhood to adolescence,[66] and problems with peer relations seem to be a core feature of the deficits preceding schizophrenia.[67]

6.7.2 Social impairment as an endophenotype for schizophrenia

Childhood social deficits have been considered to be a possible endophenotype for schizophrenia. Data from the Maudsley Twin and Family Study of Schizophrenia showed that individuals who developed schizophrenia were significantly impaired in childhood and adolescent social adjustment compared with healthy controls, and that their unaffected first degree relatives showed qualitatively similar abnormalities.[68] The data comparing monozygotic and dizygotic twin pairs suggest that the common link is due to genetic rather than shared environment,[69] although unique environmental factors contributed to the variance in the association between social abilities and risk of schizophrenia. An additive interaction effect has also been shown. Weiser et al. reported that individuals who lived in a densely populated region and had premorbid social and cognitive deficits had nine-fold risk of developing schizophrenia compared with those who did not have such deficits.[69]

6.7.3 Social cognition

The cognitive processes subserving social functioning are referred to collectively as social cognition. Fundamental to social cognition is 'theory of mind', the ability to understand that others have beliefs, desires, information, and intentions that may differ from our own. Similar to autism, there is deficit in theory of mind in schizophrenia,[70] something that could tie together the social and behavioural characteristics already reviewed. A recent prospective study from the ALSPAC Birth Cohort has reported increased risk of psychotic experiences in adolescence for autistic traits at ages 4 and 7 years.[71]

6.7.4 **Association between social impairment and functional outcome**

Social impairment in schizophrenia is important because it affects functional outcome,[72] appears to be resistant to treatment, and persists after psychotic symptoms are effectively treated.[73] Similar to motor developmental delay and obstetric complications, the evidence suggests that deficits in social functioning are a marker of vulnerability to schizophrenia but are neither a necessary nor a sufficient part of the causal pathway(s) to the illness.

6.8 **Childhood psychotic symptoms as precursor of schizophrenia**

Poulton et al. have shown that children in the Dunedin birth cohort who reported psychotic symptoms at age 11 years were five to 16 times more likely to develop schizophreniform disorder by age 26 years.[74] Recently, increased risk of psychotic disoder at age 18 years has been shown among individuals reporting psychotic experiences at age 12/13 years in the ALSPAC birth cohort.[75] Research over the last decade has shown that psychotic symptoms are widespread in the general population in all ages,[76,77] and may be related with psychotic as well as other mental disorders.

6.8.1 **Prevalence of childhood psychotic symptoms**

Recent work suggests that psychotic symptoms are more widespread in early compared with late childhood: median prevalence 17% at ages 9–12 years and 7.5% at ages 13–18 years.[77] Longitudinal studies have shown a decline in the incidence of psychotic symptoms in young people over time,[78,79] suggesting that in most children these symptoms are transient.

6.8.2 **Association of childhood psychotic symptoms with schizophrenia**

As well as increased risk of adult psychosis, childhood psychotic symptoms have been linked with a number of risk factors for adult schizophrenia. For example, in the Avon Longitudinal Study of Parents and Children (ALSPAC) birth cohort psychotic symptoms at age 12/13 years have been associated with prenatal maternal infection and increased birth complications,[80] low birth weight,[81] and poorer performance on IQ tests at age 8 years[82]—important findings that require replication. Physiological studies provide evidence for common underlying mechanisms for psychotic symptoms seen in healthy people and in schizophrenia.[83] Together, these findings support the idea that childhood psychotic symptoms may provide a high risk paradigm for studying the developmental trajectory to psychosis (the 'symptomatic' high risk approach).[84,85] However, the true nature of the relationship (both temporal and aetiological) between these symptoms and adult psychotic illness needs to be studied further.

6.8.3 **Links with other mental disorders and future directions**

Several population-based studies have shown that in children and young adults psychotic symptoms are often associated with anxiety and depression.[86–88] One study has reported that psychotic experiences at age 20 years predict a range of (non-psychotic) mental disorders at 30 years' follow-up.[89] These findings suggest that childhood psychotic symptoms should be considered beside other symptoms, such as depression and anxiety, as markers of general psychological disturbance in young people. This is important from both clinical and research perspectives. As these symptoms often cause serious psychological distress and functional impairment; they need assessment and, in some cases, specialist management.

6.9 **Other early-life risk factors**

6.9.1 **Paternal age at conception**

Population-based cohort studies have associated advancing paternal age with increased risk of schizophrenia in offspring.[90] A recent meta-analysis found that, compared with offspring of fathers aged 25–29 years (reference group), the risk of schizophrenia is significantly increased in offspring of fathers aged ≥30 years; the highest risk was observed in offspring of fathers aged ≥50 years (relative risk: 1.6).[91] This equates to a population attributable risk for schizophrenia of 10% for paternal age ≥30 years. Maternal age is not associated with risk.

6.9.2 **Time and place of birth**

About 10% excess of winter/spring birth has been reported among those who develop schizophrenia as adults. This finding is remarkably consistent in the northern hemisphere[92] and, to some extent, the southern hemisphere.[93] Putative explanations include seasonal variation in environmental factors, such as micronutrients, and excess of viral and other infections during winter and spring.[94] Another consistent finding is higher risk of schizophrenia among those born in urban areas compared with those born in rural areas; effect size: 1.5–2.5.[95-97] Some studies attempted to tease apart effects of urban birth and urban living. One Danish population-based study found that higher risk of schizophrenia was associated with higher level of urbanization at place of birth, as well as total number of years lived in urbanized areas during the first 15 years of life.[98] It is safe to assume that urban birth is a proxy variable that encompasses a large number of possible risk factors, such as pollution, infection, stress, and reduced social capital. These findings suggest that their effects may pertain to prenatal and early years of life, as well as perhaps being cumulative over childhood.

6.9.3 **Effect of migration**

Results from the Aetiology and Ethnicity in Schizophrenia and Other Psychoses (AESOP) study confirmed that in the UK the risk of schizophrenia is considerably higher among people of African origin compared with white British people (incidence rate ratio: 9.1 in African–Caribbean; 5.8 in Black Africans).[99] This effect is independent of social class.[99,100] Risk of schizophrenia is also higher in South Asian groups in England (relative risk: 2.4).[101] Excess risk of schizophrenia has also been found among second generation immigrants from some of these ethnic groups.[102] A recent study suggests that migration during early childhood may be associated with greater risk of schizophrenia.[103] Moreover, since rates of schizophrenia in the country of origin are not elevated, disproportionately higher rates in immigrants are unlikely to be due to genetic differences. Reduced social capital, increased obstetric complication as a result of improved fetal nutrition, and decreased production of vitamin D by darker-skinned people in the northern climates are some of the possible causal explanations for these findings.[104]

6.10 **Summary**

A range of evidence from population-based studies now provides a robust framework on which to build a life course model of schizophrenia and related psychoses. New understanding of dose–response relationships between the outcome of schizophrenia and earlier motor development, general cognitive ability summarized by IQ, and social cognition suggests that risk for the disorder is increased in a brain less efficiently connected than it might have been; the developmental differences manifest in children who will develop schizophrenia when they enter the decades of risk in early adulthood are reflections of this life course process. Alongside these insights, a number of factors including obstetric insults, particularly hypoxia and deviant fetal growth, malnutrition, infection, the stress response, and inflammatory processes have been identified that may contribute to suboptimal neurodevelopment. Some almost certainly interact with genetic factors whereas others exert effects through programming of the HPA axis and epigenetic effects that determine the brain's response to later events and experiences. Finally, our understanding of the importance of psychotic experiences in the general population beyond the clinical setting is being shaped by population-based and clinical research during adolescent development. No longer are such experiences seen as portents only of schizophrenia but rather as less specific signs of a troubled mind to which we are vulnerable during the window of risk during the second to the fourth decades of the life course. The past twenty-five years have seen great progress in the life course understanding of schizophrenia; we hope that the next quarter century will see resolution of remaining problems and translation into the arenas of treatment and prevention.

References

1 Gottesman II, Sheilds J. *Schizophrenia: the epigenetic puzzle*. New York: Cambridge University Press; 1982.

2 Khandaker GM, Zimbron J, Lewis G, Jones PB. Prenatal maternal infection, neurodevelopment and adult schizophrenia: a systematic review of population-based studies. *Psychol Med* 2013;**43**(2): 239–257.

3 Mortensen PB, Pedersen CB, Hougaard DM, et al. A Danish National Birth Cohort study of maternal HSV-2 antibodies as a risk factor for schizophrenia in their offspring. *Schizophr Res* 2010;**122** (1–3):257–263.

4 Buka SL, Cannon TD, Torrey EF, Yolken RH. Maternal exposure to herpes simplex virus and risk of psychosis among adult offspring. *Biol Psychiatry* 2008;**63**(8):809–815.

5 Brown AS, Schaefer CA, Quesenberry CP, Jr, Shen L, Susser ES. No evidence of relation between maternal exposure to herpes simplex virus type 2 and risk of schizophrenia? *Am J Psychiatry* 2006;**163**(12):2178–2180.

6 Brown AS, Schaefer CA, Quesenberry CP, Jr, Liu L, Babulas VP, Susser ES. Maternal exposure to toxoplasmosis and risk of schizophrenia in adult offspring. *Am J Psychiatry* 2005;**162**(4): 767–773.

7 Mortensen PB, Norgaard-Pedersen B, Waltoft BL, et al. *Toxoplasma gondii* as a risk factor for early-onset schizophrenia: analysis of filter paper blood samples obtained at birth. *Biol Psychiatry* 2007;**61**(5):688–693.

8 Xiao J, Buka SL, Cannon TD, et al. Serological pattern consistent with infection with type I *Toxoplasma gondii* in mothers and risk of psychosis among adult offspring. *Microbes Infect* 2009;**11**(13):1011–1018.

9 Brown AS, Begg MD, Gravenstein S, et al. Serologic evidence of prenatal influenza in the etiology of schizophrenia. *Arch Gen Psychiatry* 2004;**61**(8):774–780.

10 Nielsen PR, Laursen TM, Mortensen PB. Association between parental hospital-treated infection and the risk of schizophrenia in adolescence and early adulthood. *Schizophr Bull* 2013;**39**(1):230–237.

11 Weizman R, Bessler H. Cytokines:stress and immunity—an overview. **In: Plotnikoff NP, Faith RE, Murgo AJ, Good RA, Boca RF**, editors. *Cytokines: stress and immunity*. Boca Raton: CRC Press; 1999. pp. 1–15.

12 Brown AS, Hooton J, Schaefer CA, et al. Elevated maternal interleukin-8 levels and risk of schizophrenia in adult offspring. *Am J Psychiatry* 2004;**161**(5):889–895.

13 Buka SL, Tsuang MT, Torrey EF, Klebanoff MA, Wagner RL, Yolken RH. Maternal cytokine levels during pregnancy and adult psychosis. *Brain Behav Immunity* 2001;**15**(4):411–420.

14 Ellman LM, Deicken RF, Vinogradov S, et al. Structural brain alterations in schizophrenia following fetal exposure to the inflammatory cytokine interleukin-8. *Schizophr Res* 2010;**121**(1–3):46–54.

15 Brown AS, Deicken RF, Vinogradov S, et al. Prenatal infection and cavum septum pellucidum in adult schizophrenia. *Schizophr Res* 2009;**108**(1–3):285–287.

16 Ellman LM, Yolken RH, Buka SL, Torrey EF, Cannon TD. Cognitive functioning prior to the onset of psychosis: the role of fetal exposure to serologically determined influenza infection. *Biol Psychiatry* 2009;**65**(12):1040–1047.

17 Brown AS, Vinogradov S, Kremen WS, et al. Prenatal exposure to maternal infection and executive dysfunction in adult schizophrenia. *Am J Psychiatry* 2009;**166**(6):683–690.

18 Susser E, Neugebauer R, Hoek HW, et al. Schizophrenia after prenatal famine. Further evidence. *Arch Gen Psychiatry* 1996;**53**(1):25–31.

19 Stein Z, Susser M, Saenger G, Marolla F. *Famine and human development: the Dutch Hunger Winter of 1944–45.* New York: Oxford University Press; 1975.

20 Wahlbeck K, Forsen T, Osmond C, Barker DJ, Eriksson JG. Association of schizophrenia with low maternal body mass index, small size at birth, and thinness during childhood. *Arch Gen Psychiatry* 2001;**58**(1):48–52.

21 Brown AS, Susser ES. Prenatal nutritional deficiency and risk of adult schizophrenia. *Schizophr Bull* 2008;**34**(6):1054–1063.

22 Khandaker GM, Dibben CR, Jones PB. Does maternal body mass index during pregnancy influence risk of schizophrenia in the adult offspring? *Obes Rev* 2012;**13**(6):518–527.

23 Van Lieshout RJ, Taylor VH, Boyle MH. Pre-pregnancy and pregnancy obesity and neurodevelopmental outcomes in offspring: a systematic review. *Obes Rev* 2011;**12**(5):e548–559.

24 Cannon M, Jones PB, Murray RM. Obstetric complications and schizophrenia: historical and meta-analytic review. *Am J Psychiatry* 2002;**159**(7):1080–1092.

25 Boog G. Obstetrical complications and further schizophrenia of the infant: a new methodological threat to the obstetrician? *J Gynecol Obstet Biol Reprod* 2003;**32**:720–727.

26 Boksa P, El-Khodor BF. Birth insult interacts with stress at adulthood to alter dopaminergic function in animal models: possible implications for schizophreniaand other disorders. *Neurosci Biobehav Rev* 2003;**27**:91–101.

27 Cannon TD, Yolken R, Buka S, Torrey EF. Decreased neurotrophic response to birth hypoxia in the etiology of schizophrenia. *Biol Psychiatry* 2008;**64**(9):797–802.

28 Cannon TD, Rosso IM, Hollister JM, Bearden CE, Sanchez LE, Hadley T. A prospective cohort study of genetic and perinatal influences in the etiology of schizophrenia. *Schizophr Bull* 2000;**26**(2):351–366.

29 Gooding D IW. Schizophrenia through the lens of a developmental psychopathology perspective. **In:** Cicchetti DC, editor. *Developmental psychopathology.* New York: John Wiley & Sons; 1995.

30 Cornblatt B, Obuchowski M. Update of high risk research: 1987–1997. *Int Rev Psychiatry* 1997;**9**: 437–447.

31 Dickson H, Laurens KR, Cullen AE, Hodgins S. Meta-analyses of cognitive and motor function in youth aged 16 years and younger who subsequently develop schizophrenia. *Psychol Med* 2012;**42**(4):743–755.

32 Fish B. Infant predictors of the longitudinal course of schizophrenic development. *Schizophr Bull* 1987;**13**(3):395–409.

33 Welham J, Isohanni M, Jones P, McGrath J. The antecedents of schizophrenia: a review of birth cohort studies. *Schizophr Bull* 2009;**35**(3):603–623.

34 Niemi LT, Suvisaari JM, Tuulio-Henriksson A, Lonnqvist JK. Childhood developmental abnormalities in schizophrenia: evidence from high-risk studies. *Schizophr Res* 2003;**60**(2–3):239–258.

35 Jones P, Rodgers B, Murray R, Marmot M. Child development risk factors for adult schizophrenia in the British 1946 birth cohort. *Lancet* 1994;**344**(8934):1398–1402.

36 Isohanni M, Jones PB, Moilanen K, et al. Early developmental milestones in adult schizophrenia and other psychoses. A 31-year follow-up of the Northern Finland 1966 birth cohort. *Schizophr Res* 2001;**52**(1–2):1–19.

37 Clarke MC, Tanskanen A, Huttunen M, et al. Increased risk of schizophrenia from additive interaction between infant motor developmental delay and obstetric complications: evidence from a population-based longitudinal study. *Am J Psychiatry* 2011;**168**(12):1295–1302.

38 Ridler K, Veijola JM, Tanskanen P, et al. Fronto-cerebellar systems are associated with infant motor and adult executive functions in healthy adults but not in schizophrenia. *Proc Natl Acad Sci US A* 2006;**103**(42):15651–15656.

39 Khandaker GM, Zimbron J, Dalman C, Lewis G, Jones PB. Childhood infection and adult schizophrenia: a meta-analysis of population-based studies. *Schizophr Res* 2013;**39**(1):230–237.

40 Abrahao AL, Focaccia R, Gattaz WF. Childhood meningitis increases the risk for adult schizophrenia. *World J Biol Psychiatry* 2005;**6**(Suppl 2): 44–48.

41 Clarke MC, Tanskanen A, Huttunen M, Whittaker JC, Cannon M. Evidence for an interaction between familial liability and prenatal exposure to infection in the causation of schizophrenia. *Am J Psychiatry* 2009;**166**(9):1025–1030.

42 Stefansson H, Ophoff RA, Steinberg S, et al. Common variants conferring risk of schizophrenia. *Nature* 2009;**460**(7256):744–747.

43 Shi J, Levinson DF, Duan J, et al. Common variants on chromosome 6p22.1 are associated with schizophrenia. *Nature* 2009;**460**(7256):753–757.

44 Meyer U, Feldon J. Epidemiology-driven neurodevelopmental animal models of schizophrenia. *Prog Neurobiol* 2010;**90**(3):285–326.

45 Smith SE, Li J, Garbett K, Mirnics K, Patterson PH. Maternal immune activation alters fetal brain development through interleukin-6. *J Neurosci* 2007;**27**(40):10695–10702.

46 Seckl JR, Holmes MC. Mechanisms of disease: glucocorticoids, their placental metabolism and fetal 'programming' of adult pathophysiology. *Nat Clin Pract Endocrinol Metab* 2007;**3**(6):479–488.

47 Khandaker GM, Dibben CR, Jones PB. Prenatal maternal influenza and schizophrenia in offspring: what does this tell us about fetal programming of chronic disease? *J Pediatr Infect Dis* 2012:7(2): 61–68.

48 Janeway CA, Travers P, Walport M, Shlomchik MJ. *Immunobiology: the immune system in health and disease.* 5th ed. New York: Garland Science; 2001.

49 Dantzer R, O'Connor JC, Freund GG, Johnson RW, Kelley KW. From inflammation to sickness and depression: when the immune system subjugates the brain. *Nat Rev Neurosci* 2008;**9**(1):46–56.

50 Hickie IB, Banati R, Stewart CH, Lloyd AR. Are common childhood or adolescent infections risk factors for schizophrenia and other psychotic disorders? *Med J Aust* 2009;**190**(4 Suppl):S17–21.

51 Bayer TA, Falkai P, Maier W. Genetic and non-genetic vulnerability factors in schizophrenia: the basis of the "two hit hypothesis". *J Psychiatr Res* 1999;**33**(6):543–548.

52 Maynard TM, Sikich L, Lieberman JA, LaMantia AS. Neural development, cell-cell signaling, and the "two-hit" hypothesis of schizophrenia. *Schizophr Bull* 2001;**27**(3):457–476.

53 Khandaker GM, Barnett JH, White IR, Jones PB. A quantitative meta-analysis of population-based studies of premorbid intelligence and schizophrenia. *Schizophr Res* 2011;**132**(2–3):220–227.

54 Murray RM, Lewis SW. Is schizophrenia a neurodevelopmental disorder? *BMJ Clin Res Ed* 1987;**295**(6600):681–682.

55 Weinberger DR. Implications of normal brain development for the pathogenesis of schizophrenia. *Arch Gen Psychiatry* 1987;**44**(7):660–669.

56 David AS, Malmberg A, Brandt L, Allebeck P, Lewis G. IQ and risk for schizophrenia: a population-baseed cohort study. *Psychol Med* 1997;**27**(6):1311–1323.

57 Gold JM, Goldberg RW, McNary SW, Dixon LB, Lehman AF. Cognitive correlates of job tenure among patients with severe mental illness. *Am J Psychiatry* 2002;**159**(8):1395–1402.

58 Carlsson R, Nyman H, Ganse G, Cullberg J. Neuropsychological functions predict 1- and 3-year outcome in first-episode psychosis. *Acta Psychiatr Scand* 2006;**113**(2):102–111.

59 Leeson VC, Barnes TR, Hutton SB, Ron MA, Joyce EM. IQ as a predictor of functional outcome in schizophrenia: a longitudinal, four-year study of first-episode psychosis. *Schizophr Res* 2009;**107**(1): 55–60.

60 van Winkel R, Myin-Germeys I, De Hert M, Delespaul P, Peuskens J, van Os J. The association between cognition and functional outcome in first-episode patients with schizophrenia: mystery resolved? *Acta Psychiatr Scand* 2007;**116**(2):119–124.

61 Cannon M, Caspi A, Moffitt TE, et al. Evidence for early-childhood, pan-developmental impairment specific to schizophreniform disorder: results from a longitudinal birth cohort. *Arch Gen Psychiatry* 2002;**59**(5):449–456.

62 Cannon M, Jones P, Gilvarry C, et al. Premorbid social functioning in schizophrenia and bipolar disorder: similarities and differences. *Am J Psychiatry* 1997;**154**(11):1544–1550.

63 Done DJ, Crow TJ, Johnstone EC, Sacker A. Childhood antecedents of schizophrenia and affective illness: social adjustment at ages 7 and 11. *BMJ* 1994;**309**(6956):699–703.

64 Tarbox SI, Pogue-Geile MF. Development of social functioning in preschizophrenia children and adolescents: a systematic review. *Psychol Bull* 2008;**134**(4):561–583.

65 Bearden CE, Rosso IM, Hollister JM, Sanchez LE, Hadley T, Cannon TD. A prospective cohort study of childhood behavioral deviance and language abnormalities as predictors of adult schizophrenia. *Schizophr Bull* 2000;**26**(2):395–410.

66 Davidson M, Reichenberg A, Rabinowitz J, Weiser M, Kaplan Z, Mark M. Behavioral and intellectual markers for schizophrenia in apparently healthy male adolescents. *Am J Psychiatry* 1999;**156**(9): 1328–1335.

67 Rutter M, Kim-Cohen J, Maughan B. Continuities and discontinuities in psychopathology between childhood and adult life. *J Child Psychol Psychiatry Allied Discipl* 2006;**47**(3–4):276–295.

68 Picchioni MM, Walshe M, Toulopoulou T, et al. Genetic modelling of childhood social development and personality in twins and siblings with schizophrenia. *Psychol Med* 2010;**40**(8): 1305–1316.

69 Weiser M, van Os J, Reichenberg A Social and cognitive functioning, urbanicity and risk for schizophrenia. *Br J Psychiatry* 2007;**191**:320–324.

70 Brune M. Social cognition and behavior in schizophrenia. In: Brüne MR, Ribbert H, Schiefenhövel W editors. *The social brain: evolution and pathology*. Chichester: Wiley; 2003. pp. 277–313.

71 Bevan Jones R, Thapar A, Lewis G, Zammit S. The association between early autistic traits and psychotic experiences in adolescence. *Schizophr Res* 2012;**135**(1–3):164–169.

72 Horan WP, Green MF, Degroot M, et al. Social cognition in schizophrenia, Part 2: 12-month stability and prediction of functional outcome in first-episode patients. *Schizophr Bull* 2012;**38**(4):865–872.

73 Addington J, Young J, Addington D. Social outcome in early psychosis. *Psychol Med* 2003;**33**(6):1119–1124.

74 Poulton R, Caspi A, Moffitt TE, Cannon M, Murray R, Harrington H. Children's self-reported psychotic symptoms and adult schizophreniform disorder: a 15-year longitudinal study. *Arch Gen Psychiatry* 2000;**57**(11):1053–1058.

75 Zammit S, Kounali D, Cannon M, et al. Psychotic experiences and psychotic disorders at age 18 in relation to psychotic experiences at age 12 in a longitudinal population-based cohort study. *Am J Psychiatry* 2013;**170**(7):742–750.

76 van Os J, Linscott RJ, Myin-Germeys I, Delespaul P, Krabbendam L. A systematic review and meta-analysis of the psychosis continuum: evidence for a psychosis proneness–persistence–impairment model of psychotic disorder. *Psychol Med* 2009;**39**(2):179–195.

77 **Kelleher I, Connor D, Clarke MC, Devlin N, Harley M, Cannon M.** Prevalence of psychotic symptoms in childhood and adolescence: a systematic review and meta-analysis of population-based studies. *Psychol Med* 2012;**42**(9):1857–1863.

78 **Rubio JM, Sanjuan J, Florez-Salamanca L, Cuesta MJ.** Examining the course of hallucinatory experiences in children and adolescents: a systematic review. *Schizophr Res* 2012;**138**(2–3): 248–254.

79 **De Loore E, Gunther N, Drukker M, et al.** Persistence and outcome of auditory hallucinations in adolescence: a longitudinal general population study of 1800 individuals. *Schizophr Res* 2011;**127**(1–3):252–256.

80 **Zammit S, Odd D, Horwood J, et al.** Investigating whether adverse prenatal and perinatal events are associated with non-clinical psychotic symptoms at age 12 years in the ALSPAC birth cohort. *Psychol Med* 2009;**39**(9):1457–1467.

81 **Thomas K, Harrison G, Zammit S, et al.** Association of measures of fetal and childhood growth with non-clinical psychotic symptoms in 12-year-olds: the ALSPAC cohort. *Br J Psychiatry* 2009;**194**(6):521–526.

82 **Horwood J, Salvi G, Thomas K, et al.** IQ and non-clinical psychotic symptoms in 12-year-olds: results from the ALSPAC birth cohort. *Br J Psychiatry* 2008;**193**(3):185–191.

83 **Howes OD, Shotbolt P, Bloomfield M, et al.** Dopaminergic function in the psychosis spectrum: an [18F]-DOPA imaging study in healthy individuals with auditory hallucinations. *Schizophr Bull* 2013;**39**(4):807–814.

84 **Kelleher I, Cannon M.** Psychotic-like experiences in the general population: characterizing a high-risk group for psychosis. *Psychol Med* 2011;**41**(1):1–6.

85 **Murray GK, Jones PB.** Psychotic symptoms in young people without psychotic illness: mechanisms and meaning. *Br J Psychiatry* 2012;**201**:4–6.

86 **Nishida A, Tanii H, Nishimura Y, et al.** Associations between psychotic-like experiences and mental health status and other psychopathologies among Japanese early teens. *Schizophr Res* 2008;**99** (1–3):125–133.

87 **Varghese D, Scott J, Welham J, et al.** Psychotic-like experiences in major depression and anxiety disorders: a population-based survey in young adults. *Schizophr Bull* 2011;**37**(2):389–393.

88 **Polanczyk G, Moffitt TE, Arseneault L, et al.** Etiological and clinical features of childhood psychotic symptoms: results from a birth cohort. *Arch Gen Psychiatry* 2010;**67**(4):328–338.

89 **Rossler W, Hengartner MP, Ajdacic-Gross V, Haker H, Gamma A, Angst J.** Sub-clinical psychosis symptoms in young adults are risk factors for subsequent common mental disorders. *Schizophr Res* 2011;**131**(1–3):18–23.

90 **Malaspina D, Harlap S, Fennig S, et al.** Advancing paternal age and the risk of schizophrenia. *Arch Gen Psychiatry* 2001;**58**(4):361–367.

91 **Miller B, Messias E, Miettunen J, et al.** Meta-analysis of paternal age and schizophrenia risk in male versus female offspring. *Schizophr Bull* 2011;**37**(5):1039–1047.

92 **Davies G, Welham J, Chant D, Torrey EF, McGrath J.** A systematic review and meta-analysis of Northern Hemisphere season of birth studies in schizophrenia. *Schizophr Bull* 2003;**29**(3):587–593.

93 **McGrath JJ, Welham JL.** Season of birth and schizophrenia: a systematic review and meta-analysis of data from the Southern Hemisphere. *Schizophr Res* 1999;**35**(3):237–242.

94 **Torrey EF, Miller J, Rawlings R, Yolken RH.** Seasonality of births in schizophrenia and bipolar disorder: a review of the literature. *Schizophr Res* 1997;**28**(1):1–38.

95 **Lewis G, David A, Andreasson S, Allebeck P.** Schizophrenia and city life. *Lancet* 1992;**340**(8812): 137–140.

96 **Marcelis M, Navarro-Mateu F, Murray R, Selten JP, Van Os J.** Urbanization and psychosis: a study of 1942–1978 birth cohorts in The Netherlands. *Psychol Med* 1998;**28**(4):871–879.

97 Mortensen PB, Pedersen CB, Westergaard T, et al. Effects of family history and place and season of birth on the risk of schizophrenia. *N Engl J Med* 1999;**340**(8):603–608.

98 Pedersen CB, Mortensen PB. Evidence of a dose–response relationship between urbanicity during upbringing and schizophrenia risk. *Arch Gen Psychiatry* 2001;**58**(11):1039–1046.

99 Fearon P, Kirkbride JB, Morgan C, et al. Incidence of schizophrenia and other psychoses in ethnic minority groups: results from the MRC AESOP Study. *Psychol Med* 2006;**36**(11):1541–1550.

100 Kirkbride JB, Barker D, Cowden F, et al. Psychoses, ethnicity and socio-economic status. *Br J Psychiatry* 2008;**193**(1):18–24.

101 Kirkbride JB, Errazuriz A, Croudace TJ, et al. Incidence of schizophrenia and other psychoses in England, 1950–2009: a systematic review and meta-analyses. *PLoS One* 2012;7(3):e31660.

102 Coid JW, Kirkbride JB, Barker D, et al. Raised incidence rates of all psychoses among migrant groups: findings from the East London first episode psychosis study. *Arch Gen Psychiatry* 2008;**65**(11): 1250–1258.

103 Veling W, Hoek HW, Selten JP, Susser E. Age at migration and future risk of psychotic disorders among immigrants in the Netherlands: a 7-year incidence study. *Am J Psychiatry* 2011;**168**(12): 1278–1285.

104 Eaton WW, Chen C-Y, Bromet EJ. Epidemiology of schizophrenia. In: Tsuang MT, Tohen M, Jones PB, editors. *Textbook of psychiatric epidemiology*. 3rd ed. Chichester: Wiley–Blackwell; 2011. pp. 263–287.

Chapter 7

Bipolar disorder

Leslie Hulvershorn and John Nurnberger, Jr.

7.1 Introduction

Bipolar disorder (BP) is characterized by episodes of mania/hypomania and depression. As defined by DSM-IV-TR,[1] a manic episode is a distinctly elevated or irritable mood, which must last for at least one week and represents a change from an individual's baseline mood. Mania, and its less severe form, hypomania, are marked by several of the following mood and behaviour changes: inflated self-esteem, a decreased need for sleep, talkativeness, a flight of ideas, distractibility, increased activity, and impulsivity. In BP, the depressed mood state is defined as it is for unipolar major depression, with five of nine possible depressive symptoms occurring on a daily basis over at least a 2-week period. The disorder affects 2–4% of the US population (1% BP Type I, 1% BP Type II and 2% BP-NOS (BP not otherwise specified))[2] and is the sixth leading cause of disability among all medical causes worldwide.[3] BP frequently impairs quality of life: at least one type of work, social or family life disability affects more than half of individuals with BP, whereas more than one-third are affected by two of these disabilities.[4]

BP often presents with depressive episodes in the mid–late teens, commonly resulting in misdiagnosis of unipolar depression in the early course of the disorder.[5,6] Recent research with a large epidemiological sample (National Epidemiologic Survey on Alcohol and Related Conditions) revealed that approximately 1 in 25 individuals with unipolar depression transitioned to BP during the study's 3-year follow-up period.[7] Demographic risk factors associated with this transition included younger age, Black race/ethnicity, and less than a high school education. Environmental stressors that predicted the transition to BP included a history of child abuse and past-year problems with one's social support group. In a large sample of adults seeking treatment for depression, 16% met diagnostic criteria for BP.[8]

Numerous research groups have demonstrated that the earliest mood episodes in an individual's life are longest in duration.[9] The index mood episode has been documented to range from 30 to 60 months, whereas later episodes tend to last less than 10 months.[10] In an attempt to explain such findings, Post[11] postulated in his influential 'kindling hypothesis' of mood disorders that psychosocial stressors play a greater role in initial mood episodes, but that later episodes are more autonomous and less tied to life events. Further refinement of that theory, in the form of the behavioural activating system dysregulation model,[12] proposed that in vulnerable individuals, excessive activation of this system could precipitate (hypo)manic symptoms, whereas deactivation could produce depressive symptoms. Later empirical research has supported this model's application to BP and has been recently reviewed.[13] As an alternative, the social rhythm disruption theory proposed that, again in vulnerable individuals, affective episodes are triggered by life events which disrupt routine environmental cues such as meal or sleep times and routine social interactions.[14] These disruptions further trigger changes in social and circadian rhythms, resulting in the onset of episodes. Thus, theoretical accounts of the emergence of BP episodes converge on the interaction between life stressors and vulnerability (e.g. early life stress, genetics) both during the onset of BP as well as later in life. However, why episodes have their onset in late adolescence/early adulthood and decrease in duration throughout life largely remains incompletely explained by these models. Here, we begin by addressing risk for the later development in BP through the life course, starting with prenatal risk in the form of inborn genetics. We move through neonatal and eventually child and adolescent risk studies. Finally, we consider the disorder itself as it presents in childhood, adolescence, adulthood, and old age. We conclude with a discussion of limitations of the current science and future directions for the field.

7.2 **Risk for the development of bipolar disorder**

7.2.1 **Prenatal risk**

Whereas symptoms of BP have not been shown to manifest as early as infancy, risk for the development of this disorder can be viewed as present prenatally in the form of genetic risk. In recent years, it has become clear that psychiatric disorders such as BP, like other widespread medical conditions, result from complex genetic factors and interactions. Genetic and epidemiological studies of BP are reviewed in this prenatal risk section.

7.2.1.1 Clinical epidemiology: family, twin, and adoption studies

Family studies of BP have continually demonstrated aggregation of illness in relatives.[15] For example, in one study 25% of relatives of BP probands were found to have BP or unipolar illness compared with 20% of relatives of unipolar probands and 7% of relatives of healthy subjects (Table 7.1; Figure 7.1).[16] These studies also suggested that the various forms of mood disorder appear to be related in a hierarchical way; relatives of BP probands are more likely to express BP than relatives of other probands, yet they exhibit major depression more often than BP.

In terms of mode of inheritance, analyses of families have generally favoured multi-factorial inheritance,[17] which implies a mixture of multiple genetic and environmental factors acting together to cause illness, rather than the impact of a single gene, as occurs in Huntington's disease. Twin studies for BP also show consistent evidence for heritability. Bienvenu et al. summarize three recent twin studies of BP and calculated a heritability of 85%.[18] This rate of heritability in BP is higher than in other psychiatric illnesses and most complex medical conditions.

Several adoption studies have been performed examining these relationships in BP and the results have been consistent with hypotheses that genetic effects significantly explain illness variance in cases and families.[19] Namely, BP probands growing up in an adoptive family will have more biological relatives with mood disorder than control probands growing up in an adoptive family.

Table 7.1 Lifetime risk for bipolar disorder in different groups

Controls	Relatives of probands with depression	Relatives of probands with bipolar disorder	Relatives of probands with acute schizoaffective disorder	Identical twin with bipolar disorder
0.5–1%	3%	8%	17%	80%

Reproduced from Nurnberger J, General genetics of bipolar disorder. In: Strakowski SM editor, *The bipolar brain: integrating neuroimaging and genetics*, Oxford University Press, New York, Copyright © 2012, by permission of Oxford University Press.

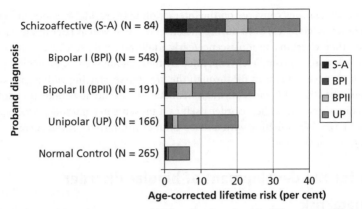

Figure 7.1 Risk of mood disorders among relatives of probands with different specific mood-disorder diagnoses and relatives of controls.

Reproduced from Nurnberger J, *General genetics of bipolar disorder*. In: Strakowski SM editor, *The Bipolar Brain: Integrating Neuroimaging and Genetics*, Oxford University Press, New York, Copyright © 2012, by permission of Oxford University Press. Source: data from Gershon ES et al., A family study of schizoaffective, Bipolar I, Bipolar II, unipolar and normal control probands, *Archives of General Psychiatry*, Volume 39, Number 10, pp. 1157–1167, Copyright © 1982.

7.2.1.2 Association/candidate gene studies

Studies of numerous candidate gene studies have been reported in the literature for BP. Several genes have emerged with replicated findings or positive meta-analyses from multiple studies and are reviewed by Seifuddin et al.[20] As genetic techniques continue to improve, it is likely that some of these genes will turn out to play a significant role in conferring risk for BP, whereas others will be only peripherally involved, or will be false positives.

7.2.1.3 Genome-wide association studies

Complex traits, such as height and risk for type II diabetes, have now been analysed extensively with genome-wide association studies (GWAS), but success required samples in the tens of thousands or even hundreds of thousands.[21] GWAS methods have now proven to be useful in psychiatric disorders, with several loci meeting stringent criteria in BP.[22,23] The presently accepted standard is $P \leq 5 \times 10e-8$ for a single nucleotide polymorphism association with illness in a GWAS study,[24] based on empirical probability of a type I error. Since the effect size of variants associated with psychiatric disorders is generally quite small (odds ratios of 1.1–1.2 are the norm), achieving P-values that meet this threshold requires very large sample sizes. Loci identified in GWAS investigations include: ANK3, CACNA1C, NCAN, ODZ4).

7.2.1.4 Copy number variation

Rare copy number variations (CNVs; small deletions and duplications in certain chromosomal areas) have been reported to be associated with BP in a number of studies in recent years (see review by Malhotra et al.[25]). CNVs may now be detected using dedicated microchips, and thus these studies are expected to be more commonly performed in the future.

7.2.1.5 Epigenetic studies/gene expression studies

Ogden et al.[26] used a convergent approach that integrated brain gene expression data from a pharmacogenomic mouse model with human data. These findings suggest that genes associated with the experiences of pleasure and pain in animals may play a role in emotional expression in humans. Le-Niculescu et al.[27] expanded this work by including data from GWAS as well as postmortem gene expression studies and expression studies in lymphocytes (and other lines of evidence including animal models). The candidate genes determined to be most likely involved in BP pathogenesis were ARNTL (aryl hydrocarbon receptor nuclear translocator-like, a circadian gene), BDNF, ALDH1A1 (an aldehyde dehydrogenase), and KLF12 (a zinc finger transcriptional repressor).

In sum, genetic risk for BP has been identified in adult samples and particularly suggests abnormalities affecting calcium channels and factors involved in neuronal growth and development. In addition to genes that an individual is born with, genetic changes that occur throughout life appear also to differ between individuals with and without BP. Future work linking these genetic changes to environmental influences is needed to disentangle causes for mood episodes seen in BP.

7.2.2 **Early life risk factors**

Risk for the development of BP in adulthood has been studied as early as the neonatal period. In a systematic review, perinatal adversities were not found to represent risk factors for BP.[28] However, in a more recently reported study of a population-based Swedish cohort, investigators determined that, compared with term babies, babies born at 32–36 weeks were 2.7 times more likely to develop BP, while those born at less than 32 weeks were 7.4 times more likely.[29] Suboptimal growth and low Apgar scores were not found to be associated with later development of BP or other mental illnesses.[29] Anomalous brain development, possibly mediated by epigenetic/gene expression changes associated with prematurity, may underlie this increase in BP risk.

Several cohorts of high risk child or adolescent offspring of adults with BP have been studied. In a sample of longitudinally followed Amish youth with and without parents with BP-I, the 'pre-school' behaviours/symptoms that most identified children with BP-I from well children in control samples were: sensitivity, crying, hyper-alertness, anxiety/worry, and somatic complaints.[30] During school years, parents reported mood (sad) and energy changes (low, not high), decreased sleep, and fearfulness as key symptoms.[30] By 17 years of age, offspring of individuals with BP in another American cohort showed a 23.4% lifetime prevalence of major affective disorders (BP and unipolar), compared with 4.4% in controls.[31] BP was seen in 8.5% and 0% of probands and controls, respectively.[31] In this study and one other, children with anxiety disorders or externalizing disorders were found to be at increased risk for development of an adolescent mood disorder.[31,32] Similar findings of high rates of mood and disruptive behaviour disorders in offspring of parents with BP-I were also seen in a smaller sample.[33] In the Bipolar Offspring Study (BIOS), offspring of parents with BP showed higher rates of BP spectrum disorders, anxiety disorders, and disruptive behaviour disorders, although most offspring did not manifest BP.[34]

In a community sample of youth with sub-threshold BP symptoms, 2% of adolescents converted to BP-I when reinterviewed during adulthood, but 41% had developed at least one episode of major depressive disorder (MDD).[35] In another epidemiological sample,[36] those with sub-threshold BP at baseline in adolescence were more likely to progress to BP-I during follow-up than those who initially presented with MDD (7.2% vs 1.7%). Using the same sample, the authors also found that whereas sub-threshold BP symptoms were common in the 14–17-year age group, new onset sub-threshold BP symptoms were rare after age 22 years.[37] However, the onset of manic symptoms was associated with cannabis use and novelty seeking, but novelty seeking predicted a lack of recurrence of episodes, when followed forward 8 years. In the same sample, the onset of depressive symptoms was associated with a family history of depression. Attention deficit/hyperactivity disorder and harm avoidance traits were associated with persistence of depressive symptoms, whereas trauma and a family history of depression predicted a lack of recurrence of episodes upon follow-up.

Among youth recruited with a distinct period of elevated, expansive, or irritable mood and two other DSM-IV manic symptoms (BP-NOS) into the Course and Outcome of Bipolar Youth (COBY) study, 45% converted to either BP-I or BP-II during a 5-year period.[38] The strongest predictor of conversion was a family history of mania or hypomania. Similarly, in a community sample, Stringaris et al.[39] described episodes that meet the symptom and impairment criteria of DSM-IV BP-I or BP-II but are of shorter duration (also termed BP-NOS), are as widespread, and lead to functional impairment. However, the particularly poor agreement between parent- and child-reported episodes and the fact that the episodes did not increase in duration as the participants aged cast some doubt on the validity of BP-NOS and whether it was on a continuum with BP-I and BP-II.[40]

In addition to direct study of BP symptoms in currently ill or at-risk populations, investigators have attempted to find paediatric endophenotypes that may herald a later onset of BP illness. An endophenotype is a biological characteristic that may substitute for a diagnosis. The advantage is that an endophenotype may be closer to the underlying pathophysiology of the illness and therefore may be more easily demonstrated to be associated with specific genetic markers. Endophenotypes related to sleep, brain activation and volume, and to neurotransmitter function have been studied in the context of BP[41–43] and have even been used to differentiate BP from other psychotic disorders.[44] In addition, in both offspring of individuals with BP as well as adolescents with BP, blood samples revealed elevations in proinflammatory marker levels in blood serum.[45] Although preliminary, these studies suggest that the BP disease course is either impacted by a proinflammatory state and/or precipitates such a state. A limitation of many of the endophenotypes studied so far is that they are difficult to measure and unlikely to be applied to large samples. Some of the brain imaging and peripheral blood markers may now be appropriate for larger-scale testing.

7.3 Bipolar disorder: across the lifespan

7.3.1 Child and adolescent onset

Diagnosis of BP in childhood has become controversial in the USA and several other countries over the past decade because rates of diagnosis have increased markedly.[46] Research into the phenomenology of paediatric BP has revealed that a shift in the diagnostic boundaries likely underlies this increase, rather than a true increase in disorder prevalence.[47] Childhood-onset BP is thought to be a valid, but much more rare, form of the disorder than that which more usually emerges in adolescence or adulthood. Data from the NIMH Genetics Initiative suggests that about 5% of first manic episodes occur prior to age 12 years (Figure 7.2). Among children presenting with episodic hypomania/mania, Stringaris et al. identified an undercontrolled dimension that was associated with significant impairment and a low risk exuberant dimension.[48] Early onset probands have increased morbid risk of illness in relatives than late onset illness, at least in some datasets.[49] In the large STEP-BD sample of adults with BP-I, Perlis et al.[50] found that those with onset before age 13 years (by retrospective report) experienced earlier recurrence of mood episodes after initial remission, fewer days of euthymia, and greater impairment in functioning and quality of life over a 2-year follow-up period.

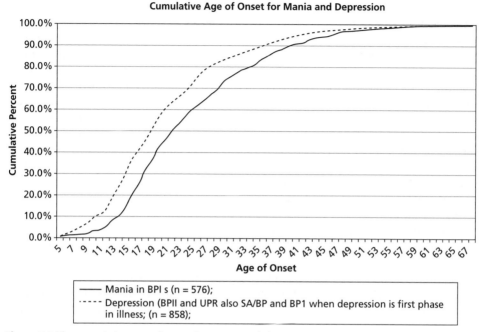

Figure 7.2 The cumulative age of onset for mania and depression in bipolar and unipolar mood disorders.

Reproduced from Nurnberger J, General genetics of bipolar disorder. In: Strakowski SM editor, *The Bipolar Brain: Integrating Neuroimaging and Genetics*, Oxford University Press, New York, Copyright © 2012, with permission from Oxford University Press. Source: data from the NIMH Genetics Initiative Study as described in Dick DM et al., Genomewide linkage analyses of bipolar disorder: a new sample of 250 pedigrees from the National Institute of Mental, Health Genetics Initiative, *American Journal of Human Genetics*, Volume 73, Issue 1, pp. 107–114, and Erratum in *American Journal of Human Genetics*, Volume 73, Issue 4, pp. 979, Copyright © 2003 by The American Society of Human Genetics. All rights reserved.

The median age of onset for major depression in BP is 19 years and the median age of onset for mania is 22 years (Figure 7.2). Thus, the onset of mood episodes in adolescence is widespread. Models of the life course of BP suggest that the emergence of depression, initially in the form of sub-threshold symptoms, frequently has its onset in early–mid adolescence and precedes mania.[51] Brief episodes of several days in duration with non-specific sleep difficulty and mood instability are also thought to be widespread in adolescence, prior to the onset of major mood episodes.[51] The onset of discrete mood episodes during early/mid adolescence is associated with greater severity of depression and mania, greater number of episodes, more days depressed, more days of ultradian cycling, and fewer euthymic days in adulthood, compared with individuals with BP whose mood episodes began in adulthood.[52]

7.3.2 **Adulthood**

The life phase during which symptoms of BP are most usually observed is adulthood. BP depressive episodes in medication-treated samples have been reported to last 2.8–4.3 months, whereas manic episodes are typically shorter, with average durations reported from 2 to 4 months.[10] As an individual experiences a greater number of lifetime mood episodes, the cycle length (time from the onset of one episode to the onset of the next) decreases, such that individuals with frequent episodes tend to have more episodes across their lifespan.[10] Tremendous variability exists in the number of lifetime mood episodes in BP. Across studies, 0–55% have one lifetime episode, whereas 2–69% have more than seven.[10]

Intrinsic predictors of BP mood episodes in adults have focused on cognitive and interpersonal style. Such work has established that dysfunctional cognitions in response to stressful situations increase an individual's risk for having a mood episode.[53,54] Researchers have debated whether or not dysfunctional cognitions in BP arise from stressful life situations[55] or whether such cognitions result in such situations.[56] Thus, social or other disadvantages could promote the development of dysfunctional cognitions and therefore BP mood episodes. Individuals with unresponsive early life caregivers,[57] low social supports,[58] and individuals in interpersonally dysfunctional environments[59] have been shown to be more at risk for the development of BP episodes. Some work also suggests a longer recovery from mood episodes in these disadvantaged environmental circumstances.[60] Across nearly two-dozen studies, childhood maltreatment has been strongly associated with an earlier onset of BP, suicidality, and co-occuring substance use disorders.[61]

Sub-threshold symptoms, persistence of symptoms, postpartum onset, and factors associated with suicide have all been studied in large samples of adults with BP. Sub-threshold symptoms in adults with BP have been found to be common and impairing, and are associated with conversion to threshold BP-I or -II.[62,63] Among adults hospitalized with BP-I or -II with psychosis, 73% returned to premorbid functioning at 4-year follow-up.[64] However, nearly half of the sample were rehospitalized prior to follow-up. Concurrent depressive symptoms, childhood psychopathology, and younger age at onset all predicted worse outcomes. In a large Danish sample, a psychiatric episode in the immediate postpartum period significantly predicted conversion to BP, suggesting that presentation of mental illness in this period is a marker for bipolarity.[65] Finally, a large French sample of adults with BP (attempters: 382; non-attempters: 708) evidenced eight risk factors associated with lifetime suicide attempts: multiple hospitalizations, depressive or mixed polarity of first episode, presence of stressful life events before illness onset, younger age at onset, no free intervals between episodes, female sex, higher number of previous episodes, and 'cyclothymic temperament'.[66]

7.3.3 **'Old age'**

While typically thought of as a disorder of young adults, BP mania in the elderly is not rare.[67] Mania accounts for 5–12% of psychiatric admissions in the elderly.[68] McDonald et al.[69] report a 20% prevalence of BP mania in elderly psychiatric patients, with a higher proportion of females presenting in later compared to mid or early life.[69] The majority of elderly patients with mania had a history of multiple prior depressive episodes.[70] Unlike BP seen in younger individuals, only about 30% of cases of mania in the elderly had a family history of affective illness.[71] Evidence of age-related cerebrovascular and related cognitive impairments were widespread among geriatric BP individuals.[69,72] Dementia is seen at increased rates in individuals with a history of BP compared to individuals with chronic health conditions, even when adjusting for age, gender, and drug and alcohol use.[73] The larger the number of lifetime mood episodes, the greater the risk for dementia.[74] Thus, as individuals with BP age, their risk for dementia and other milder forms of cognitive impairments increases. Given that the majority of cases of BP do present prior to old age and that cognitive impairments cloud the diagnostic picture, geriatric BP is more often unrecognized.[75]

Further complexity is added by the fact that drug interactions and increased sensitivities to treatments that are renally or hepatically metabolized are widespread in elderly patients.[76]

7.4 **Discussion**

7.4.1 **Methodological limitations**

Epidemiological studies have focused on measurable social and psychological factors that predate, precipitate, and perpetuate BP across the lifespan. Biological markers of BP illness have become increasingly studied, particularly in compounds found in blood samples (e.g. markers of inflammation and neurodevelopment) and images obtained from structural and functional magnetic resonance imaging (MRI). With the exception of some genetic studies, biological factors have been examined in smaller, clinically referred, cross-sectional samples, primarily in adolescence and mid-adulthood. Biological factors that likely play a significant role in the development of BP have not been integrated into the large-scale studies already discussed. Thus, our empirical knowledge of the neurobiology of the life course of BP cannot yet be fully integrated into that of the social and environmental factors.

7.4.2 **Summary**

Despite the lack of large-scale research on the interaction of biological, social and environmental factors that shape BP, the life course approach has already led to major changes in the treatment of mood disorders. Decades ago, treatment was focused on addressing acute symptoms of mood episodes, whereas now the emphasis has shifted to prophylaxis.[77] For example, maintaining patients with BP on their medications for a longer period, after their symptoms have resolved, has likely decreased the number of hospitalizations for mania, as well as suicides.[78,79] Public policies that prioritize the research and delivery of preventive interventions to youth early in the course of BP will likely continue to advance the entire life course of individuals living with BP.

7.4.3 **Future directions**

We believe that there remains a major need for biomarkers of vulnerability and course of illness for BP. Biomarkers of vulnerability might include genetic risk panels and functional MRI abnormalities in persons with a family history of BP. Such markers are now being tested, but are not yet ready for clinical use. Biomarkers of course of illness might include neuroinflammatory markers (e.g. interleukins) and markers of neuronal development (e.g. BDNF) that parallel or precede symptom changes. Clinical markers, such as early indicators of sleep disturbance and childhood psychiatric diagnoses, may also be important as early predictors of course. It is also useful in many cases for persons with mood disorders to track their own mood, hours of sleep and activity, life events, and medication changes over time. With widespread use of the Internet, such information may be rapidly communicated to an individual's family or treatment providers. Innovations harnessing newly available technology may prove to be increasingly helpful and efficient as an aid to clinical monitoring.

References

1 **American Psychiatric Association.** Task Force on DSM-IV. *Diagnostic and statistical manual of mental disorders.* 4th ed. Text revision. Washington, DC: American Psychiatric Association; 2000.
2 **Merikangas KR, Akiskal HS, Angst J, et al.** Lifetime and 12-month prevalence of bipolar spectrum disorder in the National Comorbidity Survey replication. *Arch Gen Psychiatry* 2007;**64**(5):543–552.

3 Murray C, Lopez A. *A comprehensive assessment of mortality and disability from diseases, injuries, and risk factors in 1990 and projected to 2020*. Cambridge, MA: Harvard University Press; 1996.

4 Gutierrez-Rojas L, Jurado D, Gurpegui M. Factors associated with work, social life and family life disability in bipolar disorder patients. *Psychiatry Res* 2011;**186**(2–3):254–260.

5 Stensland MD, Schultz JF, Frytak JR. Diagnosis of unipolar depression following initial identification of bipolar disorder: a common and costly misdiagnosis. *J Clin Psychiatry* 2008;**69**(5):749–758.

6 Baca-Garcia E, Perez-Rodriguez MM, Basurte-Villamor I, et al. Diagnostic stability and evolution of bipolar disorder in clinical practice: a prospective cohort study. *Acta Psychiatr Scand* 2007;**115**(6): 473–480.

7 Gilman SE, Dupuy JM, Perlis RH. Risks for the transition from major depressive disorder to bipolar disorder in the National Epidemiologic Survey on Alcohol and Related Conditions. *J Clin Psychiatry* 2012;**73**(6):829–836.

8 Angst J, Azorin JM, Bowden CL, et al. Prevalence and characteristics of undiagnosed bipolar disorders in patients with a major depressive episode: the BRIDGE study. *Arch Gen Psychiatry* 2011;**68**(8):791–798.

9 Roy-Byrne P, Post RM, Uhde TW, Porcu T, Davis D. The longitudinal course of recurrent affective illness: life chart data from research patients at the NIMH. *Acta Psychiatr Scand Suppl* 1985;**317**:1–34.

10 Goodwin FK, Redfield Jamison K. *Manic-depressive illness: bipolar disorders and recurrent depression*. 2nd ed. Oxford: Oxford University Press; 2007.

11 Post RM. Transduction of psychosocial stress into the neurobiology of recurrent affective disorder. *Am J Psychiatry* 1992;**149**(8):999–1010.

12 Gray JA. Brain systems that mediate both emotion and cognition. *Cognition and Emotion* 1990;**4**: 269–288.

13 Bender RE, Alloy LB. Life stress and kindling in bipolar disorder: review of the evidence and integration with emerging biopsychosocial theories. *Clin Psychol Rev* 2011;**31**(3):383–398.

14 Ehlers CL, Frank E, Kupfer DJ. Social zeitgebers and biological rhythms. A unified approach to understanding the etiology of depression. *Arch Gen Psychiatry* 1988;**45**(10):948–952.

15 Faraone SV, Kremen WS, Tsuang MT. Genetic transmission of major affective disorders: quantitative models and linkage analyses. *Psychol Bull* 1990;**108**(1):109–127.

16 Gershon ES, Hamovit J, Guroff JJ, et al. A family study of schizoaffective, bipolar I, bipolar II, unipolar, and normal control probands. *Arch Gen Psychiatry* 1982;**39**(10):1157–1167.

17 Nurnberger JI, Jr. Implications of multifactorial inheritance for identification of genetic mechanisms in major psychiatric disorders. *Psychiatr Genet* 2002;**12**(3):121–126.

18 Bienvenu OJ, Davydow DS, Kendler KS. Psychiatric 'diseases' versus behavioral disorders and degree of genetic influence. *Psychol Med* 2011;**41**(1):33–40.

19 Nurnberger JI, Jr, Berrettini W. *Psychiatric genetics*. London: Chapman & Hall; 1998.

20 Seifuddin F, Mahon PB, Judy J, et al. Meta-analysis of genetic association studies on bipolar disorder. *Am J Med Genet B Neuropsychiatr Genet* 2012;**159B**(5):508–518.

21 Lango Allen H, Johansson S, Ellard S, et al. Polygenic risk variants for type 2 diabetes susceptibility modify age at diagnosis in monogenic HNF1A diabetes. *Diabetes* 2010;**59**(1):266–271.

22 Psychiatric GWAS Consortium Bipolar Disorder Working Group. Large-scale genome-wide association analysis of bipolar disorder indentifies a new susceptibility locus near ODZ4. *Nat Genet* 2011;**43**: 977–983.

23 Cichon S, Muhleisen TW, Degenhardt FA, et al. Genome-wide association study identifies genetic variation in neurocan as a susceptibility factor for bipolar disorder. *Am J Hum Genet* 2011;**88**(3):372–381.

24 Altshuler D, Daly MJ, Lander ES. Genetic mapping in human disease. *Science* 2008;**322**(5903):881–888.

25 Malhotra D, McCarthy S, Michaelson JJ, et al. High frequencies of de novo CNVs in bipolar disorder and schizophrenia. *Neuron* 2011;**72**(6):951–963.

26 Ogden CA, Rich ME, Schork NJ, et al. Candidate genes, pathways and mechanisms for bipolar (manic-depressive) and related disorders: an expanded convergent functional genomics approach. *Mol Psychiatry* 2004;**9**(11):1007–1029.

27 Le-Niculescu H, Patel SD, Bhat M, et al. Convergent functional genomics of genome-wide association data for bipolar disorder: comprehensive identification of candidate genes, pathways and mechanisms. *Am J Med Genet B Neuropsychiatr Genet* 2009;**150B**(2):155–181.

28 Scott J, McNeill Y, Cavanagh J, Cannon M, Murray R. Exposure to obstetric complications and subsequent development of bipolar disorder: systematic review. *Br J Psychiatry* 2006;**189**:3–11.

29 Nosarti C, Reichenberg A, Murray RM, et al. Preterm birth and psychiatric disorders in young adult life. *Arch Gen Psychiatry* 2012;**69**(6):E1–8.

30 Egeland JA, Endicott J, Hostetter AM, Allen CR, Pauls DL, Shaw JA. A 16-year prospective study of prodromal features prior to BPI onset in well Amish children. *J Affect Disord* 2012;**142**(1–3):186–192.

31 Nurnberger JI, Jr, McInnis M, Reich W, et al. A high-risk study of bipolar disorder. Childhood clinical phenotypes as precursors of major mood disorders. *Arch Gen Psychiatry* 2011;**68**(10):1012–1020.

32 Duffy A, Alda M, Hajek T, Grof P. Early course of bipolar disorder in high-risk offspring: prospective study. *Br J Psychiatry* 2009;**195**(5):457–458.

33 Zappitelli MC, Bordin IA, Hatch JP, et al. Lifetime psychopathology among the offspring of Bipolar I parents. *Clinics (Sao Paulo)* 2011;**66**(5):725–730.

34 Goldstein BI, Shamseddeen W, Axelson DA, et al. Clinical, demographic, and familial correlates of bipolar spectrum disorders among offspring of parents with bipolar disorder. *J Am Acad Child Adolesc Psychiatry* 2010;**49**(4):388–396.

35 Lewinsohn PM, Klein DN, Seeley JR. Bipolar disorder during adolescence and young adulthood in a community sample. *Bipolar Disord* 2000;**2**(3 Pt 2):281–293.

36 Zimmerman M, Ruggero CJ, Chelminski I, Young D. Psychiatric diagnoses in patients previously overdiagnosed with bipolar disorder. *J Clin Psychiatry* 2010;**71**(1):26–31.

37 Tijssen MJ, van Os J, Wittchen HU, et al. Prediction of transition from common adolescent bipolar experiences to bipolar disorder: 10-year study. *Br J Psychiatry* 2010;**196**(2):102–108.

38 Axelson DA, Birmaher B, Strober MA, et al. Course of subthreshold bipolar disorder in youth: diagnostic progression from bipolar disorder not otherwise specified. *J Am Acad Child Adolesc Psychiatry* 2011;**50**(10):1001–1016 e3.

39 Stringaris A, Santosh P, Leibenluft E, Goodman R. Youth meeting symptom and impairment criteria for mania-like episodes lasting less than four days: an epidemiological enquiry. *J Child Psychol Psychiatry* 2010;**51**(1):31–38.

40 Stringaris A, Baroni A, Haimm C, et al. Pediatric bipolar disorder versus severe mood dysregulation: risk for manic episodes on follow-up. *J Am Acad Child Adolesc Psychiatry* 2010;**49**(4):397–405.

41 Hasler G, Drevets WC, Gould TD, Gottesman, II, Manji HK. Toward constructing an endophenotype strategy for bipolar disorders. *Biol Psychiatry* 2006;**60**(2):93–105.

42 Matsuo K, Kopecek M, Nicoletti MA, et al. New structural brain imaging endophenotype in bipolar disorder. *Mol Psychiatry* 2012;**17**(4):412–420.

43 Johannesen JK, O'Donnell BF, Shekhar A, McGrew JH, Hetrick WP. Diagnostic specificity of neurophysiological endophenotypes in schizophrenia and bipolar disorder. *Schizophr Bull* 2012 Aug 27 [Epub ahead of print].

44 Milanovic SM, Thermenos HW, Goldstein JM, et al. Medial prefrontal cortical activation during working memory differentiates schizophrenia and bipolar psychotic patients: a pilot FMRI study. *Schizophr Res* 2011;**129**(2–3):208–210.

45 Goldstein BI, Collinger KA, Lotrich F, et al. Preliminary findings regarding proinflammatory markers and brain-derived neurotrophic factor among adolescents with bipolar spectrum disorders. *J Child Adolesc Psychopharmacol* 2011;**21**(5):479–484.

46 Moreno C, Laje G, Blanco C, Jiang H, Schmidt AB, Olfson M. National trends in the outpatient diagnosis and treatment of bipolar disorder in youth. *Arch Gen Psychiatry* 2007;**64**(9):1032–1039.

47 Leibenluft E. Severe mood dysregulation, irritability, and the diagnostic boundaries of bipolar disorder in youths. *Am J Psychiatry* 2011;**168**(2):129–142.

48 Stringaris A, Stahl D, Santosh P, Goodman R. Dimensions and latent classes of episodic mania-like symptoms in youth: an empirical enquiry. *J Abnorm Child Psychol* 2011;**39**(7):925–937.

49 Faraone SV, Su J, Tsuang MT. A genome-wide scan of symptom dimensions in bipolar disorder pedigrees of adult probands. *J Affect Disord* 2004;**82**(Suppl 1):S71–78.

50 Perlis RH, Dennehy EB, Miklowitz DJ, et al. Retrospective age at onset of bipolar disorder and outcome during two-year follow-up: results from the STEP-BD study. *Bipolar Disord* 2009;**11**(4):391–400.

51 Duffy A, Alda M, Hajek T, Sherry SB, Grof P. Early stages in the development of bipolar disorder. *J Affect Disord* 2010;**121**(1–2):127–135.

52 Post RM, Leverich GS, Kupka RW, et al. Early-onset bipolar disorder and treatment delay are risk factors for poor outcome in adulthood. *J Clin Psychiatry* 2010;**71**(7):864–872.

53 Reilly-Harrington NA, Alloy LB, Fresco DM, Whitehouse WG. Cognitive styles and life events interact to predict bipolar and unipolar symptomatology. *J Abnorm Psychol* 1999;**108**(4):567–578.

54 Scott J, Stanton B, Garland A, Ferrier IN. Cognitive vulnerability in patients with bipolar disorder. *Psychol Med* 2000;**30**(2):467–472.

55 Alloy LB, Abramson LY, Walshaw PD, Keyser J, Gerstein RK. A cognitive vulnerability–stress perspective on bipolar spectrum disorders in a normative adolescent brain, cognitive, and emotional development context. *Dev Psychopathol* 2006;**18**(4):1055–1103.

56 Van der Gucht E, Morriss R, Lancaster G, Kinderman P, Bentall RP. Psychological processes in bipolar affective disorder: negative cognitive style and reward processing. *Br J Psychiatry* 2009;**194**(2): 146–151.

57 Morriss RK, van der Gucht E, Lancaster G, Bentall RP. Adult attachment in bipolar 1 disorder. *Psychol Psychother* 2009;**82**(Pt 3):267–277.

58 Johnson L, Lundstrom O, Aberg-Wistedt A, Mathe AA. Social support in bipolar disorder: its relevance to remission and relapse. *Bipolar Disord* 2003;**5**(2):129–137.

59 Schwannauer M, Noble A, Fraser G. Behavioural risk of bipolar disorder in an analogue population: the role of cognitive, developmental and interpersonal factors. *Clin Psychol Psychother* 2011;**18**(5): 411–417.

60 Johnson SL, Meyer B, Winett C, Small J. Social support and self-esteem predict changes in bipolar depression but not mania. *J Affect Disord* 2000;**58**(1):79–86.

61 Daruy-Filho L, Brietzke E, Lafer B, Grassi-Oliveira R. Childhood maltreatment and clinical outcomes of bipolar disorder. *Acta Psychiatr Scand* 2011;**124**(6):427–434.

62 Regeer EJ, Krabbendam L, de Graaf R, ten Have M, Nolen WA, van Os J. A prospective study of the transition rates of subthreshold (hypo)mania and depression in the general population. *Psychol Med* 2006;**36**(5):619–627.

63 Fiedorowicz JG, Endicott J, Leon AC, Solomon DA, Keller MB, Coryell WH. Subthreshold hypomanic symptoms in progression from unipolar major depression to bipolar disorder. *Am J Psychiatry* 2011;**168**(1):40–48.

64 Carlson GA, Kotov R, Chang SW, Ruggero C, Bromet EJ. Early determinants of four-year clinical outcomes in bipolar disorder with psychosis. *Bipolar Disord* 2012;**14**(1):19–30.

65 Munk-Olsen T, Laursen TM, Meltzer-Brody S, Mortensen PB, Jones I. Psychiatric disorders with postpartum onset: possible early manifestations of bipolar affective disorders. *Arch Gen Psychiatry* 2012;**69**(4):428–434.

66 Azorin JM, Kaladjian A, Adida M, et al. Risk factors associated with lifetime suicide attempts in bipolar I patients: findings from a French National Cohort. *Compr Psychiatry* 2009;**50**(2):115–120.

67 **Yassa R, Nair V, Nastase C, Camille Y, Belzile L.** Prevalence of bipolar disorder in a psychogeriatric population. *J Affect Disord* 1988;**14**(3):197–201.

68 **Snowdon J.** A retrospective case-note study of bipolar disorder in old age. *Br J Psychiatry* 1991;**158**:485–490.

69 **McDonald WM.** Epidemiology, etiology, and treatment of geriatric mania. *J Clin Psychiatry* 2000;**61** Suppl 13:3–11.

70 **Tohen M, Shulman KI, Satlin A.** First-episode mania in late life. *Am J Psychiatry* 1994;**151**(1):130–132.

71 **Shulman KI, Tohen M.** Unipolar mania reconsidered: evidence from an elderly cohort. *Br J Psychiatry* 1994;**164**(4):547–549.

72 **Shulman KI.** Neurologic comorbidity and mania in old age. *Clin Neurosci* 1997;**4**(1):37–40.

73 **Kessing LV, Nilsson FM.** Increased risk of developing dementia in patients with major affective disorders compared to patients with other medical illnesses. *J Affect Disord* 2003;**73**(3):261–269.

74 **Nilsson FM, Kessing LV, Sorensen TM, Andersen PK, Bolwig TG.** Affective disorders in neurological diseases: a case register-based study. *Acta Psychiatr Scand* 2003;**108**(1):41–50.

75 **Sajatovic M, Blow FC, Ignacio RV.** Psychiatric comorbidity in older adults with bipolar disorder. *Int J Geriatr Psychiatry* 2006;**21**(6):582–587.

76 **Tueth MJ, Murphy TK, Evans DL.** Special considerations: use of lithium in children, adolescents, and elderly populations. *J Clin Psychiatry* 1998;**59**(Suppl 6):66–73.

77 **Geddes JR, Burgess S, Hawton K, Jamison K, Goodwin GM.** Long-term lithium therapy for bipolar disorder: systematic review and meta-analysis of randomized controlled trials. *Am J Psychiatry* 2004;**161**(2):217–222.

78 **Wyatt RJ.** Risks of withdrawing antipsychotic medications. *Arch Gen Psychiatry* 1995;**52**(3):205–208.

79 **Cipriani A, Pretty H, Hawton K, Geddes JR.** Lithium in the prevention of suicidal behavior and all-cause mortality in patients with mood disorders: a systematic review of randomized trials. *Am J Psychiatry* 2005;**162**(10):1805–1819.

Chapter 8

Applying a life course perspective to depression

Sasha Rudenstine

8.1 Introduction

Depression is one of the most prevalent forms of psychopathology today. The World Health Organization estimates that depression affects 121 million people worldwide and is a leading cause of disability-adjusted life years for men and women aged 15–44 years.[1] Moreover, studies have found that the lifetime prevalence of any affective disorder is ~20% and the 12-month prevalence of major depressive disorder, specifically, is 10.3%.[2,3] Depression places a substantial burden on individuals affected as well as on society. For example, 80% of individuals with moderate to severe depression report that their depressive symptoms hinder their daily functioning.[4] The cost to human life is also great. Ninety per cent of individuals who commit suicide have a psychiatric disorder and affective disorders are the most prevalent.[5,6] The exorbitant economic burden of depression on society compounds the human suffering. In 2000 alone, the economic burden (e.g. costs pertaining to treatment, workforce, and suicide) totalled US$83 billion.[7]

Major depression (MD), broadly defined by extreme sadness, hopelessness, thoughts of death, and lack of energy and interest, is a chronic condition that afflicts individuals throughout the course of their life.[8,9] The common relapsing and recurring trajectory of MD makes it a burdensome and complicated disease.[10] For example, following an initial depressive episode 50–60% of individuals will have a second episode. Among this group, 70–80% will have a third episode, and 90% of people with a history of three episodes will experience a fourth episode.[8,9]

There is abundant rationale for considering depression from a life course perspective. For decades, depression subtypes have been classified by symptom manifestation.[9] However, given the overlap in symptom expression across all classifications of depression, these distinctions do not inform clinical interventions.[11] Accordingly, clinicians from different theoretical orientations have long proposed defining the differences in depression by the life experiences that cause depression's onset and manifestation over time.[11] In applying a life course perspective to depression, Blatt and Maroudas suggested that depression is not simply a 'clinical disorder', but 'an affect state that ranges from a mild and appropriate transient reaction to difficult life events, to a profound and sustained disabling clinical disorder involving dysphoria, distorted cognition, and neurovegetative disturbances.'[11]

Moreover, the origins of MD are complex and it is now widely recognized that MD is influenced both by genetic and by environmental factors.[12] Life course epidemiology provides a useful lens through which we can study how these determinants intersect over time. Although this chapter focuses specifically on MD, much of the discussion is relevant to all depressive disorders including depression, not otherwise specified (NOS), and dysthymic disorder.

8.2 **Applying a life course approach**

The link among early familial relationships, the environment, and biology as conjoint influences on child development has long been recognized.[13] Significant advances in neuroscience and molecular biology over the past decade provide evidence for how early life experiences are biologically imprinted on to the developing brain and thus affect physical and mental health throughout the life course.[14] We reference three conceptual frameworks that are useful background to a foundational understanding of the role of life course epidemiology in helping us understand MD: sensitive periods, accumulation of risk, and trajectories of risk.

8.2.1 **Sensitive periods**

Sensitive periods are developmental stages when the brain is particularly vulnerable to environmental disruptions.[15] During such periods, experiences have the potential to alter developmental processes that may adversely affect later physical and mental health.[15] For example, prolonged or recurring adverse experiences in early childhood result in stress later in life being 'toxic' versus being 'positive' or 'tolerable'.[15] Toxic stress refers to 'excessive or prolonged activation of the physiological stress response systems [hypothalamic–pituitary–adrenal (HPA) axis], in the absence of the buffering protection afforded by stable, responsive relationships'.[16] The examination of how environmental disruptions in childhood modify neurobiological and genetic development and consequently foster adult psychopathology has direct implications for both individual treatment and overall population health.

8.2.2 **Accumulation of risk**

Normal brain development can also be interrupted by the cumulative damage caused by recurring adverse experiences. Therefore, while MD may follow exposure to a single stressful event at any point in life, the accumulation of stressful events over a life course can permanently alter biological mechanisms and significantly increase one's risk of depression onset and recurrence.[16] Attention to an individual's history of stressful events, as a result, illuminates one's vulnerability to depression as well as the persistence of depression over time (discussed further in Section 8.3).

8.2.3 **Recurring trajectory of depression over the life course**

Major depressive episodes may resolve spontaneously and the disorder typically follows a relapsing and remitting trajectory, and the aetiology of a single episode of depression is likely different from the causal factors of subsequent episodes.[8]

Just as there are many different pathways that can lead to adult depression, risk factors for depression change throughout life. A life course perspective applied to longitudinal studies highlights some of the antecedent causes of MD episodes. The presence of depressive and anxiety symptoms in childhood, including as early as toddlerhood, increases the risk for adult depression.[17–19] Furthermore, the best predictors of recurring adult depression are having a history of a depressive episode and younger age at first onset.[17]

8.3 **Risk factors for depression**

This section provides an overview of the most studied risk factors of MD and how they independently alter an individual's susceptibility to depression over the life course.

8.3.1 **Age**

Whereas depression can manifest at any point over the life course, prospective data suggest that the age of onset for major depression is most often at or before age 18 years.[20] Longitudinal studies of depression provide evidence that developing depression in young adulthood is a strong risk factor for persistent depression.[21]

The variables associated with individual risk of depression shift throughout the life course and are often related to age-related biological changes and the psychosocial environment. Overall, 3–5% of children and adolescents suffer from MD,[22] and the prevalence of MD among adolescents is significantly greater than among pre-schoolers and school-aged children (5–8% as compared with 1–2%, respectively).[23] Similar to MD in adulthood, child and adolescent MD will wax and wane, and subsequently increase the risk of adult depression.[24]

A handful of variables, such as increased frequency of physical and cognitive diseases, decreased social support, and chronic stress, make older adults more vulnerable to MD than younger adults.[25] Nevertheless, compared with younger adults, the overall prevalence of MD among older adults is lower than what has been reported among young and middle-aged adults.[26] Large-scale epidemiological studies suggest that the prevalence of MD among adults aged ≥65 years is between 1% and 5%.[27] Although MD may be less widespread among older adults, more than half of the older adults with MD suffered their first depressive episode after age 60 years.[26]

8.3.2 **Gender**

There exist significant gender differences in the prevalence of depression. Kessler et al.[28] found that 20–25% of women and 10–17% of men at some point in their lifetime have depression. Although gender differences in depression exist throughout the life course, they are first evident in adolescence.[3,29] Hyde et al.[29] propose that females, more than males, are at greater risk of depression during adolescence since females suffer a disproportionate number of stressors in adolescence compared with males (e.g. weight gain resulting from biological changes from puberty). Other studies suggest that women are at greater risk of depression due to gender-specific genes.[30,31] Three twin studies (the Virginia Twin Registry, the Swedish National Twin study, and the Australian Volunteer Twin Study) have documented that the heritability of depression is higher in women than in men.[32–34] Further exploration is needed to determine the role of genetics and the environment on the observed gender difference in the prevalence of depression in a population. Regardless of the root cause, women are consistently at greater risk of depression than men are throughout the life course.

8.3.3 **Socio-economic status**

The prevalence of psychiatric morbidity, including depression, is disproportionally high among individuals with low socio-economic status (SES) compared with those who fall within higher socio-economic groups.[35] A meta-analysis evaluating the relationship between SES and depression found that individuals with comparatively lower SES had a greater risk of incident and persistent depression.[36] There are several hypothesized explanations for this observation. The psychosocial environment theory suggests that people's perception of their place in the social and economic sphere will affect health via psycho-neuro-endocrine processes.[37] Another explanation is that the accumulation of stress associated with low SES results in higher rates of depression among individuals of low SES.[36,37] Although these differences are most often measured among adult populations, similar differences have been observed in children.[38]

8.3.4 **Genetics**

The role of genes in the development of MD has been the focus of substantial research over the past three decades.

Family studies have previously shown that the prevalence of depression among immediate family members (parents and siblings) of individuals diagnosed with MD is higher than the prevalence of MD in the general population (15% vs 5% respectively).[12] A meta-analysis on the genetic epidemiology of depression confirmed that there is a strong association between MD in first-degree relatives.[39] Adoption and twin studies confirm that genes are an important, but not an independent, variable in risk of depression. Sullivan et al.[39] concluded that the heritability of MD is between 31% and 42%, which is significantly less than the heritability of other psychopathology, such as bipolar disorder and schizophrenia.

The risk of MD is likely shaped by many genes that jointly make up the small percentage of the genetic risk. As for all complex genetic diseases, the influence of genetics on depression is best understood through the sensitivity threshold model rather than the classic Mendelian inheritance model. The sensitivity threshold model stipulates that 'the "disease susceptibility" variable is distributed continuously in the population, so that only those individuals who surpass a certain threshold manifest disorder'.[12] Linkage studies have identified several genes on different chromosomes associated with depression.[12] Association studies have identified six genes (APOE, DR4D, GNB3, MTHFR, SLC6A3, and SLC6A4) as significantly associated with MD.[40]

There is little question that the aetiology of MD is rooted in the interaction of environmental factors on several minor effect genes.[41] Multiple genes are therefore risk factors for MD in the context of severe life stressors;[12,42] this is discussed in more detail in Section 8.4.

8.3.5 **Stress**

Stressors come in many forms and will increase the risk of depression onset.[15,17] More specifically, the onset of a depressive episode typically follows within one month of exposure to stressful events.[43,44] Yet, it is equally important to emphasize that most people will successfully cope with stressful life events without suffering lasting impairment.[8,45] An individual's resilience or vulnerability in the face of stressful life events is associated with a range of factors, such as genetics and early life experiences that modify the effect that stress may have on depression onset and recurring episodes.[46]

Introduced by Post,[47] the 'kindling hypothesis' suggests that stressful life events are indicative of the initial episodes of MD and are less predictive of recurring episodes. Other studies have found that whereas recurring episodes of MD can be triggered by mild stressors, more severe life events precede depression's onset.[48] This latter finding is best explained by the 'sensitization hypothesis' which argues that a history of stressful life events reduces the amount of stress necessary to generate future depressive episodes.[49] Stated differently, the 'wear and tear' of stress throughout the life course diminishes resilience to future strain. McGonagle and Kessler[50] found that chronic stress, as compared with acute stress, was more strongly associated with severe depressive symptoms, and Muscatell et al.[51] found that lower global functioning was associated with exposure to severe life events prior to first onset.

While stressful life events are a widely recognized risk factor for adverse physical and mental health there is considerable evidence that some people are not only more vulnerable to stress, but also have disproportionate exposure to adverse experiences.[43,45] For example, Hammen[52] found that women with a history of depression were more likely than women with no such history to contribute to negative life events. To explain this finding, Hammen[43] defined events as dependent or independent. Dependent events are those experiences 'to which a person has contributed', whereas independent events are 'fateful', out of the person's control (p. 297). In this manner, whereas a stressful event (e.g. death of a parent) may trigger depression, the 'dependent' event category suggests that an individual's actions (e.g. inappropriate conduct at work) may produce adverse life events (e.g. unemployment) which in turn may lead to depressive symptoms.[43,44] Furthermore, the stress generation of depression model suggests that individuals at high risk of depression are more likely than individuals at low risk of depression to create negative events in their lives.[52]

8.3.6 Cognitive styles

An individual's 'ideology' or personality is an important variable in one's risk for depression as it directly relates to how s/he makes sense of experiences. Similarly, how events are evaluated and subsequently processed affects an individual's self-perception.[53] Therefore, if an experience affirms a negative self-image it will likely trigger depressive reactions.[53] Along these lines, Blatt[54] and others have argued that adverse childhood experiences nurture the development of a negative self-schema, which not only becomes a lens through which future events are interpreted, but also increases the susceptibility for depression following stressors. Beck et al.[55] referred to a negative self-image and the consequent maladaptive or faulty appraisal of events as cognitive vulnerability to depression.

Beevers[53] argues that a dual process model, which involves associative and reflective processing, underlies the cognitive vulnerability to depression model. Associative processing refers to the preconscious and automatic interpretation of events informed by comparable prior experiences. Reflective processing involves an individual consciously applying information to deduce an interpretation of his experience. When cognitive resources are limited, such as in the context of stress, reflective processing may be limited. Therefore information processing is initially guided by prior experience and secondarily, when possible, modified by the current context. As such, in the context of heightened stress, depression-vulnerable individuals lack the cognitive capacity for reflective processing and they default to their predisposition for negative thoughts. Similarities exist between Beevers' dual process model and the kindling effect in as much as an individual's vulnerability for depression increases with each stressor via the reinforcing of one's associative memory.

8.4 Gene–environment interactions: major depression as a multifactorial disorder

Section 8.3 reviewed some of the factors that independently affect our risk of depression. The aetiology of MD, however, is dynamic and a result of the continuous interaction of these factors across the life course.

Historically we have known that genes and our environments contribute to our vulnerability and resilience to depression. Studying a cohort of female twins, Kendler et al.[56] assessed the role of stress on MD among individuals with similar genetic and childhood environments. In this study, stressful life events increased a person's risk of developing MD irrespective of his/her genetic predisposition. Additionally, adverse life events were stronger predictors of MD among individuals with a genetic predisposition for MD than among those with low genetic risk. More recently, studies assessing gene–environment interactions have empirically shown the complex aetiology of depression. Karg et al.[57] published a meta-analysis of 54 studies confirming that the *5-HTTLPR* allele (found on the *SLC64A* gene) does moderate the relationship between stress and depression. Specifically, they note that the most robust association is between the *5-HTTLPR* allele and childhood maltreatment, followed by medical conditions and stressful life events, respectively. Furthermore, of the identified genes associated with MD, *SLC6A4* is the most studied due to the widely believed association between stress and depression.[12] Echoing these findings, Hyde et al.'s model of depression states that biological and cognitive vulnerabilities for depression necessitate the interaction with stressful life events.[29]

The interaction between stress and the *5-HTTLPR* allele does not guarantee that an individual will develop depression.[12] Several studies have identified variables that modify this particular gene–environment interaction. One such finding suggests that exposure to adverse events in early childhood may result in permanent cerebral modifications, such as to the HPA axis, which subsequently increases one's vulnerability to stress in adulthood.[58] Other findings establish that familial genetic risk of depression modifies the risk of depression after stressful events.[12] Prenatal maternal stress during sensitive periods of fetal development may also permanently modify the infants' stress response in much the same way that cumulative stress in childhood or adulthood may lead to HPA axis dysregulation.[14]

Hyde et al.[29] apply an integrative model to explain gender differences in depression; it is also a useful lens for looking more broadly at the aetiology of depression. They consider the interaction of biological, affective, and cognitive vulnerability as well as the environment, in particular the presence of negative life events. Furthermore, they propose that the presence of one vulnerability, whether it be biological, environmental, affective, or cognitive, will invariably increase an individual's overall risk of MD. Figure 8.1 illustrates the potential cyclical nature of depression and the continual interaction between risk and protective factors in determining depression onset, duration, and recurrence.

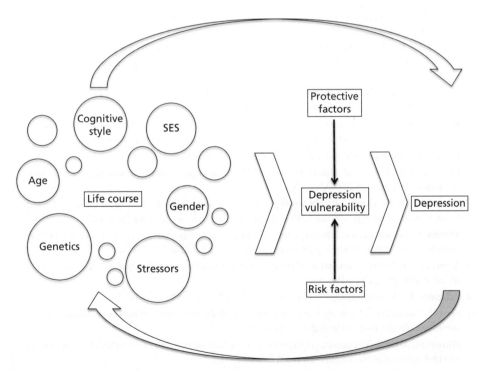

Figure 8.1 Conceptual framework for understanding the multifactorial aetiology of depression over the life course.

8.6 **Summary**

Bowlby[59] wrote that 'development turns at each and every stage of the journey on an interaction between the organism as it has developed up to that moment and the environment in which it then finds itself.' This dynamic perspective on development is the only viable lens through which to examine the complexity of depression. Longitudinal epidemiological studies of depression would benefit from a life course approach that integrates the breadth of factors underlying this burdensome disease.

Longitudinal studies and clinical observations consistently find that depression is a cyclical disease that, once present, re-emerges sporadically in relation to the biological and environmental context. Every depressive episode increases the risk of future depression; the younger the onset, the greater the potential for developing a chronic condition. The trajectories of depression are thus determined by the risk factors discussed in this chapter, including age, gender, SES, genetics, stress, and cognitive styles, and by protective factors such as early intervention treatments. Moreover, prevention efforts may benefit as the aetiology of depression is better defined. For example, screening for postpartum depression may help to deter the intergenerational transmission of depression given the significant effect that maternal depression may have on children.[60] By considering the environmental and biological contributors to depression we will more effectively be able to prescribe appropriate treatments. Thus, a life course approach to research and practice offers a lens through which we can more precisely dissect the interrelating mechanisms that mitigate or enhance vulnerability for depression.

References

1 **World Health Organization**. *Mental health: depression*. Geneva: WHO; 2012. <http://www.who.int/mental_health/management/depression/definition/en/>

2 **Kessler RC, Berglund PA, Demler O, Jin R, Merikangas KR, Walters EE**. Lifetime prevalence and age-of-onset distributions of DSM-IV disoders in the national comorbidity survey replication. *Arch Gen Psychiatry* 2005;**62**(6):593–602.

3 **Kessler RC, Magee WJ**. Childhood adversities and adult depression: basic patterns of association in a US national survey. *Psychol Med* 1993;**23**(3):679–690.

4 **Pratt LA, Brody DJ**. *Depression in the United States household population, 2005–2006*. Maryland: Centers for Disease Control; 2008. <http://www.cdc.gov/nchs/data/databriefs/db07.htm>

5 **Hawton K, Heeringen KV**. Suicide. *Lancet* 2009;**373**:1372–1381.

6 **Cavanagh JTO, Carson AJ, Sharpe M, Lawrie SM**. Psychological autopsy studies of suicide: a systematic review. *Psychol Med* 2003;**33**(3):395–405.

7 **Greenberg PE, Kessler RC, Birnbaum HG, et al**. The economic burden of depression in the United States: how did it change between 1990 and 2000? *J Clin Psychiatry* 2003;**64**:1465–1475.

8 **Monroe SM, Harkness KL**. Life stress, the "kindling" hypothesis, and the recurrence of depression: considerations from a life stress perspective. *Psychol Rev* 2005;**112**(2):417–445.

9 **American Psychiatric Association**. *Diganostic and statistical manual of mental disorders, text revision—4th ed*. Washington, DC: APA; 2000.

10 **Palazidou E**. The neurobiology of depression. *Br Med Bull* 2012;**101**:127–145.

11 **Blatt SJ, Maroudas C**. Convergence among psychoanalytic and cognitive: behavioral theories of depression. *Psychoanalytic Psychol* 1992;**9**:157–190.

12 **Mitjans M, Arias B**. The genetics of depression: what information can new methodologic aproaches provide? *Actas españolas de psiquiatría* 2012;**40**(2):70–83.

13 **Baltes PB, Reese HW, Lipsitt LP**. Life-span developmental psychology. *Ann Rev Psychol* 1980;**31**:65–110.

14 Bale TL, Baram TZ, Brown AS, et al. Early life programming and neurodevelopmental disorders. *Biol Psychiatry* 2010;**68**(4):314–319.

15 Heim C, Binder EB. Current research trends in early life stress and depression: review of human studies on sensitive periods, gene–environment interactions, and epigenetics. *Exp Neurol* 2012;**233**(1):102–111.

16 Garner AS, Shonkoff, JP, Siegel BS, et al. American Academy of Pediatrics. Early childhood adversity, toxic stress, and the role of the pediatrician: translating developmental science into lifelong health. *Pediatrics* 2012;**129**(e):224–231.

17 Colman I, Ataullahjan A. Life course perspectives on the epidemiology of depression. *Rev Can Psychiatrie* 2010;**55**(10):622–632.

18 Cote SM, Boivin M, Liu X, Nagin DS, Zoccolillo M, Tremblay RE. Depression and anxiety symptoms: onset, developmental course and risk factors during early childhood. *J Child Psychol Psychiatry* 2009;**50**(10):1201–1208.

19 Caspi A, Moffitt TE, Newman DL, Silva PA. Behavioral observations at age 3 years predict adult psychaitric disorders: longitudinal evidence from a birth cohort. *Arch Gen Psychiatry* 1996;**53**:1033–1039.

20 Kim-Cohen J, Caspi A, Moffit TE, Harrington H, Milne BJ, Poulton R. Prior juvenile diagnosis in adults with mental disorder. *Arch Gen Psychiatry* 2003;**60**:709–717.

21 Korten NC, Comijs HC, Lamers F, Penninx BW. Early and late onset depression in young and middle aged adults: differential symptomatology, characteristics and risk factors? *J Affect Disord* 2012;**138**(3):259–267.

22 Bhatia SK, Bhatia SC. Childhood and adolescent depression. *Am Acad Fam Physicians* 2007;**75**(1): 73–80.

23 Son SE, Kirchner JT. Depression in children and adolescents. *Am Acad Fam Physicians* 2000;**62**(10):2297–2308.

24 Pine DS, Cohen E, Cohen P, Brook J. Adolescent depressive symptoms as predictors of adult depression: moodiness or mood disorder? *Am J Psychiatry* 1999;**156**:133–135.

25 Blazer DG, 2nd, Hybels CF. Origins of depression in later life. *Psychol Med* 2005;**35**(9):1241–1252.

26 Fiske A, Wetherell JL, Gatz M. Depression in older adults. *Annu Rev Clin Psychol* 2009;5:363–389.

27 Hasin DS, Goodwin RD, Stinson FS, Grant BF. Epidemiology of major depressive disorder: results from the National Epidemiologic Survey on Alcoholism and Related Conditions. *Arch Gen Psychiatry* 2005;**62**:1097–1106.

28 Kessler RC, McGonagle KA, Zhao S, et al. Lifetime and 12-month prevalence of DSM-III-R psychaitric disorders in the United States. *Arch Gen Psychiatry* 1994;**51**:8–19.

29 Hyde JS, Mezulis AH, Ambramson LY. The ABCs of depression: integrating affective, biological, and cognitive models to explain the emergence of the gender difference in depression. *Psychol Rev* 2008;**115**(2):291–313.

30 Holmans P, Zubenko GS, Crowe RR, et al. Genome-wide significant linkage to recurrent, early-onset major depressive disorder on chromosome 15q. *Am J Hum Genet* 2004;**74**:1154–1167.

31 Abkevich V, Camp NJ, Hensel CH, et al. Predisposition locus for major depression at chromosome 12q22–12q23.2. *Am J Hum Genet* 2003;**73**:1271–1281.

32 Kendler KS, Gatz M, Gardner CO, Pedersen NL. A Swedish national twin study of lifetime major depression. *Am J Psychiatry* 2006;**163**(1):109–114.

33 Bierut LJ, Heath AC, Phil D, et al. Major depressive disorder in a community-based twin sample. *Arch Gen Psychiatry* 1999;**56**:557–563.

34 Kendler KS, Gardner CO, Neale MC, Prescott CA. Genetic risk factors for major depressin in men and women: similar or different heritabilities and same or partly distinct genes? *Psychol Med* 2001;**31**:605–616.

35 van der Waerden JE, Hoefnagels C, Hosman CM. Psychosocial preventive interventions to reduce depressive symptoms in low-SES women at risk: a meta-analysis. *J Affect Disord* 2011;**128**(1–2):10–23.

36 **Lorant V.** Socioeconomic inequalities in depression: a meta-analysis. *Am J Epidemiol* 2003;**157**(2): 98–112.

37 **Lynch J, Smith GD, Hillemeier M, Shaw M, Raghunathan T, Kaplan G.** Income inequality, the psychosocial environment, and health: comparisons of wealthy nations. *Lancet* 2001;**358**(9277):194–200.

38 **Lupien SJ, King S, Meaney MJ, McEwen BS.** Child's stress hormone levels correlate with mother's socioeconomic status and depressive state. *Biol Psychiatry* 2000;**48**(10):976–980.

39 **Sullivan PF, Neale MC, Kendler KS.** Genetic epidemiology of major depression: review and meta-analysis. *Am J Psychiatry* 2000;**157**(10):1552–1562.

40 **Lopez-Leon S, Janssens AC, Gonzalez-Zuloeta Ladd AM, et al.** Meta-analyses of genetic studies on major depressive disorder. *Mol Psychiatry* 2008;**13**(8):722–785.

41 **Lohoff FW.** Overview of the genetics of major depressive disorder. *Curr Psychiatry Rep* 2010;**12**(6): 539–546.

42 **Caspi A, Sugden K, Moffitt TE, et al.** Influence of life stress on depression: moderation by a polymorphism in the 5-HTT gene. *Science* 2005;**301**(5631):386–389.

43 **Hammen C.** Stress and depression. *Annu Rev Clin Psychol* 2005;**1**:293–319.

44 **Liu RT, Alloy LB.** Stress generation in depression: a systematic review of the empirical literature and recommendations for future study. *Clin Psychol Rev* 2010;**30**(5):582–593.

45 **Keers R, Uher R.** Gene–environment interaction in major depression and antidepressant treatment response. *Curr Psychiatry Rep* 2012;**14**(2):129–137.

46 **Kendler KS, Karowski LM, Prescott CA.** Causal relationship between stressful life events and the onset of major depression. *Am J Psychiatry* 1999;**156**(6):837–841.

47 **Post RM.** Transduction of psychosocial stress into the neurobiology of recurrent affective disorder. *Am J Psychiatry* 1992;**129**(8):999–1010.

48 **You S, Conner KR.** Stressful life events and depressive symptoms: influences of gender, event severity, and depression history. *J Nerv Ment Dis* 2009;**197**(11):829–833.

49 **Dienes KA, Hammen C, Henry RM, Cohen AN, Daley SE.** The stress sensitization hypothesis: understanding the course of bipolar disorder. *J Affect Disorders* 2006;**95**(1–3):43–49.

50 **McGonagle KA, Kessler RC.** Chronic stress, acute stress, and depressive symptoms. *Am J Community Psychol* 1990;**18**:681–706.

51 **Muscatell KA, Slavich GM, Monroe SM, Gotlib IH.** Stressful life events, chronic difficulties, and the symptoms of clinical depression. *J Nerv Ment Dis* 2009;**197**(3):154–160.

52 **Hammen C.** Generation of stress in the course of unipolar depression. *J Abnorm Psychol* 1991;**100**: 555–561.

53 **Beevers CG.** Cognitive vulnerability to depression: a dual process model. *Clin Psychol Rev* 2005;**25**(7):975–1002.

54 **Blatt SJ.** The destructiveness of perfectionism: implications for the treatment of depression. *Am Psychologist* 1995;**50**(12):1003–1020.

55 **Beck AT, Rush AJ, Shaw BF, Emery G.** *Cognitive therapy of depression.* New York: Guilford; 1979.

56 **Kendler KS, Kessler RC, Walters EE, et al.** Stressful life events, genetic liability, and onset of an episode of major depression in women. *Am J Psychiatry* 1995;**152**(6):833–842.

57 **Karg K, Burmeister M, Shedden K, Sen S.** The serotonin transporter promoter variant (5-HTTLPR), stress, and depression meta-analysis revisited: evidence of genetic moderation. *Arch Gen Psychiatry* 2011;**68**(5):444–454.

58 **Heim C, Nemeroff CB.** Neurobiology of early life stress: clinical studies. *Semin Clin Neuropsychiatry* 2002;**7**(2):147–159.

59 **Bowlby J.** *Attachment and loss: separation.* New York: Basic Books; 1973.

60 **Patel M, Bailey RK, Jabeen S, Ali S, Barker NC, Osiezagha K.** Postpartum depression: a review. *J health care poor underserved* 2012;**23**(2):534–542.

Chapter 9

Life course epidemiology of anxiety disorders

Renee D. Goodwin, Katja Beesdo-Baum, Susanne Knappe, and Dan J. Stein

9.1 Introduction

Thought to be the most widespread and earliest occurring mental disorders,[1,2] anxiety disorders are associated with social, academic, and occupational impairment in childhood, and increased risk of a range of mental health problems throughout development and into adulthood.[3-5] While there is substantial overlap in the correlates, predictors and long-term outcomes associated with anxiety disorders in childhood and adolescence, there is also convincing evidence that each of these conditions has distinct correlates.[6-7]

In this review, we will examine the prevalence, correlates/risk factors, and treatment of specific phobia, generalized anxiety disorder (GAD), panic disorder (PD), social phobia, and obsessive–compulsive disorder over the life course. Post-traumatic stress disorder (PTSD) is covered in detail in Chapter 10. We will then discuss implications of a life course approach on the epidemiology of anxiety disorders for clinical work, public health, and future research.

9.2 Specific phobia

9.2.1 Prevalence, onset, and natural course

Specific phobia is characterized by a marked and persistent fear of clearly discernible, circumscribed objects or situations such as animals, insects, storms, heights, elevators, water, blood, injections, etc. Exposure to such objects or situations usually provokes an immediate anxiety response and the phobic stimuli are frequently avoided.

Specific phobia is the most widespread anxiety disorder with a 12-month prevalence of 12% and lifetime prevalence of 15%.[8,9] It is the earliest of all forms of anxiety disorder with the core incidence period occurring in childhood and early adolescence.[10] The DSM-IV specifies various subtypes of specific phobia: animal, situational, natural environmental, blood/injection/injury, and other. Retrospective data from cross-sectional studies suggest a considerable persistence of specific phobia (12-month prevalence to lifetime prevalence ratios of ~80%), which is highest among all the anxiety disorders.[9] Ten-year prospective–longitudinal data from adolescents and young adults show that specific phobia (41%) is the anxiety disorder with the highest 'homotypic' stability (same disorder at later points in time) other than PTSD (50%).[11] Stability rates for specific phobia subtypes were also considerable (22% for environment and animal type and 34% for blood–injection–injury type), but the overall high persistence/stability is also attributable to the fact that different types of specific fears and phobias co-occur.[12]

9.2.2 **Correlates and risk factors**

There is little evidence for demographic correlates, such as systematic variation by countries, cultures, urbanicity, or education,[11,13] with the exception of gender and age. On the other hand, studies show that specific phobia is associated with high levels of psychiatric comorbidity.[13,14] The findings that specific phobias (a) are early onset disorders, (b) have high comorbidity with many forms of mental disorders that usually occur later in life, and (c) have high rates for 'heterotypic' continuity (other disorders later in the life course[11]) suggests that specific phobias may be early risk factors for a sequence of subsequent psychopathology.[15]

9.2.3 **Public health and treatment approaches**

Specific phobia is not generally considered a pressing public health problem in itself—especially among youth it is thought that this problem is developmentally transient and fairly constricted to a circumscribed phobic object or situation. Yet, given (i) the high prevalence, (ii) the early onset, (iii) the high persistence, and (iv) evidence of risk for development of subsequent mental disorders, specific phobias are a good potential target for early intervention and possibly secondary prevention of comorbid psychopathological complications. Specific phobias can be effectively treated with cognitive behavioural therapy (CBT), particularly exposure.[11]

9.3 **Generalized anxiety disorder**

9.3.1 **Prevalence, onset, and natural course**

Generalized anxiety disorder (GAD) is characterized by excessive, uncontrollable, and persistent anxiety and worry about a number of events or activities such as work or school performance, the health of family members, finances, or minor matters.

GAD is a widespread mental disorder in the general population with a lifetime prevalence of 5.7%[16] and a 12-month prevalence of 3.1%;[17] the projected lifetime risk as of age 75 years has been estimated at 9.0%.[9] Compared with other anxiety disorders, GAD reveals a later age of onset with most cases emerging in early or middle adulthood; first onsets in older adulthood are not infrequent.[9,17] Retrospectively, few cases date onset back to childhood, which contrasts with high prevalence reports of DSM-III-R Overanxious Disorder (OAD)[18,19] which has been subsumed under the diagnosis of GAD in DSM-IV. Similar to panic disorder and agoraphobia, GAD incidence begins to increase in adolescence.[10,20] Methodologically sound data on the natural course of GAD in the general population are scarce. Extant evidence suggests that the natural course of GAD may be more appropriately characterized as 'waxing and waning', i.e. as repeated episodes of shorter durations of months or few years and intervals with few or no symptoms.[21-23]

9.3.2 **Correlates and risk factors**

Females are about twice as likely as males to be affected by GAD. GAD is particularly common among non-married individuals and among those with low socio-economic status. GAD is associated with high rates of comorbidity (up to 90% with any lifetime mental disorder). Although all types of other mental disorders can occur together with GAD (e.g. 58% anxiety disorders, 72% mood disorders, 34% substance use disorders[24]), the high comorbidity with major depression (e.g. 61%[24]) has received the most attention and raised questions as to whether GAD is an independent disorder or rather a prodrome, residual, or severity marker of depression. Several epidemiological studies have, however, found that comorbidity with depression is not higher in GAD than in other disorders.[22,25] Moreover, it has been shown that GAD without depression is at least as impairing and disabling as depression without GAD; with the most impairment and disability found among individuals with comorbid major depression and GAD.[26] GAD has been found to be a predictor for a range of other mental disorders in future years, including other anxiety disorders, depression, substance use and disruptive behaviour disorders.[10,18,27–30] Physical health problems are also frequent among individuals with GAD.[31] They often prompt help-seeking at general practitioners, where GAD is often underrecognized and undertreated.[26,32]

9.3.3 Public health and treatment approaches

Pharmacological and psychological treatments are available for GAD. Among pharmacological agents, antidepressants are recommended for GAD, but other novel agents (e.g. pregabalin) also have proven efficacy.[33] Psychological treatment, particularly CBT, is an important option[34] because it may be better tolerated by the patients[35] and because improvements generally remain stable after completion of treatment.[36,37] Nevertheless, there is room for improvement of psychological treatments for GAD given recovery rates of around 50% (70–80% in more recent innovative refinements of CBT).[37] GAD onset usually precedes major depression and some evidence suggests that early treatment may be protective.[38] In addition, despite considerable treatment-seeking in individuals with GAD, only a minority of individuals affected by GAD receive any appropriate treatment because the disorder is rarely correctly recognized and diagnosed.[26]

9.4 Panic attacks and panic disorder

9.4.1 Prevalence, onset, and natural course

Panic disorder (PD), characterized by frequent panic attacks (PA) and either accompanying anticipatory anxiety or avoidance of situations in which they are likely to occur, is estimated to be present in 0.5–1.9% of adolescents[39,40] and in 1.5–3.0% of adults in the USA, and international rates are similar.[41]

From a life course perspective, the onset of PD begins to appear in adolescence—similar to GAD and PTSD—and later than phobias. Reported rates of PD in children (pre-adolescence) are fairly low (e.g. 0.3%). Among children, there is no notable gender difference in prevalence of PA, whereas beginning in adolescence both PA and PD are more widespread in females. Further exploration is needed to understand whether panic changes—either in phenomenology or prevalence—in older age.

9.4.2 Risk factors and correlates

Risk factors for PA and PD include female gender (in adolescence and beyond), family history of depression and anxiety disorders (including panic), traumatic, stressful, or adverse early life events (e.g. child abuse, parental separation), personality traits, prior onset of childhood anxiety disorder (e.g. social phobia, specific phobia, separation anxiety disorder (SAD),[42–44] and prior onset of PA (in the absence of PD).[45] For instance, a study using data from the Baltimore Epidemiologic Catchment Area study follow-up study showed that after excluding people with histories of PA, avoidant and dependent personality traits assessed in 1981 were associated with increased risk of first onset of PD during the follow-up period (re-interviewed again in 1993–1996).[46] Behavioural inhibition[47–53] and early anxious/shy behaviours[45] have consistently been associated longitudinally with vulnerability to PA/PD. Family history of panic is a strong risk factor, and evidence from family studies suggests that family history may be associated with earlier onset of panic.[54–57]

A study using the Early Developmental Stages of Psychopathology study (EDSP) found that panic during adolescence was associated with increased risk of any anxiety disorder (odds ratio (OR): 2.8; 1.3–5.9), social phobia (OR: 2.8; 1.0–7.6), specific phobia (OR: 2.3; (1.0–5.1), GAD (OR: 10.1; 2.7–36.8), any substance use disorder (OR: 2.1; 1.0–4.4), and any alcohol use disorder (OR: 2.4; 1.2–5.1)—after adjusting for comorbid disorders[58] and that more than half of those with PA early in adolescence have more than one mental disorder[58] by early adulthood. PA and PD have also been associated with suicide-related outcomes in numerous studies, after adjustment for other psychopathology.[59] Additionally, adults with PA/PD are more likely to be divorced, separated, or widowed, younger and of lower socio-economic status. PA and PD are also strongly associated with increased physical disease including cardiovascular disease,[60–62] gastrointestinal disease,[63,64] diabetes,[65,66] and especially respiratory disease including asthma and chronic obstructive pulmonary disease.[67–71]

9.4.3 Public health and treatment approaches

PD is thought to be among the most debilitating and costly mental disorders—both in terms of work loss[72,73] and direct and indirect health care costs.[74,75] Panic attacks have also been shown to be associated with similar levels of comorbidity, disability, and costs, and are far more prevalent than PD. Despite the debilitation and distress associated with PA and PD, evidence to date suggests that only a minority receives treatment for these problems.[76] Some data, however, suggest that treatment for panic is protective against subsequent development of depression.[38,77] Current treatments for panic including pharmacological intervention and/or CBT[78–81] (i.e. antidepressants) remain uncertain.[78] Further, psychopharmacological treatments are increasingly dispensed,[79] even those without demonstrated efficacy for treating panic disorder.[80] Yet, only a small percentage of mental health professionals are trained in CBT, which is considered the most effective non-pharmacological treatment for panic.[81] This confluence of circumstances suggests a substantial unmet need for treatment for PA/PD, which contributes to the degree to which PA/PD is a major public health problem.

9.5 Social phobia

Social phobia (SP) or social anxiety disorder is characterized by a marked and persistent fear of social or performance situations in which the person is exposed to unfamiliar people or to possible scrutiny by others.[82,83] SP is associated with substantial impairment and severe distress, affecting social and academic areas, as well as impaired subjective well-being.[84]

9.5.1 Prevalence, onset, and natural course

Lifetime prevalences for SP considerably vary between 1.4%[85] and 13.3%,[79] most likely due to methodological differences between the studies. Similarly diverging, 12-month rates are usually substantially lower than lifetime rates (range: 1.3%[86] to 8.4%[87]). Mean lifetime and 12-month rates are 6.7%[88] and 2–3%,[89] and the most recent estimation from the National Comorbidity Survey—Replication (NCS-R) in the USA yielded a lifetime rate of 9.1% in adolescents aged 13–18 years,[90,91] which is fairly consistent with an estimated cumulative incidence rate of 11% from the German prospective, longitudinal Early Developmental Stages of Psychopathology Study (EDSP) in representative samples of adolescents and young adults up to age 34 years.[92]

Studies generally concur that the risk of onset for SP is greatest early in life with peak incidence in childhood and adolescence, and declines substantially thereafter. Based on prospective–longitudinal data, first onset of SP occurs in childhood or early adolescence,[84,92,93] with rare onsets after the third decade of life (<5%[92]) and without additional incidence periods during the life span. Notably, findings from cross-sectional studies often point to an onset in late adolescence and adulthood,[94,95] characterizing SP as a stable and chronic condition with mean durations of 16.3 years[96] or longer.[84,94] These differences may be in part attributable to the frequent waxing and waning course of the disorder.[97,98] Both consistently meeting the full threshold diagnostic criteria and complete (spontaneous) remission of SP is rare, and remission rates are probably one of the lowest among all anxiety disorders.[94,99,100] There is substantial comorbidity of SP with other anxiety, affective, somatoform, and substance use disorders, with SP in many, but not all, cases being the primary disorder. Hence, assessment of SP is further challenged or 'covered' by symptoms of co-occurring disorders. Some evidence exists that comorbidity is higher in generalized than in non-generalized SP.[90,97]

9.5.2 Correlates and risk factors

From prevalence estimates it is known than women are much more often affected than men and that the risk for SP increases with age. Nonetheless, women and men follow similar incidence patterns and the reasons for the preponderance of females has not yet been fully understood.[101] SP is not consistently associated with poverty or socio-economic status,[102] urbanicity[103,104] or race/ethnicity.[105] Findings on lower socio-economic status in SP may also be interpreted as a consequence of SP, as affected individuals[106–109] have lower academic achievements and impaired work performance, which in turn may promote underemployment and lower household income and subsequently lower socio-economic status.[110,111] Other risk factors for social phobia may include social traumas, such as being bullied,[102] although these findings are mixed and may also be affected by memory bias. Since the high risk phase for SP onset is located in late childhood/early adolescence, familial risk factors such as parental psychopathology and unfavourable parental rearing styles are likely particularly important for targeted prevention and intervention.[112,113] SP runs in families[114–117] and is moderately heritable.[118,119]

9.5.3 Public health and treatment approaches

SP places a substantial strain upon the health care system,[120] with only few costs related to SP-specific treatment such as psychiatric and non-psychiatric care, hospitalization, and prescription drugs. Though effective treatment is available,[121] SP has the lowest treatment rates[122] among the anxiety or mood disorders, probably because primary care physicians or psychiatrists may not detect symptoms,[123,124] affected individuals are afraid to disclose an illness condition, or because of financial strains and uncertainty over where to seek help.[125,126] The low rate of treatment seeking/service use among those with SP is thus consistent with data suggesting that SP itself is a barrier to mental health service use by its very nature. Fewer than one in five (18.48% of adolescents with social phobia) reported any anxiety treatment contact; rates were slightly increased in those with generalized SP (23.7%).[127]

9.6 Obsessions, compulsions, and obsessive–compulsive disorder

9.6.1 Prevalence, onset, and natural course

Obsessive–compulsive disorder (OCD) is characterized by recurrent intrusive thoughts (obsessions) and repeated rituals or mental acts (compulsions). OCD is estimated to have a 12-month prevalence of 1.2% and a lifetime prevalence of 2.3% in the USA[19] with similar cross-national rates.[128,129] OCD is associated with significant comorbidity and morbidity, including distress, role impairment, and decreased quality of life;[130,131] indeed, in the World Health Organization burden of disease study, OCD is ranked highly in the list of the most disabling medical conditions.[132] Although prevalence is higher in females than males, persistence of OCD is not significantly associated with gender;[133] this is one of many findings suggesting that OCD is distinctive from other anxiety disorders.[134]

The mean age of onset of OCD is 19.5 years and the age-of-onset curves differ significantly for males and females.[133] The majority of early onset cases are made up of males, with nearly one-quarter of males having onset before age 10 years. Females, on the other hand, have a high slope of onset during adolescence in epidemiological data, and may have onset during pregnancy or the puerperium in clinical reports.[135,136] Early and later onset OCD may have different psychobiological underpinnings.[137,138]

There is a relative lack of longitudinal data on long-term outcomes of OCD. In the Harvard/Brown Anxiety Disorders Research Program, a prospective, naturalistic, longitudinal study, a 15-year report found that whereas many people recover from OCD, there are low rates of remission.[139] Similarly in one 40-year follow-up report from an OCD clinic, improvement was observed in 83% of patients, although most patients continued to have clinical or subclinical symptoms,[140] with early age of onset and low social functioning at baseline associated with worse outcome.

9.6.2 Correlates and risk factors

A range of sociodemographic variables (e.g. marital status, education, race, socio-economic status), environmental variables (e.g. seasonality of birth, birth order and family size, substance abuse, life events), and other variables (e.g. intelligence levels, psychiatric comorbidity) have been investigated to determine risk factors for OCD.[141] Few such variables have, however, consistently been replicated in the literature. Family history of OCD is one exception: accumulating evidence from family, twin, and genetic studies indicates that genetic factors contribute to the pathogenesis of OCD.[142,143] Nevertheless, considerable additional work with larger sample sizes and more sophisticated methods is needed in order to outline the precise genetic risk factors for OCD.

Obsessive–compulsive disorder is associated cross-sectionally with increased comorbidity and morbidity. In the NCS-R, while depression often began after OCD (45.6%), most comorbid impulse-control (92.8%) and substance use (58.9%) disorders began at an earlier age than OCD.[137] Clinical data reveal an association between Tourette disorder and OCD.[138] In both epidemiological and clinical data, evidence emerges for a subtype of OCD characterized by male gender, early onset, comorbid tics, and perhaps comorbid impulsive symptoms.[138] Further study of comorbidity in OCD may reveal additional insights into the heterogeneity of this disorder.[144] Finally, it is important to note the association between OCD and suicidality. In the British National Psychiatric Morbidity Survey of 2000, one-quarter of participants with OCD had previously attempted suicide.[145] Further work is needed to examine suicidal behaviour in obsessive–compulsive and related disorders.

9.6.3 Public health and treatment approaches

Although OCD has only recently received attention in population studies, and although obsessive–compulsive-related disorders remain very poorly studied in such work, there is growing evidence of the public health significance of these disorders. In the past few decades there have been accumulating data on the distinctive psychobiology of OCD, and the recognition of OCD and related disorders as a separate diagnostic grouping may lead to increased efforts to measure various kinds of obsessions and compulsions as cross-cutting dimensions in epidemiological studies of psychopathology. In the interim, there has been an interesting convergence between epidemiological data on early onset OCD in males and clinical data that tic-related early onset OCD is an important subtype that deserves tailored intervention. Furthermore there is growing evidence that, whereas OCD remains underdiagnosed and undertreated,[146,147] with intervention a substantial proportion of those with disorder can recover, if not remit.

9.7 Summary: life course approach—treatment and public health implications

A life course approach to understanding adult mental health problems is particularly pertinent in the case of anxiety disorders because diagnosis in adulthood is likely to have underpinnings and detectable harbingers much earlier in life. From a prevention and early intervention perspective, it has been thought that anxiety disorders are especially likely to be overlooked or not given sufficient attention by parents, caregivers, and teachers, compared with disruptive behaviour disorders. Children suffering with anxiety are often quiet and well-behaved; they do not make as much trouble in the classroom as youngsters with externalizing behaviours frequently do. However, the disorder is still associated with impairment and distress at the time, and there is substantial risk that even those children with subclinical anxiety (e.g. PA) will go on to develop full-blown mental disorders ($\rangle$50% met criteria for at least one DSM-IV disorder) by early adulthood.[58] As such, early intervention with anxiety—an area that has received little research attention compared with other mental disorders—may be conceptualized as a way to prevent future onset of anxiety disorders and potentially decrease the risk of developing other mental disorders as well.

A life course perspective may also be important in shedding light on the course of symptoms, on the development of comorbidity, and on the underlying mechanisms which are involved in onset and persistence of anxiety disorders. This perspective has proved key in understanding not only particular disorders (e.g. how PA eventually turn into PD, which in turn leads to PD with agoraphobia) but also the relationship between anxiety disorders and other conditions. A full understanding of the course and comorbidity of anxiety disorders may in turn be useful in identifying causal mechanisms that underlie these conditions. Such an understanding may ultimately inform diagnostic and treatment approaches.

References

1 Kessler RC, Berglund P, Demler O, Jin R, Merikangas KR, Walters EE. Lifetime prevalence and age-of-onset distributions of DSM-IV disorders in the National Comorbidity Survey Replication. *Arch Gen Psychiatry* 2005;**62**(6):593–602.

2 Barlow DH, Pincus DB, Heinrichs N, Choate ML. Anxiety disorders. In: Stricker G, Widiger TA, Weiner IB, editors. *Handbook of psychology: clinical psychology*. Volume 8. Hoboken, NJ: Wiley; 2003. pp. 119–147.

3 Otto MW, Pollack MH, Maki KM, et al. Childhood history of anxiety disorders among adults with social phobia: rates, correlates, and comparisons with patients with panic disorder. *Depress Anxiety* 2001;**14**(4):209–213.

4 Aschenbrand SG, Kendall PC, Webb A, Safford SM, Flannery-Schroeder E. Is childhood separation anxiety disorder a predictor of adult panic disorder and agoraphobia? A seven-year longitudinal study. *J Am Acad Child Adolesc Psychiatry* 2003;**42**(12):1478–1485.

5 King SM, Iacono WG, McGue M. Childhood externalizing and internalizing psychopathology in the prediction of early substance use. *Addiction* 2004;**99**(12):1548–1559.

6 **Ollendick TH, March JS, editors.** *Phobic and anxiety disorders: a clinician's guide to effective psychoso-cial and pharmacological interventions.* Oxford: Oxford University Press; 2004.

7 **Andrews G.** The epidemiology of anxiety disorders. *Curr Opin Psychiatry* 2002;**15**(2):129–130.

8 **Beesdo-Baum K, Knappe S.** Developmental epidemiology of anxiety disorders. *Child Adolesc Psychiatr Clin N Am* 2012;**21**(3):457–478.

9 **Kessler RC, Petukhova M, Sampson NA, Zaslavsky AM, Wittchen H-U.** Twelve-month and lifetime prevalence and lifetime morbid risk of anxiety and mood disorders in the US. *Int J Method Psychiatr Res* 2012;**21**(3):169–184.

10 **Beesdo K, Pine DS, Lieb R, Wittchen HU.** Incidence and risk patterns of anxiety and depressive disorders and categorization of Generalized Anxiety Disorder. *Arch Gen Psychiatry* 2010;**67**(1): 47–57.

11 **Emmelkamp PMG, Wittchen HU.** Specific phobias. In: Andrews G, Charney DS, Sirovatka PJ, Regier DA, editors. *Stress-induced and fear circuitry disorders. Refining the research Agenda for DSM-V.* Arlington, VA: APA; 2009. pp. 77–101.

12 **Curtis GC, Magee WJ, Eaton WW, Wittchen H-U, Kessler RC.** Specific fears and phobias: epidemiol-ogy and classification. *Br J Psychiatry* 1998;**173**:212–217.

13 **LeBeau RT, Glenn D, Liao B, et al.** Specific phobia: a review of DSM-IV specific phobia and prelimi-nary recommendations for DSM-V. *Depress Anxiety* 2010;**27**(2):148–167.

14 **Wittchen H-U, Lecrubier Y, Beesdo K, Nocon A.** Relationships among anxiety disorders: patterns and implications. In: Nutt DJ, Ballenger JC, editors. *Anxiety disorders.* Oxford: Blackwell; 2003. pp. 25–37.

15 **Shear MK, Bjelland I, Beesdo K, Gloster AT, Wittchen H-U.** Supplementary dimensional assessment in anxiety disorders. *Int J Method Psychiatr Res* 2007;**16**(Suppl 1):S52–S64.

16 **Kessler RC, Berglund P, Demler O, Jin R, Merikangas KR, Walters EE.** Lifetime prevalence and age-of-onset distributions of DSM-IV disorders in the national comorbidity survey replication. [Correction.] *Arch Gen Psychiatry* 2005;**62**(7):593–602.

17 **Kessler RC, Chiu WT, Demler O, Walters EE.** Prevalence, severity, and comorbidity of 12-month DSM-IV disorders in the National Comorbidity Survey Replication. *Arch Gen Psychiatry* 2005;**62**: 617–627.

18 **Bittner A, Egger HL, Erkanli A, Costello EJ, Foley DL, Angold A.** What do childhood anxiety disor-ders predict? *J Child Psychol Psychiatry* 2007;**48**(12):1174–1183.

19 **Romano E, Tremblay RE, Vitaro F, Zoccolillo M, Pagani L.** Prevalence of psychiatric diagnoses and the role of perceived impairment: findings from and adolescent community sample. *J Child Psychol Psychiatry* 2001;**42**(4):451–461.

20 **Merikangas KR, He JP, Burstein M, et al.** Lifetime Prevalence of Mental Disorders in U.S. Adolescents: Results from the National Comorbidity Survey Replication—Adolescent Supplement (NCS-A). *J Am Acad Child Adolesc Psychiatry* 2010;**49**(10):980–989.

21 **Kessler RC, Brandenburg N, Lane M, et al.** Rethinking the duration requirement for general-ized anxiety disorder: evidence from the National Comorbidity Survey Replication. *Psychol Med* 2005;**35**(7):1073–1082.

22 **Beesdo K.** *Wie entstehen Generalisierte Ängste? Eine prospektiv-longitudinale, klinisch–epidemiologische Studie bei Jugendlichen und jungen Erwachsenen.* [The development of Generalized Anxiety. A prospective-longitudinal, clinical–epidemiologic study among adolescents and young adults]. Dresden: TUDpress; 2006.

23 **Grant BF, Hasin DS, Stinson FS, et al.** Prevalence, correlates, co-morbidity, and comparative disability of DSM-IV generalized anxiety disorder in the USA: results from the National Epidemiologic Survey on alcohol and related conditions. *Psychol Med* 2005;**35**(12):1747–1759.

24 **Kessler RC, Andrade L, Bijl R, Offord D, Demler O, Stein DJ.** The effects of co-morbidity on the onset and persistence of generalized anxiety disorder in the ICPE surveys. *Psychol Med* 2002;**32**: 1213–1225.

25 **Kessler RC.** Evidence that generalized anxiety disorder is an independent disorder. In: Nutt DJ, Rickels K, Stein DJ, editors. *Generalized anxiety disorder: symptomatology, pathogenesis and management.* London: Martin Dunitz; 2002. pp. 3–10.

26 **Wittchen H-U, Kessler RC, Beesdo K, Krause P, Höfler M, Hoyer J.** Generalized anxiety and depression in primary care: prevalence, recognition and management. *J Clin Psychiatry* 2002;**63**(8): 24–34.

27 **Pine DS, Cohen P, Gurley D, Brook J, Ma YJ.** The risk for early-adulthood anxiety and depressive disorders in adolescents with anxiety and depressive disorders. *Arch Gen Psychiatry* 1998;**55**(1):56–64.

28 **Bittner A, Goodwin RD, Wittchen HU, Beesdo K, Hofler M, Lieb R.** What characteristics of primary anxiety disorders predict subsequent major depressive disorder? *J Clin Psychiatry* 2004;**65**(5):618–626.

29 **Copeland WE, Shanahan L, Costello J, Angold A.** Childhood and adolescent psychiatric disorders as predictors of young adult disorders. *Arch Gen Psychiatry* 2009;**66**(7):764–772.

30 **Kessler RC, Gruber M, Hettema JM, Hwang I, Sampson N, Yonkers KA.** Co-morbid major depression and generalized anxiety disorders in the National Comorbidity Survey follow-up. *Psychol Med* 2008;**38**(3):365–374.

31 **Stein DJ.** Comorbidity in generalized anxiety disorder: impact and implications. *J Clin Psychiatry* 2001;**62**(Suppl 11):29–34.

32 **Munk-Jorgenson P, Allgulander C, Dahl AA, et al.** Prevalence of Generalized Anxiety Disorder in General Practice in Denmark, Finland, Norway and Sweden. *Psychiatr Serv* 2006;**57**(12):1738–1744.

33 **Allgulander C.** Generalized anxiety disorder: between now and DSM-V. *Psychiatr Clin North Am* 2009;**32**:611–628.

34 **Hunot V, Churchill R, Silva de Lima M, Teixeira V.** Psychological therapies for generalised anxiety disorder. *Cochrane Database of Syst Rev* 20071:Art. No.: CD001848.

35 **Mitte K.** Meta-analysis of cognitive–behavioral treatments for generalized anxiety disorder: a comparison with pharmacotherapy. *Psychol Bull* 2005;**131**(5):785–795.

36 **Hoyer J, Beesdo K, Gloster AT, Höfler M, Runge J, Becker ES.** Worry exposure versus applied relaxation in the treatment of generalized anxiety disorder. *Psychother Psychosom* 2009;**78**:106–115.

37 **Hoyer J, Gloster AT.** Psychotherapy for generalized anxiety disorder: don't worry, it works! *Psychiatr Clin North Am* 2009;**32**:629–640.

38 **Goodwin RD, Gorman JM.** Psychopharmacologic treatment of generalized anxiety disorder and the risk of major depression. *Am J Psychiatry* 2002;**159**(11):1935–1937.

39 **Kessler RC, Avenevoli S, Costello EJ, et al.** Prevalence, persistence, and sociodemographic correlates of DSM-IV Disorders in the National Comorbidity Survey Replication Adolescent Supplement. *Arch Gen Psychiatry* 2012;**69**(4):372–380.

40 **Canino G, Shrout PE, Rubio-Stipec M, et al.** The DSM-IV rates of child and adolescent disorders in Puerto Rico: prevalence, correlates, service use, and the effects of impairment. *Arch Gen Psychiatry* 2004;**61**(1):85–93.

41 **Weissman MM, Bland RC, Canino GJ, et al.** The cross-national epidemiology of panic disorder. *Arch Gen Psychiatry* 1997;**54**(4):305–309.

42 **Bruckl TM, Wittchen HU, Hofler M, Pfister H, Schneider S, Lieb R.** Childhood separation anxiety and the risk of subsequent psychopathology: results from a community study. *Psychother Psychosom* 2007;**76**(1):47–56.

43 **Lewinsohn PM, Holm-Denoma JM, Small JW, Seeley JR, Joiner Jr TE.** Separation anxiety disorder in childhood as a risk factor for future mental illness. *J Am Acad Child Adolesc Psychiatry* 2008;**47**(5): 548–555.

44 **Biederman J, Petty CR, Hirshfeld-Becker DR, et al.** Developmental trajectories of anxiety disorders in offspring at high risk for panic disorder and major depression. *Psychiatry Res* 2007;**153**(3):245–252.

45 **Goodwin RD, Fergusson DM, Horwood LJ.** Early anxious/withdrawn behaviours predict later internalising disorders. *J Child Psychol Psychiatry* 2004;**45**(4):874–883.

46 Bienvenu OJ, Stein MB, Samuels JF, Onyike CU, Eaton WW, Nestadt G. Personality disorder traits as predictors of subsequent first-onset panic disorder or agoraphobia. *Compr Psychiatry* 2009;**50**(3): 209–214.

47 Kagan J, Snidman N. Infant predictors of inhibited and uninhibited profiles. *Psychol Sci* 1991;**2**(1): 40–44.

48 Biederman J, Rosenbaum JF, Hirshfeld DR, et al. Psychiatric correlates of behavioral inhibition in young children of parents with and without psychiatric disorders. *Arch Gen Psychiatry* 1990;**47**(1): 21–26.

49 Hirshfeld DR, Rosenbaum JF, Biederman J, et al. Stable behavioral inhibition and its association with anxiety disorder. *J Am Acad Child Adolesc Psychiatry* 1992;**31**(1):103–111.

50 Biederman J, Rosenbaum JF, Bolduc-Murphy EA, et al. A 3-year follow-up of children with and without behavioral inhibition. *J Am Acad Child Adolesc Psychiatry* 1993;**32**(4):814–821.

51 Kagan J, Snidman N. Early childhood predictors of adult anxiety disorders. *Biol Psychiatry* 1999;**46**(11):1536–1541.

52 Rosenbaum JF, Biederman J, Hirshfeld DR, et al. Further evidence of an association between behavioral inhibition and anxiety disorders: results from a family study of children from a non-clinical sample. *J Psychiatr Res* 1991;**25**(1–2):49–65.

53 Rosenbaum JF, Biederman J, Hirshfeld DR, et al. Behavioral inhibition in children: a possible precursor to panic disorder or social phobia. *J Clin Psychiatry* 1991;**52**(Suppl):5–9.

54 Goldstein RB, Wickramaratne PJ, Horwath E, Weissman MM. Familial aggregation and phenomenology of 'early'-onset (at or before age 20 years) panic disorder. *Arch Gen Psychiatry* 1997;**54**(3): 271–278.

55 Biederman J, Rosenbaum JF, Bolduc EA, Faraone SV, Hirshfeld DR. A high risk study of young children of parents with panic disorder and agoraphobia with and without comorbid major depression. *Psychiatry Res* 1991;**37**(3):333–348.

56 Biederman J, Faraone SV, Hirshfeld-Becker DR, Friedman D, Robin JA, Rosenbaum JF. Patterns of psychopathology and dysfunction in high-risk children of parents with panic disorder and major depression. *Am J Psychiatry* 2001;**158**(1):49–57.

57 Weissman MM, Leckman JF, Merikangas KR, Gammon GD, Prusoff BA. Depression and anxiety disorders in parents and children: results from the Yale Family Study. *Arch Gen Psychiatry* 1984;**41**(9):845–852.

58 Goodwin RD, Lieb R, Hoefler M, et al. Panic attack as a risk factor for severe psychopathology. *Am J Psychiatry* 2004;**161**(12):2207–2214.

59 Sareen J, Cox BJ, Afifi TO, et al. Anxiety disorders and risk for suicidal ideation and suicide attempts: a population-based longitudinal study of adults. *Arch Gen Psychiatry* 2005;**62**(11):1249–1257.

60 Sardinha A, Araujo CG, Soares-Filho GL, Nardi AE. Anxiety, panic disorder and coronary artery disease: issues concerning physical exercise and cognitive behavioral therapy. *Expert Rev Cardiovasc Ther* 2011;**9**(2):165–175.

61 Goodwin RD, Davidson KW, Keyes K. Mental disorders and cardiovascular disease among adults in the United States. *J Psychiatr Res* 2009;**43**(3):239–246.

62 Vural M, Acer M, Akbas B. The scores of Hamilton depression, anxiety, and panic agoraphobia rating scales in patients with acute coronary syndrome. *Anadolu kardiyoloji dergisi* (Anatolian Journal of Cardiology) 2008;**8**(1):43–47.

63 Gros DF, Antony MM, McCabe RE, Lydiard RB. A preliminary investigation of the effects of cognitive behavioral therapy for panic disorder on gastrointestinal distress in patients with comorbid panic disorder and irritable bowel syndrome. *Depress Anxiety* 2011;**28**(11):1027–1033.

64 Logue MW, Bauver SR, Kremen WS, et al. Evidence of overlapping genetic diathesis of panic attacks and gastrointestinal disorders in a sample of male twin pairs. *Twin Res Hum Genet* 2011;**14**(1):16–24.

65 de Ornelas Maia AC, Braga AD, Brouwers A, Nardi AE, de Oliveira ESAC. Prevalence of psychiatric disorders in patients with diabetes types 1 and 2. *Compr Psychiatry* 2012;**53**(8):1169–1173.

66 Lin EH, Korff MV, Alonso J, et al. Mental disorders among persons with diabetes—results from the World Mental Health Surveys. *J Psychosom Res* 2008;**65**(6):571–580.

67 Lydiard RB. Increased prevalence of functional gastrointestinal disorders in panic disorder: clinical and theoretical implications. *CNS Spectrums* 2005;**10**(11):899–908.

68 Slaughter JR, Jain A, Holmes S, Reid JC, Bobo W, Sherrod NB. Panic disorder in hospitalized cancer patients. *Psychooncology* 2000;**9**(3):253–258.

69 Perna G, Bertani A, Politi E, Colombo G, Bellodi L. Asthma and panic attacks. *Biol Psychiatry* 1997;**42**(7):625–630.

70 Goodwin RD, Pine DS, Hoven CW. Asthma and panic attacks among youth in the community. *J Asthma* 2003;**40**(2):139–145.

71 Porzelius J, Vest M, Nochomovitz M. Respiratory function, cognitions, and panic in chronic obstructive pulmonary patients. *Behav Res Ther* 1992;**30**(1):75–77.

72 de Graaf R, Tuithof M, van Dorsselaer S, Ten Have M. Comparing the effects on work performance of mental and physical disorders. *Soc Psychiatry Psychiatr Epidemiol* 2012;**47**(11):1873–1883.

73 Smit F, Cuijpers P, Oostenbrink J, Batelaan N, de Graaf R, Beekman A. Costs of nine common mental disorders: implications for curative and preventive psychiatry. *J Mental Health Policy Econ* 2006;**9**(4):193–200.

74 Batelaan N, Smit F, de Graaf R, van Balkom A, Vollebergh W, Beekman A. Economic costs of full-blown and subthreshold panic disorder. *J Affect Disorder* 2007;**104**(1–3):127–136.

75 Hu TW. Perspectives: an international review of the national cost estimates of mental illness, 1990–2003. *J Mental Health Policy Econ* 2006;**9**(1):3–13.

76 Andrews G, Henderson S, Hall W. Prevalence, comorbidity, disability and service utilisation. Overview of the Australian National Mental Health Survey. *Br J Psychiatry* 2001;**178**:145–153.

77 Goodwin R, Olfson M. Treatment of panic attack and risk of major depressive disorder in the community. *Am J Psychiatry* 2001;**158**(7):1146–1148.

78 Donovan MR, Glue P, Kolluri S, Emir B. Comparative efficacy of antidepressants in preventing relapse in anxiety disorders—a meta-analysis. *J Affect Disorders* 2010;**123**(1–3):9–16.

79 Kessler RC, Demler O, Frank RG, et al. Prevalence and treatment of mental disorders, 1990 to 2003. *N Engl J Med* 2005;**352**(24):2515–2523.

80 Comer JS, Mojtabai R, Olfson M. National trends in the antipsychotic treatment of psychiatric outpatients with anxiety disorders. *Am J Psychiatry* 2011;**168**(10):1057–1065.

81 Ost LG. Cognitive behavior therapy for anxiety disorders: 40 years of progress. *Nord J Psychiatry* 2008;**62**(Suppl 47):5–10.

82 American Psychiatric Association. *Diagnostic and statistical manual of mental disorders.* 4th ed. Washington DC: APA; 1994.

83 American Psychiatric Association. *Diagnostic and statistical manual of mental disorders. Text revision.* 4th ed. (DSM-IV-TR). Washingston, DC: APA; 2000.

84 Wittchen HU, Fehm L. Epidemiology and natural course of social fears and social phobia. *Acta Psychiatr Scand Suppl* 2003(**417**):4–18.

85 Lewinsohn PM, Hops H, Roberts RE, Seeley JR, Andrews JA. Adolescent psychopathology: I. Prevalence and incidence of depression and other DSM-III-R disorders in high school students. *J Abnorm Psychol* 1993;**102**(1):133–144.

86 Fergusson DM, Horwood LJ, Lynskey MT. Prevalence and comorbidity of DSM-III-R diagnoses in a birth cohort of 15 year olds. *J Am Acad Child Adolesc Psychiatry* 1993;**32**(6):1127–1134.

87 Newman DL, Moffitt TE, Caspi A, Magdol L, Silva PA, Stanton WR. Psychiatric disorder in a birth cohort of young adults: prevalence, comorbidity, clinical significance, and new case incidence from ages 11 to 21. *J Consult Clin Psychol* 1996;**64**(3):552–562.

88 **Fehm L, Pelissolo A, Furmark T, Wittchen HU**. Size and burden of social phobia in Europe. *Eur Neuropsychopharmacol* 2005;**15**(4):453–462.

89 **Lampe L, Slade T, Issakidis C, Andrews G**. Social phobia in the Australian National Survey of Mental Health and Well-Being (NSMHWB). *Psychol Med* 2003;**33**:637–646.

90 **Burstein M, He JP, Kattan G, Albano AM, Avenevoli S, Merikangas KR**. Social phobia and subtypes in the national comorbidity survey-adolescent supplement: prevalence, correlates, and comorbidity. *J Am Acad Child Adolesc Psychiatry* 2011;**50**(9):870–880.

91 **Merikangas KR, He JP, Burstein M, et al**. Lifetime prevalence of mental disorders in U.S. adolescents: results from the National Comorbidity Survey Replication—Adolescent Supplement (NCS-A). *J Am Acad Child Adolesc Psychiatry* 2010;**49**(10):980–989.

92 **Beesdo K, Bittner A, Pine DS, et al**. Incidence of social anxiety disorder and the consistent risk for secondary depression in the first three decades of life. *Arch Gen Psychiatry* 2007;**64**(8):903–912.

93 **Magee WJ, Eaton WW, Wittchen HU, McGonagle KA, Kessler RC**. Agoraphobia, simple phobia, and social phobia in the National Comorbidity Survey. *Arch Gen Psychiatry* 1996;**53**(2):159–168.

94 **Keller MB**. Social anxiety disorder clinical course and outcome: Review of Harvard/Brown Anxiety Research Project (HARP) findings. *J Clin Psychiatry* 2006;**67**(Suppl 12):14–19.

95 **Wittchen HU, Fehm L**. Epidemiology, patterns of comorbidity, and associated disabilities of social phobia. *Psychiatr Clin North Am* 2001;**24**(4):617–641.

96 **Grant BF, Hasin DS, Blanco C, et al**. The epidemiology of social anxiety disorder in the United States: Results from the National Epidemiologic Survey on Alcohol and Related Conditions. *J Clin Psychiatry* 2005;**66**(11):1351–1361.

97 **Wittchen HU, Stein MB, Kessler RC**. Social fears and social phobia in a community sample of adolescents and young adults: prevalence, risk factors and co-morbidity. *Psychol Med* 1999;**29**(2):309–323.

98 **Merikangas KR, Avenevoli S, Acharyya S, Zhang H, Angst J**. The spectrum of social phobia in the Zurich cohort study of young adults. *Biol Psychiatry* 2002;**51**(1):81–91.

99 **Becker ES, Türke V, Neumer S, Soeder U, Krause P, Margraf J**. Incidence and prevalence rates of mental disorders in a community sample of young women: results of the "Dresden Study". In: Manz R, Kirch W, editors. *Public health research and practice: report of the Public Health Reserach Association Saxony*. Volume II. Regensburg: S. Roederer; 2000. pp. 259–291.

100 **Essau CA, Conradt J, Petermann F**. Course and outcome of anxiety disorders in adolescents. *J Anxiety Disord* 2002;**16**(1):67–81.

101 **Craske MG**. *Origins of phobias and anxiety disorders: why more women than men?* Oxford: Elsevier; 2003.

102 **Ranta K, Kaltiala-Heino R, Pelkonen M, Marttunen M**. Associations between peer victimization, self-reported depression and social phobia among adolescents: the role of comorbidity. *J Adolesc* 2009;**32**(1):77–93.

103 **de Graaf R, Bijl RV, Smit F, Vollebergh WA, Spijker J**. Risk factors for 12-month comorbidity of mood, anxiety, and substance use disorders: findings from the Netherlands Mental Health Survey and Incidence Study. *Am J Psychiatry* 2002;**159**(4):620–629.

104 **Hybels CF, Blazer DG, Kaplan BH**. Social and personal resources and the prevalence of phobic disorder in a community population. *Psychol Med* 2000;**30**(3):705–716.

105 **Bourdon KH, Boyd JH, Rae DS, Burns BJ, Thompson JW, Locke BZ**. Gender differences in phobias: results of the ECA community survey. *J Anxiety Disorder* 1988;**2**:227–241.

106 **Lepine JP**. The epidemiology of anxiety disorders: prevalence and societal costs. *J Clin Psychiatry* 2002;**63**(Suppl 14):4–8.

107 **Acarturk C, Smit F, de Graaf R, van Straten A, Ten Have M, Cuijpers P**. Economic costs of social phobia: a population-based study. *J Affect Disorders* 2009;**115**(3):421–429.

108 **Katzelnick DJ, Kobak KA, DeLeire T, et al**. Impact of generalized social anxiety disorder in managed care. *Am J Psychiatry* 2001;**158**(12):1999–2007.

109 Wittchen HU, Beloch E. The impact of social phobia on quality of life. *Int Clin Psychopharmacol* 1996;**11**(Suppl 3):15–23.

110 Davidson JR, Hughes DL, George LK, Blazer DG. The epidemiology of social phobia: findings from the Duke Epidemiological Catchment Area Study. *Psychol Med* 1993;**23**(3):709–718.

111 Leon AC, Portera L, Weissman MM. The social costs of anxiety disorders. *Br J Psychiatry Suppl* 1995(27):19–22.

112 Knappe S, Beesdo-Baum K, Wittchen HU. Familial risk factors in social anxiety disorder: calling for a family-oriented approach for targeted prevention and early intervention. *Eur Child Adolesc Psychiatry* 2010;**19**(12):857–871.

113 Murray L, de Rosnay M, Pearson J, et al. Intergenerational transmission of social anxiety: the role of social referencing processes in infancy. *Child Dev* 2008;**79**(4):1049–1064.

114 Fyer AJ. Heritability of social anxiety: a brief review. *J Clin Psychiatry* 1993;**54** Suppl:10–12.

115 Knappe S, Beesdo K, Fehm L, Hofler M, Lieb R, Wittchen HU. Do parental psychopathology and unfavorable family environment predict the persistence of social phobia? *J Anxiety Disord* 2009;**23**(7):986–994.

116 Lieb R, Wittchen HU, Hofler M, Fuetsch M, Stein MB, Merikangas KR. Parental psychopathology, parenting styles, and the risk of social phobia in offspring: a prospective-longitudinal community study. *Arch Gen Psychiatry* 2000;**57**(9):859–866.

117 Merikangas KR, Lieb R, Wittchen HU, Avenevoli S. Family and high-risk studies of social anxiety disorder. *Acta Psychiatr Scand Suppl* 2003(**417**):28–37.

118 Kendler KS, Myers J, Prescott CA. The etiology of phobias: an evaluation of the stress–diathesis model. *Arch Gen Psychiatry* 2002;**59**(3):242–248.

119 Kendler KS, Myers J, Prescott CA, Neale MC. The genetic epidemiology of irrational fears and phobias in men. *Arch Gen Psychiatry* 2001;**58**(3):257–265.

120 Alonso J, Angermeyer MC, Bernert S, et al. Disability and quality of life impact of mental disorders in Europe: results from the European Study of the Epidemiology of Mental Disorders (ESEMeD) project. *Acta Psychiatr Scand Suppl* 2004;(420):38–46.

121 Acarturk C, Cuijpers P, van Straten A, de Graaf R. Psychological treatment of social anxiety disorder: a meta-analysis. *Psychol Med* 2009;**39**(2):241–254.

122 Issakidis C, Andrews G. Service utilisation for anxiety in an Australian community sample. *Soc Psychiatry Psychiatr Epidemiol* 2002;**37**(4):153–163.

123 Dalrymple KL, Zimmerman M. Screening for social fears and social anxiety disorder in psychiatric outpatients. *Compr Psychiatry* 2008;**49**(4):399–406.

124 Dalrymple KL, Zimmerman M. Treatment-seeking for social anxiety disorder in a general outpatient psychiatry setting. *Psychiatry Res* 2011;**187**(3):375–381.

125 Goodwin RD, Fitzgibbon ML. Social anxiety as a barrier to treatment for eating disorders. *Int J Eat Disord* 2002;**32**(1):103–106.

126 Olfson M, Guardino M, Struening E, Schneier FR, Hellman F, Klein DF. Barriers to the treatment of social anxiety. *Am J Psychiatry* 2000;**157**(4):521–527.

127 Merikangas KR, He JP, Burstein M, et al. Service utilization for lifetime mental disorders in U.S. adolescents: results of the National Comorbidity Survey—Adolescent Supplement (NCS-A). *J Am Acad Child Adolesc Psychiatry* 2011;**50**(1):32–45.

128 Ruscio AM, Stein DJ, Chiu WT, Kessler RC. The epidemiology of obsessive–compulsive disorder in the National Comorbidity Survey Replication. *Mol Psychiatry* 2010;**15**(1):53–63.

129 Fontenelle LF, Mendlowicz MV, Versiani M. The descriptive epidemiology of obsessive–compulsive disorder. *Prog Neuropsychopharmacol Biol Psychiatry* 2006;**30**(3):327–337.

130 Weissman MM, Bland RC, Canino GJ, et al. The cross national epidemiology of obsessive compulsive disorder. The Cross National Collaborative Group. *J Clin Psychiatry* 1994;(**55** Suppl):5–10.

131 **Mogotsi M, Kaminer D, Stein DJ.** Quality of life in the anxiety disorders. *Harv Rev Psychiatry* 2000;8(6):273–282.

132 **Stein D, Allen A, Bobes J, et al.** Quality of life in obsessive–compulsive disorder. *CNS Spectr* 2000;5(Suppl 4):37–39.

133 **Murray C, Lopez A.** *Global burden of disease: a comprehensive assessment of mortality and morbidity from diseases, injuries and risk factors in 1990 and projected to 2020.* Volume I. Boston: Harvard School of Public Health; 1996.

134 **Stein DJ, Fineberg NA, Bienvenu OJ, et al.** Should OCD be classified as an anxiety disorder in DSM-V? *Depress Anxiety* 2010;27(6):495–506.

135 **McGuinness M, Blissett J, Jones C.** OCD in the perinatal period: is postpartum OCD (ppOCD) a distinct subtype? A review of the literature. *Behav Cogn Psychother* 2011;39(3):285–310.

136 **Williams KE, Koran LM.** Obsessive-compulsive disorder in pregnancy, the puerperium, and the premenstruum. *J Clin Psychiatry* 1997;58(7):330–334; quiz 335–336.

137 **Hemmings SM, Kinnear CJ, Lochner C, et al.** Early- versus late-onset obsessive–compulsive disorder: investigating genetic and clinical correlates. *Psychiatry Res* 2004;128(2):175–182.

138 **Leckman JF, Denys D, Simpson HB, et al.** Obsessive–compulsive disorder: a review of the diagnostic criteria and possible subtypes and dimensional specifiers for DSM-V. *Depress Anxiety* 2010;27(6): 507–527.

139 **Marcks BA, Weisberg RB, Dyck I, Keller MB.** Longitudinal course of obsessive–compulsive disorder in patients with anxiety disorders: a 15-year prospective follow-up study. *Compr Psychiatry* 2011;52(6):670–677.

140 **Skoog G, Skoog I.** A 40-year follow-up of patients with obsessive–compulsive disorder [see comments]. *Arch Gen Psychiatry* 1999;56(2):121–127.

141 **Fontenelle LF, Hasler G.** The analytical epidemiology of obsessive–compulsive disorder: risk factors and correlates. *Prog Neuropsychopharmacol Biol Psychiatry* 2008;32(1):1–15.

142 **Hemmings SM, Stein DJ.** The current status of association studies in obsessive–compulsive disorder. *Psychiatr Clin North Am* 2006;29(2):411–444.

143 **Pauls DL.** The genetics of obsessive–compulsive disorder: a review. *Dialogues Clin Neurosci* 2010;12(2):149–163.

144 **Lochner C, Hemmings SM, Kinnear CJ, et al.** Cluster analysis of obsessive–compulsive spectrum disorders in patients with obsessive–compulsive disorder: clinical and genetic correlates. *Compr Psychiatry* 2005;46(1):14–19.

145 **Torres AR, Prince MJ, Bebbington PE, et al.** Obsessive–compulsive disorder: prevalence, comorbidity, impact, and help-seeking in the British National Psychiatric Morbidity Survey of 2000. *Am J Psychiatry* 2006;163(11):1978–1985.

146 **Blanco C, Olfson M, Stein DJ, Simpson HB, Gameroff MJ, Narrow WH.** Treatment of obsessive–compulsive disorder by U.S. psychiatrists. *J Clin Psychiatry* 2006;67(6):946–951.

147 **Hollander E, Stein D, Broatch J, Himelein C, Rowland C.** A pharmacoeconomic and quality of life study of obsessive–compulsive disorder. *CNS Spectr* 1997;2:16–25.

Chapter 10

Epidemiology of post-traumatic stress disorder

Nicole R. Nugent, Ruth Brown, Kelcey Stratton, and Ananda B. Amstadter

10.1 Introduction

This chapter uses a life course approach to summarize the distribution and patterns of exposure to traumatic events and development of post-traumatic stress disorder (PTSD). First, the literature is summarized in respect of samples from the USA, starting with childhood/adolescence and ending with older age. Next, consistent with the importance of considering culture and context, as well as developmental course processes, patterns of PTSD in other countries are addressed. The chapter concludes with a discussion of the important contextual role of type of trauma exposure (e.g. combat, disasters).

10.2 Traumatic stress and PTSD across the life course

10.2.1 Childhood/adolescence

Few general population studies have examined the prevalence of trauma exposure and PTSD among youth, particularly young children. Three nationally representative studies suggest that the lifetime prevalence of DSM-IV-defined PTSD among children and adolescents ranges from 5% to 7% and that 6-month prevalence ranges from 3.7% to 6.3%.[1-3] Consistent sex differences have supported a higher prevalence in girls (6.3–8.0%) compared with boys (2.3–3.7%).[2,3] By contrast with national samples, The Great Smoky Mountains Study of Youth[4] yielded a notably low 3-month prevalence of 0.02% among 1,015 youth aged 9–13 years according to DSM-III-R PTSD criteria. However, this study used a two-stage screening based on externalizing behaviour, an approach that may underrepresent overall prevalence.

Although the pattern of trauma and victimization is complex, with rates of specific types of victimization differing as a function of gender and developmental stage, adolescence appears to be a time of increased risk for exposure to a range of traumatic events.[5] Whereas some studies suggest that trauma-exposed children are more vulnerable to the effects of trauma than adults,[6] others report lower conditional risk.[7-9] The National Comorbidity Survey Replication—Adolescent Supplement2 found that the prevalence of PTSD increased across three age groups (13–14 years: 3.7%; 15–16 years: 5.1%; 17–18 years: 7.0%), possibly reflecting age-related increases in victimization likelihood. Youth who experience multiple traumas, violent and sexual traumas, anxiety disorders, and family adversity were also at elevated risk for PTSD symptoms.[3] In addition to PTSD, trauma exposure in childhood is associated with anxiety, depression, substance use, eating disorders, and increased risk of later trauma.[3]

An important consideration in research exploring child risk for trauma and PTSD is evidence of intergenerational transmission of trauma.[10] This transmission of risk for both trauma exposure and subsequent PTSD may operate via a variety of mechanisms (e.g. genetic transmission, shared environment such as socio-economic context, influences of past victimization on parenting behaviours, and temperament).

Child-specific factors may also affect PTSD prevalence estimates.[11] For example, most studies have relied solely on youth self-report of trauma and symptoms. Young children may have difficulty identifying and reporting on their own emotional states or behavioural patterns, especially with regard to child-specific PTSD symptoms (e.g. disorganized behaviour, repetitive trauma-related play).[12] These differences make comparison of rates of PTSD between youth and adults difficult to interpret. Indeed, studies have found that DSM-IV criteria may underdiagnose PTSD in very young children and have recommended reducing the number of symptoms required for diagnosis.[13]

10.2.2 Emerging adulthood

Although no general population studies have been conducted on PTSD specifically in emerging adults, Breslau et al. have conducted two regional studies in suburban[14] and urban-dwelling[15] samples. The period from late adolescence to emerging adulthood was found to be a time of increased risk for exposure to traumas, with lifetime prevalence of PTSD ranging from 7.1% to 9.2%.[5,15] Relative to other trauma types, victims of assaultive violence evidenced the highest probability for developing PTSD. This effect was strongest for women, particularly those who experienced sexual assault and rape. Social, economic, and environmental factors may also play a role in risk for trauma, as young males in urban areas were at significantly higher risk for exposure to assaultive violence than the suburban sample.[14,15]

10.2.3 Adulthood

The majority of epidemiological studies have examined PTSD prevalence in adults aged ≥18 years. The St Louis and North Carolina sites of the Epidemiologic Catchment Area Survey (ECA)[16–18] were the earliest population-based surveys to assess PTSD. These studies found lifetime prevalence rates around 1% according to DSM-III criteria for PTSD. By contrast, the National Comorbidity Survey (NCS),[19] the first nationally representative epidemiological study, found a lifetime DSM-III-R prevalence rate of 7.8%. Differences in population, sampling, assessment, and change in diagnostic criteria from DSM-III to DSM-III-R complicate interpretation of differences in prevalence. However, a subsequent all-female study (National Women's Study),[20] using the DSM-III-R, found a lifetime prevalence of 12.3%.

Two national epidemiological studies using the DSM-IV resulted in estimates similar to those based on the DSM-III-R. The replication of the NCS[21] reported a lifetime prevalence of 6.8% (9.7% of women, 3.6% of men) following DSM-IV criteria. The largest population-based sample to include assessment of PTSD to date comes from the second wave of the National Epidemiologic Survey on Alcohol and Alcoholism,[22] which reported a lifetime prevalence of 6.4%.

10.2.4 Older adulthood

Many large-scale epidemiological studies have either excluded older adults from the sample or have not separately examined the prevalence of PTSD in older adults. The NCS-R found significantly lower rates of 12-month PTSD for people aged ≥65 years (65–74 years: 0.6%; ≥75 years: 0.2%) compared with people aged <64 years.[23] Lifetime PTSD rates were similarly lower in older participants (65–74 years: 2.1%; ≥75 years: 1.1%). Consistent with other research, women aged ≥65 years exhibited higher rates of PTSD (2.5%) compared with men (0.4%).[23] Although more empirical investigation is needed, several factors could account for the low rates including matu-rational and/or cohort differences in coping with adversity, mental-health-related differences in health/survival, and underreporting due to loss of memory or stigma.

10.2.5 Summary of PTSD across the life course

Although diagnostic criteria, sampling, and assessment strategies have varied across studies, life-time prevalence estimates across studies using DSM-III-R and later criteria have yielded similar point estimates with notable patterns emerging from the studies. First, risk for trauma exposure increases with age, with highest risk evident in late adolescence/emerging adulthood.[5,15,19] Rates of lifetime PTSD show similar increases across childhood/adolescence (5–7%), emerging adult-hood (7–9%), and adulthood (6–12%). Relatedly, rates may be impacted by evidence that early trauma may confer risk for subsequent revictimization. Nationally representative surveys,[24] as well as meta-analytic studies,[25] support increased PTSD risk among individuals with prior trauma history, with evidence of a dose–response relationship between number of prior traumas and PTSD symptom severity.[26] The effect of cumulative trauma exposure may be particularly robust in children and adolescents.[27] Second, although men are more likely to experience trauma, women are twice as likely to experience PTSD.[14,19,22] Third, those who experience interpersonal and/or assaultive violence are more likely to experience PTSD than other types of trauma.[3,20]

10.3 Post-traumatic stress in non-US countries

Although we have so far focused on the US epidemiology, research conducted in other countries can help to inform our understanding of the roles of cultural and contextual factors.

10.3.1 PTSD in high income countries

Studies conducted in other high income nations have generally reported lower prevalence esti-mates of both trauma and PTSD compared to US studies. The European Study of Epidemiology of Mental Disorders[28] surveyed adults from Spain, Italy, Germany, The Netherlands, Belgium, and France, and found that 63.6% of respondents endorsed exposure to at least one traumatic event.[28] Although lifetime prevalence of PTSD was not determined, past-year prevalence was 1.1% (0.5% of men, 1.7% of women), with some variability by country, ranging from 0.6% in Spain to 2.6% in The Netherlands. Studies focused on specific regions offer further estimates of PTSD in Western Europe. For example, in a study of young adults in Munich, 26% of men and 17.7% of women reported exposure to a trauma,[9] and lifetime PTSD was reported by <1% of men and 2.2% of women. Consistent with US data, estimates from a representative sample in The Netherlands found that 80.7% of the sample had a lifetime history of trauma exposure, with a lifetime PTSD prevalence of 7.4% and a past-year prevalence of 3.3%.[29]

In a study of Australian adults, 64.5% of men and 49.5% of women reported lifetime trauma exposure, and 12-month prevalence of PTSD was 1.3%.[30] Interestingly, this study did not repli-cate the sex difference reported in many other studies. By contrast, results from a random sample of adults in Winnipeg, Canada, estimated that 2.7% of women and 1.2% of men met criteria for PTSD in the past month.[31]

Koenen et al.[32] conducted one of the few longitudinal cohort studies, in Dunedin, New Zealand, to explore the life course effects of childhood risk factors on lifetime trauma and PTSD assessed at age 26 years. Childhood externalizing, maternal distress, and loss of a parent were associated with increased risk for both trauma exposure and PTSD in adulthood. Risk for PTSD at 26 years of age was also associated with low IQ and with a cumulative burden of chronic environmental adversity. Furthermore, early childhood factors of low IQ, antisocial behaviour, and poverty predicted PTSD secondary to traumas occurring in adulthood.

10.3.2 Post-traumatic stress in low income countries

There are few epidemiological studies of mental health in low income countries. An epidemiological study in Mexico found that lifetime prevalence of trauma exposure and PTSD was 76% and 11.2%, respectively.[33] Risk for PTSD was highest among persons of lower socio-economic status and women. By contrast, the rate of trauma exposure and PTSD was much lower in Chile, in which 39.7% of the population reported exposure to a traumatic event, and the lifetime prevalence of PTSD was 4.4% (men: 2.5%; women: 6.2%;).[34] In a national epidemiological study in Lebanon, 12-month prevalence of PTSD was 2.0%.[35] Evidence from these studies supports the general pattern of PTSD prevalence determined elsewhere; namely, PTSD risk is increased among women, individuals of lower socio-economic status, and survivors of assaultive violence.

10.4 Post-traumatic stress in special populations

There is ample evidence that the risk for exposure to certain types of trauma varies across the life course and that type of trauma is related to differential risk for PTSD.[19,20,22,30] Thus when considering patterns of PTSD prevalence, it can be helpful to research communities of individuals who have experienced a common trauma.

10.4.1 Political conflict and terrorism

Civilian experiences with political conflict and terrorism, civil unrest, and mass violence can have lasting psychological effects. An epidemiological survey in Algeria, Cambodia, Ethiopia, and Gaza assessed exposure to conflict-related traumas and rates of mental health disorders in a community sample.[36] Exposure to armed conflict-related violence was high, ranging from 59.3% in Gaza to 91.9% in Algeria. PTSD was the most common mental health disorder in conflict-exposed individuals and lifetime rates of PTSD were highest in Algeria (37.4%) and Cambodia (28.4%), where exposure to violence was greatest.[36]

In the USA, mass violence and terrorism are also shown to have a lasting impact. Among adults living in Manhattan during the 11 September 2001 terrorist attacks, 7.5% of current PTSD is related to the attacks.[37] Six months after the 1995 bombing of the Federal Building in Oklahoma City, the rate of disaster-related PTSD was 34.3%.[38] Like natural disasters, political conflicts and terrorism are associated with a significant public health burden.

10.4.2 Natural disasters

Epidemiological studies of post-disaster distress have shown that disaster severity and level of exposure to disaster-related stressors (i.e. loss, injury), rather than type of disaster event, is associated with for PTSD.[39] For example, following the 2004 Florida hurricane season, current PTSD was estimated at 3.6%, and PTSD risk was associated with displacement from one's home.[40] However, rates of current PTSD after the more severe Hurricane Katrina were much higher (16.3%;41). Hurricane-related stressors involving physical illness/injury and physical adversity were most associated with PTSD among individuals living in the New Orleans metropolitan area (30.3%), whereas stressors related to financial loss were associated with PTSD in other affected areas (12.5%).

Examples from other selected natural disaster studies show current rates of PTSD ranging from 2.4% in Australian adults following the 2003 brush fires[42] to 9.7% in adults who survived flooding in Hunan, China.[43] Following the 2004 Southeast Asian earthquake-tsunami, PTSD prevalence was 33.6% and 21.6% at 3 and 6 months post disaster.[44]

10.4.3 Combat veterans

Military personnel may be exposed to a variety of physical dangers and psychological stressors during service. A range of PTSD prevalence estimates has been reported for the three major US combat operations of the past several decades: the Vietnam War, the Persian Gulf War, and the wars in Iraq and Afghanistan (Table 10.1). The Vietnam Experience Study,[45] one of the first epidemiological studies of mental health among veterans, determined that 2.2% of veterans met current DSM-III criteria for PTSD and 14.7% met lifetime criteria for the disorder. By contrast, the National Vietnam Veterans Readjustment Survey (NVVRS)[46] reported much higher rates of PTSD, based on DSM-III-R criteria. However, a re-analysis of the NVVRS data adjusted for documentation of combat-related trauma exposure and impairment in functioning, and concluded that rate of lifetime PTSD in this sample was 18.7%, and that rate of current PTSD was 9.1%.[47] Additional reports of mental health in Vietnam War veterans have produced variable rates of PTSD which appear to depend, in part, on the intensity of combat.[48]

With regard to subsequent military operations, a population estimate of 10.1% for current PTSD prevalence has been reported for veterans of the Gulf War.[49] Rates of PTSD increased with higher exposure to combat stress, with upper estimates of 22.6% for veterans who reported the highest levels of combat exposure. By contrast, the Iowa Persian Gulf War Study estimated a much lower rate (2.0%) of past year PTSD among combat veterans.[50] Based on self-report measures, estimates of past month PTSD prevalence in the military operations in Iraq and Afghanistan ranged from 6.2% to 11.5% after deployment to Afghanistan and from 12.2% to 18% after deployment to Iraq.[51]

10.5 Summary and conclusions

As PTSD is conditional on exposure to a traumatic experience, the prevalence of PTSD will necessarily vary as a function of patterns of exposure, with lifetime likelihood of experiencing trauma(s) increasing over time. However, research has demonstrated (a) that the experience of trauma increases risk of subsequent trauma and (b) a cumulative impact of trauma, whereby risk of PTSD is increased by multiple traumas. Thus, early trauma experience can have lasting and possibly multiplicative effects on later functioning over the life course. Longitudinal cohort designs, including multigenerational investigations, are needed to understand how the risk factors of trauma exposure and PTSD, as well as how trauma and PTSD may themselves influence subsequent outcomes, may change over the life course.

The challenge to life course research is the availability of developmentally appropriate assessments for PTSD, particularly for young children, that allow for comparisons across developmental stages. This challenge is further complicated by changes over time in the definition of trauma and of PTSD. To date, changing definitions of a 'Criterion A trauma' (see Box 10.1) have shifted prevalence rates over time. Further, as PTSD symptoms have been shown to decrease over time, it would not be surprising to find differences across studies as a function of assessment timing. Given these factors, it is remarkable to find consistency reported here regarding rates and risk factors for PTSD. On the whole, US community samples suggest lifetime rates of PTSD around 10%, which is slightly higher than the estimates in most non-US studies; however, this could be

Table 10.1 Epidemiological studies of post-traumatic stress disorder organized by sample characteristics

Study	Key publications	Year of data collection	Sample selection methods	Instrument(s)/ interview	Lifetime assessment of trauma (Y/N)	Age (years)	N (women/ men)	Ethnicity/ race	Trauma types assessed	PTSD prevalence	Other key findings
National Studies (USA and Canada)											
National Comorbidity Study (NCS)	Kessler et al.[19]	1990–1992	Stratified, multistage area probability sample of the USA	CIDI and a version of the Revised DIS	Y	15–54	N = 5,877, 52.2% women	W = 76.3%, AA = 11.4%, H = 9.0%, O = 3.3%	12 types of DSM-III-R traumas	7.8%, lifetime	PTSD highly comorbid with another type of DSM-III-R lifetime disorder; women at least twice as likely to have lifetime PTSD compared with men. Lifetime prevalence higher in previously married women; for men, prevalence higher among married versus never married
National Women's Study	Resnick et al.[20]	Not reported	Random digit-dialling (RDD), multistage area probability sample of the US adult women	NWS-PTSD	Y	M = 44.9 (18.4)	N = 4,008, 100% women	W = 85.2%, AA = 11.6%, O = 3.2%	DSM-III-R; most severe assessed	12.3%, lifetime; 4.6%, 6-month	68.9% of the women reported at least one type of traumatic event; crime victims had higher rates of lifetime and current PTSD. Rate of PTSD among the women with assault history that had both life threat and injury was more than double that observed in the women who had neither life threat nor injury during their assault

Table 10.1 (continued) Epidemiological studies of post-traumatic stress disorder organized by sample characteristics

Study	Key publications	Year of data collection	Sample selection methods	Instrument(s)/ interview	Lifetime assessment of trauma (Y/N)	Age (years)	N (women/ men)	Ethnicity/ race	Trauma types assessed	PTSD prevalence	Other key findings
National Survey of Adolescents	Kilpatrick et al.[3,53]	1995	RDD, multistage area probability sample of the US adolescents	Telephone interview. Modified NWS-PTSD	N	12–17	N = 3,907, 49% women	W = 72%, AA = 15%, A = 1%, H = 8%, NA = 4%	DSM-III-R	3.7% for boys, 6-month; 6.3% for girls, 6-month	PTSD had high comorbidity with major depressive episode; African-American or Hispanic ethnicity and older age associated with PTSD; interpersonal violence was strong predictor of comorbid diagnoses. PTSD predicted drug use
National Comorbidity Study— Replication	Kessler et al.[21,54,55]	2001–2003	Nationally representative household survey of English speakers based on probability sampling	Face-to-face interviews	N	18–44	N = 9,282; PTSD assessed in subsample of N = 5,692	W = 72.8%, AA = 12.4%, H = 11.1%, O = 3.8%	DSM-IV	6.8% lifetime; 3.5%, 12-month	36.6% classified as 'serious', 33.1% as 'moderate' PTSD
National Comorbidity Survey Replication— Adolescent Supplement	Merikangas et al.[2,57]; Kessler et al.[56]	2001–2004	Adolescents residing in households from the NCS-R sample	Face-to-face interviews. CIDI. Parent present in house, but not in same room	Y	13–18	N = 10,148, 48.7% women	W = 65.6%, AA = 15.1%, H = 14.4%, O = 5.0%	DSM-IV	5%, lifetime	Higher for women (8.0%) than men (2.3%). Overall prevalence increased with age: 13–14 years (3.7%), 15–16 years (5.1%), and 17–18 years (7.0%)

Table 10.1 (continued) Epidemiological studies of post-traumatic stress disorder organized by sample characteristics

Study	Key publications	Year of data collection	Sample selection methods	Instrument(s)/ interview	Lifetime assessment of trauma (Y/N)	Age (years)	N (women/ men)	Ethnicity/ race	Trauma types assessed	PTSD prevalence	Other key findings
NESARC	Pietrzak et al.[22]; Roberts et al.[10]	2004–2005	Housing unit sampling frame using Census Supplementary Survey	Face-to-face interviews. AUDADIS-IV	Y	≥20	N = 34,653	W = 58%, AA = 19%, A = 3%, H = 18%	DSM-IV	6.4%, lifetime; 6.6%, sub-threshold	Rates higher for women than men (8.6% vs 4.1%, lifetime); PTSD more frequent among younger, previously married, lower income individuals; less frequent among never married and Asian/ Hawaiian/Pacific Islanders. Longer duration of symptoms among those who reported direct (vs indirect) trauma exposure. PTSD and partial PTSD related to elevated Axis I comorbidity, lifetime suicide attempts, past month functional impairment. Asians experienced lower risk of trauma exposure and lower risk for PTSD than Whites; although Blacks had lower trauma exposure than Whites, risk for PTSD was higher than for Whites

Table 10.1 (continued) Epidemiological studies of post-traumatic stress disorder organized by sample characteristics

Study	Key publications	Year of data collection	Sample selection methods	Instrument(s)/ interview	Lifetime assessment of trauma (Y/N)	Age (years)	N (women/ men)	Ethnicity/ race	Trauma types assessed	PTSD prevalence	Other key findings
National Survey of Adolescents—Replication	McCauley et al.[1]	2005	RDD, multistage area probability sample of the US adolescents. Oversampling of urban dwelling adolescents	Telephone interview. Modified NWS-PTSD	Y	12–17	N = 3,614, 48.8% women	W = 69%, AA = 13%, H = 10%, O = 5%	DSM-IV	7%, lifetime	6.7% of the adolescents had misused prescription drugs in the last year. Witnessing violence was the only traumatic event that was a significant risk factor for non-medical use of prescription drugs (NMUPD). Delinquent behaviour also predicted NMUPD
Regional Studies											
NIMH Epidemiologic Catchment Area (ECA)—St Louis catchment area	Helzer et al.[17]	1982	Stratified area sampling	Face-to-face interview. DIS for DSM-III	Y	Not reported	N = 2,493, 61.3% women	Not reported	DSM-III trauma	1%, lifetime	Rates of PTSD higher in women (1.3%) than men (0.5%); physical attack associated with higher rates of PTSD (3.5%) in civilians; PTSD occurred in 20% of veterans wounded in Vietnam; PTSD predicted by behavioural problems before the age of 15 years. Individuals with PTSD are twice as likely to have another disorder as those without it

Table 10.1 (continued) Epidemiological studies of post-traumatic stress disorder organized by sample characteristics

Study	Key publications	Year of data collection methods	Sample selection methods	Instrument(s)/ interview	Lifetime assessment of trauma (Y/N)	Age (years)	N (women/ men)	Ethnicity/ race	Trauma types assessed	PTSD prevalence	Other key findings
NIMH Epidemiologic Catchment Area (ECA)— North Carolina catchment area	Davidson et al.[16]	Not reported	Stratified area sampling	Face-to-face interview. DIS for DSM-III	Y	18–95	N = 2,985 54.4% women	W = 62.7%	DSM-III	1.3%, lifetime; 0.44%, 6-month	Sub-threshold PTSD = 6.6%. PTSD associated with childhood instability, family history of psychiatric illness, psychiatric comorbidity, physical health problems
Detroit Traumatic Events and PTSD in Young Adults	Breslau et al.[14]	1989	Random sample of young adults in a large health maintenance organization in south-east Michigan	Face-to-face interview in their homes. DIS revised to cover DSM-III-R diagnoses	Y	21–30	N = 1,007, 61.7% women	W = 80.7%	DSM-III-R criteria. 'Most-stressful' trauma assessed	9.2%, lifetime	Exposure to trauma more frequent in men than in women, but higher PTSD rate in women than men; rate of PTSD according to traumatic event did not vary greatly among most types of events (11.6–24%), except for women who reported being raped (80%). Risk factors included female sex, neuroticism, early childhood separation, pre-existing psychiatric disorders (not including substance use disorders), and familial history of anxiety disorders and antisocial behaviour

Table 10.1 (continued) Epidemiological studies of post-traumatic stress disorder organized by sample characteristics

Study	Key publications	Year of data collection	Sample selection methods	Instrument(s)/ interview	Lifetime assessment of trauma (Y/N)	Age (years)	N (women/ men)	Ethnicity/ race	Trauma types assessed	PTSD prevalence	Other key findings
The Great Smokey Mountains Study of Youth	Costello et al.[4]	Not reported	Screening-stratified sampling design in Southern Appalachian region of North Carolina	Face-to-face interview conducted with children and parents. CAPA	N	9–13	N = 1,015	W = 90%, AA = 8%, H <1%, A <1%, Mixed Race = 1%	DSM-III-R	0.02% ± 0.96 overall; 0.05 ± 1.60% for girls, 0 for boys	Fewer than 5 cases in the sample met diagnostic criteria for PTSD. Sample was selected based on positive screen for externalizing symptoms plus 10% of non-positive sample
Canadian PTSD Community Survey	Stein et al.[31]	1994	RDD, 2-stage probability sample. Winnipeg, Canada	Telephone interview. Modified PTSD Symptom Scale	Y	≥18	N = 1,002, 52.3% women	Not reported	DSM-IV. Current most severe	Women = 2.7%, 1-month; men = 1.2%, 1-month	Prevalence of partial PTSD: women = 3.4%, men = 0.3%. Those with partial PTSD exhibited clinically meaningful impairment
1996 Detroit Area Survey of Trauma	Breslau et al.[5]	1996	RDD	Computer-assisted telephone interview. Modified DIS for DSM-IV and CIDI	Y	18–45	N = 2,181, 51.4% women	W = 71%; Non-White = 28%	DSM-IV. Assessed (1) 'most stressful' and (2) a computer randomly selected trauma	Only conditional probabilities reported: (1) 13.6% for worst event, (2) 9.2% for randomly selected trauma	Exposure to any trauma: 89.6%. Conditional probability of PTSD higher for women (13.0%) than men (6.2%). Men twice as likely to be exposed to assaultive violence. Highest probability of PTSD associated with assaultive violence: 20.9%

Table 10.1 (continued) Epidemiological studies of post-traumatic stress disorder organized by sample characteristics

Study	Key publications	Year of data collection	Sample selection methods	Instrument(s)/ interview	Lifetime assessment of trauma (Y/N)	Age (years)	N (women/ men)	Ethnicity/ race	Trauma types assessed	PTSD prevalence	Other key findings
Mid-Atlantic epidemiological sample	Breslau and Anthony[58]; Breslau et al.[15]	2000–2002	All first-graders from five different urban areas within a school district were chosen to represent variations in ethnicity, housing, income, and other US census characteristics	A face-to-face interview by trained non-clinician interviewers. CIDI	Y	19–23 (M = 21)	N = 1,698, 53.2% women	AA = 71.0%, W = 29.0%	DSM-IV traumas. 'Most stressful' assessed for PTSD	7.1%, lifetime; Women = 7.9% Men = 6.3%	Rates of assaultive violence or injury peaked at 16–17 years; overall conditional probability of PTSD from trauma: 8.8%; highest conditional probability associated with assaultive violence (15.1%). Women had significantly higher conditional risk from assaultive violence (23.5%) than men (7.1%); social environment may affect exposure to traumas, especially assaultive violence
Event-specific studies											
PTSD in American Legionnaires with Combat Experience in Vietnam	Snow et al.[59]	1984	Random selection from The American Legion roster in Colorado, Indiana, Minnesota, Maryland, Ohio, and Pennsylvania	Self-report questionnaire. 18-item survey based on PTSD criteria from the DSM-III	N	Not reported	N = 2,858, 100% men	Not reported	Combat exposure, as well as any other lifetime trauma exposure	1.8–15%, current	PTSD symptoms more likely to occur in those with higher levels of combat trauma exposure. Exposure to traumatic stress may also be related to depression or other behavioural outcomes.

Table 10.1 (continued) Epidemiological studies of post-traumatic stress disorder organized by sample characteristics

Study	Key publications	Year of data collection	Sample selection methods	Instrument(s)/ interview	Lifetime assessment of trauma (Y/N)	Age (years)	N (women/ men)	Ethnicity/ race	Trauma types assessed	PTSD prevalence	Other key findings
PTSD in Vietnam War Twin Veterans	Goldberg et al.[48]	1987	Mail, telephone, or in-person interviews offered to members of the Vietnam Era Twin Registry database	12-item survey based on PTSD criteria from the DSM-III	N (post-combat only)	Not reported	N = 4,184 (2,092 monozygotic twin pairs), 100% male	Not reported	Combat exposure	For twins discordant for South East Asia (SEA) service: Served in SEA = 16.8%, 6-month; Did not serve in SEA = 5%, 6-month	Rates of 6-month PTSD among twin pairs in which neither twin served in SEA = 5.1%; in which both twins served in SEA = 12.9%. Greater combat exposure associated with higher prevalence of PTSD symptoms
National Vietnam Veterans Readjustment Study	Kulka et al.[46,60,61]; Schlenger et al.[62]; Weiss et al.[63]	1988	Veterans: stratified random sample from military records. Civilians: probability household sampling, state nurse directories	Face-to-face interviews. Mississippi Scale for Combat-Related PTSD, SCID, MMPI PTSD scale, Impact of Event Scale, Stress Response Rating Scale	Y	19–25+ at time of entry to Vietnam	N = 1,532 Vietnam theatre veterans, 27% women	W = 87%, AA = 11% (population estimates)	Combat-related trauma	Vietnam theatre veterans: men = 15.2%, women = 8.5%, current; men = 30.6%, women = 26.9%, lifetime	Significant differences in prevalence by ethnicity: 27.9% among Hispanic, 20.6% among African-American, 13.7% among Caucasian/other ethnicity. PTSD significantly higher for those exposed to high levels of war zone stress. Rates of partial PTSD: men = 11.1%, women = 7.8%, current; men = 22.5%, women = 21.2%, lifetime

Table 10.1 (continued) Epidemiological studies of post-traumatic stress disorder organized by sample characteristics

Study	Key publications	Year of data collection	Sample selection methods	Instrument(s)/ interview	Lifetime assessment of trauma (Y/N)	Age (years)	N (women/ men)	Ethnicity/ race	Trauma types assessed	PTSD prevalence	Other key findings
Centers for Disease Control Vietnam Experience Study (VES)	Centers for Disease Control[45]	Not reported	Random sample of male army veterans who served during Vietnam era (Vietnam-deployed and non-deployed).	Computer-assisted telephone interview; a subsample was selected for face-to-face interview. DIS	N	M = 37.4 (at interview); M = 19.8 (at enlistment)	N = 4,462 selected for face-to-face psychological evaluation, 100% men	W = 81.8%	Combat-related trauma	Vietnam-deployed veterans = 14.7%, lifetime; 2.2% past month	Higher incidence of PTSD associated with combat exposure, tactical military occupation. Veterans with PTSD more likely to have comorbid psychiatric diagnosis: 66% comorbid with anxiety or depression; 39% comorbid with alcohol abuse or dependence
Gulf War Veterans	Kang et al.[49]	1995–1996	Stratified random sampling method	Self-report PCL	N	M = 31.7 (non-Gulf veterans), M = 30.4 (Gulf veterans)	N = 20,917, 20% women	W = 75.1% (non-Gulf veterans); W = 73.7% (Gulf veterans)	Combat-related experiences versus non-combat related experiences	Gulf veterans = 12.1%, current (population estimate = 10.1%); non-Gulf veterans = 4.3%, current (population estimate = 4.2%)	Prevalence of PTSD increased with deployment status and stressor intensity. Veterans with PTSD more likely to be female, older, non-White, in the enlisted ranks, and in the Army and National Guard

Table 10.1 (continued) Epidemiological studies of post-traumatic stress disorder organized by sample characteristics

Study	Key publications	Year of data collection	Sample selection methods	Instrument(s)/ interview	Lifetime assessment of trauma (Y/N)	Age (years)	N (women/ men)	Ethnicity/ race	Trauma types assessed	PTSD prevalence	Other key findings
Survivors of Widespread Fire	Parslow and Jorn[42]	1999–2004	Random selection using electoral rolls, trauma-specific sample was identified as part of a larger longitudinal study	Trauma Screening Questionnaire	N	M = 26.7 (1.5)	N = 1,599, 52% women	Not reported	Exposure to bushfire	2.4% met the criteria for PTSD; 37.8% sub-threshold PTSD symptoms	PTSD symptoms of re-experiencing and arousal were inversely associated with certain neurocognitive functions, including word recall, digit span, coding speed, and verbal intelligence, as assessed 3 years before the trauma. Greater verbal working memory capacity was associated with lower risk of PTSD re-experiencing or arousal symptoms
Post-9/11 terrorist attacks	Galea et al.[37]	2001	RDD, Manhattan residents living south of 110th St.	Telephone interview. NWS-PTSD	N	M = 42 (15)	N = 988, 52% women	W = 71%, AA = 5%, A = 7%, H = 12%, O = 2%	PTSD associated with 9/11 terrorist attacks	7.5%, 30-day	Significant predictors of PTSD included: Hispanic ethnicity, >2 stressors in past 12 months, a panic attack during or soon after attacks, living in close proximity to attack site, loss of possessions due to attacks

Table 10.1 (continued) Epidemiological studies of post-traumatic stress disorder organized by sample characteristics

Study	Key publications	Year of data collection	Sample selection methods	Instrument(s)/ interview	Lifetime assessment of trauma (Y/N)	Age (years)	N (women/ men)	Ethnicity/ race	Trauma types assessed	PTSD prevalence	Other key findings
Combat duty in Iraq and Afghanistan	Hoge et al.[51]	2003	Three active duty army units and one active duty marine corps unit selected for assessment before or after deployment; participants volunteered during recruitment briefings	Self-report PCL	N	18–40+	N = 6,201, 1% women	W = 67%, AA = 10%, H = 13%, O = 8%	Combat-related experiences; any self-identified traumatic event	Before deployment = 5.0–9.4%, past month. After deployment to Iraq = 12.2–19.9%, past month. After deployment to Afghanistan = 6.2–1.5%, past month	Rates of reported combat experience were much higher in soldiers who had been deployed to Iraq than to Afghanistan; strong relation between combat experiences and PTSD. Prevalence rate ranges vary depending on strictness of PTSD criteria

Table 10.1 (continued) Epidemiological studies of post-traumatic stress disorder organized by sample characteristics

Study	Key publications	Year of data collection	Sample selection methods	Instrument(s)/ interview	Lifetime assessment of trauma (Y/N)	Age (years)	N (women/ men)	Ethnicity/ race	Trauma types assessed	PTSD prevalence	Other key findings
2004 Florida hurricanes	Acierno et al.[40]	2005	RDD in 33 counties that were in the direct path of at least one of the hurricanes	Computer-assisted telephone interviews. NWS-PTSD.	N	M = 49.6 (18.4)	N = 1,452, 51.9% women	W = 76%, AA = 11%, H = 9%, A = 2%, NA = 1%, Bi-Racial = 0.3%	Exposure to any trauma (PTSD-general) and exposure to hurricane-specific trauma	PTSD general = 3.6%, 9-month; PTSD hurricane = 1.4%, 9-month	Most participants were older adults, who are likely to report psychopathology symptoms at a lower rate than the general population. GAD and PTSD shared hurricane exposure risk factors; increased risk of psychological problems associated with previous exposure to PTEs, significant displacement, and low social support preceding the hurricane

Table 10.1 (continued) Epidemiological studies of post-traumatic stress disorder organized by sample characteristics

Study	Key publications	Year of data collection	Sample selection methods	Instrument(s)/ interview	Lifetime assessment of trauma (Y/N)	Age (years)	N (women/ men)	Ethnicity/ race	Trauma types assessed	PTSD prevalence	Other key findings
Rape survivors, National Institute of Justice study	Kilpatrick et al.[64]	2007	RDD for general population sample, college women sample selected from the American Student List	Computer-assisted telephone interview. NWS-PTSD	Y (rape only)	College women, M = 20.1 (3.2); general population, M = 46.6 (17.9)	N = 5,001 (N = 2,000 college women), 100% women	Full sample: W = 75%; AA = 11%; H = 6%; A = 6%	Drug/alcohol-related rape, forcible rape, incapacitated rape	General population = 6–29%, 6-month, and 13–46%, lifetime; college women = 9–46%, 6-month, and 15–53%, lifetime	Women who had been raped were significantly more likely to have lifetime diagnosis of PTSD and/or major depression; more likely to have repeated occasions of binge drinking, prescription drug misuse, and marijuana or other illicit drug use in the past year. They were more likely to have current PTSD, major depression, and substance abuse

DSM-III(IV), *Diagnostic and statistical manual of mental disorders*, 3rd (4th) edition; PTSD, post-traumatic stress disorder; PTE, potentially traumatic event; RDD, random digit dialling; AUDADIS-IV, Alcohol Use Disorder and Associated Disabilities Interview Schedule-DSM-IV Version; CAPA, Child and Adolescent Psychiatric Assessment; CIDI, World Mental Health Composite International Diagnostic Interview; DIS, Diagnostic Interview Schedule; MMPI, Minnesota Multiphasic Personality Inventory; NWS-PTSD, National Women's Study—PTSD Module; PCL, 17-item National Center for PTSD Checklist; SCID, Structured Clinical Interview for DSM Disorders; W, White/Caucasian; AA, African-American/Black; A, Asian/Pacific Islander; H, Hispanic; NA, Native American/Alaskan Native; O, other race/ethnicity.

Box 10.1: The evolution of post-traumatic stress disorder (PTSD) criteria in the *Diagnostic and statistical manual of mental disorders* (DSM)

Historical and theoretical considerations

◆ The PTSD diagnosis was initially somewhat controversial for its inclusion of a criterion that required exposure to an external event.

◆ The definition of a traumatic event, a necessary but not sufficient aspect of the diagnosis, has been the subject of revisions over time.

◆ Changes in PTSD criteria have had implications for resulting prevalence estimates across time and across studies.

DSM-III (1980)

◆ The American Psychiatric Association first added PTSD to the third edition of the DSM.

◆ Required exposure to a 'trauma' such as war or natural disaster that is 'outside the range of usual experience and that would be markedly distressing to almost anyone' (Criterion A).

◆ PTSD was defined by the presence of symptoms of re-experiencing (Criterion B), avoidance (Criterion C), physiological arousal (Criterion D), and impairment continuing for at least one month post trauma.

DSM-III-R (1987)

◆ Criterion A was broadened to include experiences involving 'serious threat' to self or others, as well as witnessing harm to others.

DSM-IV (1994)

◆ More refined Criterion A with the addition of subjective response of 'intense fear, helplessness, or horror.'

◆ One of the Criterion D symptoms (physiological reactivity to reminders) was moved to Criterion B.

influenced by differences in measurement tools or other factors such as community cohesion.[52] In US and non-US studies rates increase in samples of civilian who have experienced extensive traumas such as war, political conflict and terrorism, and mass violence.

References

1 McCauley JL, Danielson CK, Amstadter AB, et al. The role of traumatic event history in non-medical use of prescription drugs among a nationally representative sample of US adolescents. *J Child Psychol Psychiatry* 2010;**51**(1):84–93.

2 Merikangas KR, He J, Burstein M, et al. Lifetime prevalence of mental disorders in U.S. adolescents: results from the National Comorbidity Survey Replication—Adolescent Supplement (NCS-A). *J Am Acad Child Adolesc Psychiatry* 2010;**49**(10):980–989.

3 Kilpatrick DG, Ruggiero KJ, Acierno R, Saunders BE, Resnick HS, Best CL. Violence and risk of PTSD, major depression, substance abuse/dependence, and comorbidity: results from the National Survey of Adolescents. *J Consult Clin Psychol* 2003;**71**(4):692–700.

4 **Costello EJ, Angold A, Burns BJ, et al.** The Great Smoky Mountains Study of Youth. Goals, design, methods, and the prevalence of DSM-III-R disorders. *Arch Gen Psychiatry* 1996;**53**(12):1129–1136.

5 **Breslau N, Kessler R, Chilcoat HD, Schultz LR, Davis GC, Andreski P.** Trauma and posttraumatic stress disorder in the community: the 1996 Detroit area survey of trauma. *Arch Gen Psychiatry* 1998;**55**:626–32.

6 **Trickey D, Siddaway AP, Meiser-Stedman R, Serpell L, Field AP.** A meta-analysis of risk factors for posttraumatic stress disorder in children and adolescents. *Clin Psychol Rev* 2012;**32**(2):122–138.

7 **Copeland WE, Keeler G, Angold A, Costello EJ.** Traumatic events and posttraumatic stress in childhood. *Arch Gen Psychiatry* 2007;**64**(5):577–584.

8 **Cuffe SP, Addy CL, Garrison CZ, et al.** Prevalence of PTSD in a community sample of older adolescents. *J Am Acad Child Adolesc Psychiatry* 1998;**37**(2):147–154.

9 **Perkonigg A, Kessler RC, Storz S, Wittchen H-U.** Traumatic events and post-traumatic stress disorder in the community: prevalence, risk factors, and comorbidity. *Acta Psychiatr Scand* 2000;**101**:46–59.

10 **Roberts AL, Galea S, Austin SB, et al.** Posttraumatic stress disorder across two generations: concordance and mechanisms in a population-based sample. *Biol Psychiatry* 2012;**72**(6):505–511.

11 **Blom M, Oberink R.** The validity of the DSM-IV PTSD criteria in children and adolescents: a review. Clin Child Psychol Psychiatry 2012;**17**(4):571–601.

12 **Cohen JA, Scheeringa MS.** Post-traumatic stress disorder diagnosis in children: challenges and promises. *Dialogues Clin Neurosci* 2009;**11**(1):91–99.

13 **Scheeringa MS, Wright MJ, Hunt JP, Zeanah CH.** Factors affecting the diagnosis and prediction of PTSD symptomatology in children and adolescents. *Am J Psychiatry* 2006;**163**:644–651.

14 **Breslau N, Davis GC, Andreski P, Peterson E.** Traumatic events and posttraumatic stress disorder in an urban population of young adults. *Arch Gen Psychiatry* 1991;**48**:216–222.

15 **Breslau N, Wilcox HC, Storr CL, Lucia VC, Anthony JC.** Trauma exposure and posttraumatic stress disorder: a study of youths in urban America. *J Urban Health* 2004;**81**(4):530–544.

16 **Davidson JR, Hughes D, Blazer DG, George LK.** Post-traumatic stress disorder in the community: an epidemiological study. *Psychol Med* 1991;**21**:713–721.

17 **Helzer JE, Robins LN, McEvoy L.** Post-traumatic stress disorder in the general population: findings of the epidemiological catchment area survey. *N Engl J Med* 1987;**317**:1630–1634.

18 **Regier DA, Myers JK, Kramer M, et al.** The NIMH Epidemiologic Catchment Area program. Historical context, major objectives, and study population characteristics. *Arch Gen Psychiatry* 1984;**41**(10):934–941.

19 **Kessler RC, Sonnega A, Bromet E, Hughes M, Nelson CB.** Posttraumatic stress disorder in the National Comorbidity Survey. *Arch Gen Psychiatry* 1995;**52**(12):1048–1060.

20 **Resnick HS, Kilpatrick DG, Dansky BS, Saunders BE, Best CL.** Prevalence of civilian trauma and posttraumatic stress disorder in a representative national sample of women. *J Consult Clin Psychol* 1993;**61**:984–991.

21 **Kessler RC, Chiu WT, Demler O, Merikangas KR, Walters EE.** Prevalence, severity, and comorbidity of 12-month DSM-IV disorders in the National Comorbidity Survey Replication. *Arch Gen Psychiatry* 2005;**62**(6):617–627.

22 **Pietrzak RH, Goldstein RB, Southwick SM, Grant BF.** Prevalence and Axis I comorbidity of full and partial posttraumatic stress disorder in the United States: results from Wave 2 of the National Epidemiologic Survey on Alcohol and Related Conditions. *J Anxiety Disorders* 2011;**25**(3):456–465.

23 **Gum AM, King-Kallimanis B, Kohn R.** Prevalence of mood, anxiety, and substance-abuse disorders for older Americans in the national comorbidity survey-replication. *Am J Geriatr Psychiatry* 2009;**17**(9):769–781.

24 **Acierno R, Resnick H, Kilpatrick DG, Saunders B, Best CL.** Risk factors for rape, physical assault, and posttraumatic stress disorder in women: examination of differential multivariate relationships. *J Anxiety Disorders* 1999;**13**(6):541–563.

25 Ozer EJ, Best SR, Lipsey TL, Weiss DS. Predictors of posttraumatic stress disorder and symptoms in adults: a meta-analysis. *Psychol Bull* 2003;**129**(1):52–73.

26 Johnson H, Thompson A. The development and maintenance of post-traumatic stress disorder (PTSD) in civilian adult survivors of war trauma and torture: a review. *Clin Psychol Rev* 2008;**28**(1):36–47.

27 Suliman S, Mkabile SG, Fincham DS, Ahmed R, Stein DJ, Seedat S. Cumulative effect of multiple trauma on symptoms of posttraumatic stress disorder, anxiety, and depression in adolescents. *Compr Psychiatry* 2009;**50**(2):121–127.

28 Darves-Bornoz JM, Alonso J, de Girolamo G, et al. Main traumatic events in Europe: PTSD in the European study of the epidemiology of mental disorders survey. *J Traum Stress* 2008;**21**(5):455–462.

29 de Vries GJ, Olff M. The lifetime prevalence of traumatic events and posttraumatic stress disorder in the Netherlands. *J Traum Stress* 2009;**22**(4):259–267.

30 Creamer M, Burgess P, McFarlane AC. Post-traumatic stress disorder: findings from the Australian National Survey of Mental Health and Well-being. *Psychol Med* 2001;**31**(7):1237–1247.

31 Stein MB, Walker JR, Hazen AL, Forde DR. Full and partial posttraumatic stress disorder: findings from a community survey. *Am J Psychiatry* 1997;**154**:1114–1119.

32 Koenen KC, Moffitt TE, Poulton R, Martin J, Caspi A. Early childhood factors associated with post-traumatic stress disorder: results from a longitudinal birth cohort. *Psychol Med* 2007;**37**:181–192.

33 Norris FH, Murphy AD, Baker CK, Perilla JL, Rodriguez FG, Rodriguez Jde J. Epidemiology of trauma and posttraumatic stress disorder in Mexico. *J Abnormal Psychol* 2003;**112**(4):646–656.

34 Zlotnick C, Johnson J, Kohn R, Vicente B, Rioseco P, Saldivia S. Epidemiology of trauma, post-traumatic stress disorder (PTSD) and co-morbid disorders in Chile. *Psychol Med* 2006;**36**(11):1523–1533.

35 Karam EG, Mneimneh ZN, Karam AN, et al. Prevalence and treatment of mental disorders in Lebanon: a national epidemiological survey. *Lancet* 2006;**367**(9515):1000–1006.

36 de Jong JT, Komproe IH, van Ommeren M, et al. Lifetime events and posttraumatic stress disorder in 4 postconflict settings. *JAMA* 2001;**286**(5):555–563.

37 Galea S, Ahern J, Resnick H, et al. Psychological sequelae of the September 11 terrorist attacks in New York City. *N Engl J Med* 2002;**346**:982–987.

38 North CS, Nixon SJ, Shariat S, et al. Psychiatric disorders among survivors of the Oklahoma City bombing. *JAMA* 1999;**282**:755–762.

39 Briere J, Elliott D. Prevalence , characteristics, and long-term sequelae of natural disaster exposure in the general population. *J Traum Stress* 2000;**13**(4):661–679.

40 Acierno R, Ruggiero KJ, Galea S, et al. Psychological sequelae of the 2004 Florida hurricanes: implications for post-disaster intervention. *Am J Public Health* 2007;**97**(Suppl 1):S103–S108.

41 Galea S, Brewin CR, Gruber M, et al. Exposure to hurricane-related stressors and mental illness after Hurricane Katrina. *Arch Gen Psychiatry* 2007;**64**(12):1427–1434.

42 Parslow RA, Jorn AF. Pretrauma and posttrauma neurocognitive functioning and PTSD symptoms in a community sample of young adults. *Am J Psychiatry* 2007;**164**(3):509–515.

43 Feng S, Tan H, Benjamin A, et al. Social support and posttraumatic stress disorder among flood victims in Hunan, China. *Ann Epidemiol* 2007;**17**(10):827–833.

44 Thavichachart N, Tangwongchai S, Worakul P, et al. Posttraumatic mental health establishment of the Tsunami survivors in Thailand. *Clin Pract Epidemiol Mental Health* 2009;**3**:5–11.

45 Centers for Disease Control. Health status of Vietnam veterans: psychosocial characteristics. *JAMA* 1988;**259**:2701–2707.

46 Kulka R, Schlenger W, Fairbank J, et al. *Trauma and the Vietnam War generation: report of the findings from the National Vietnam Veterans Readjustment Study*. New York: Brunner/Mazel; 1990.

47 Dohrenwend BP, Turner JB, Turse NA, Adams BG, Koenen KC, Marshall R. The psychological risks of Vietnam for U.S. veterans: a revisit with new data and methods. *Science* 2006;**313**(5789):979–982.

48 Goldberg J, True WR, Eisen S, Henderson W. A twin study of the effects of the Vietnam War on post-traumatic stress disorder. *JAMA* 1990;**263**(9):1227–1232.

49 Kang HK, Natelson BH, Mahan CM, Lee KY, Murphy FM. Post-traumatic stress disorder and chronic fatigue syndrome-like illness among Gulf War veterans: a population-based survey of 30,000 veterans. *Am J Epidemiol* 2003;**157**:141–148.

50 Group TIPGS. Self-reported illness and health status among Gulf War veterans. *JAMA* 1997;**277**(3):238–245.

51 Hoge CW, Castro CA, Messer SC, McGurk D, Cotting DI, Koffman RL. Combat duty in Iraq and Afghanistan, mental health problems, and barriers to care. *N Engl J Med* 2004;**351**(1):13–22.

52 Gapen M, Cross D, Ortigo K, et al. Perceived neighborhood disorder, community cohesion, and PTSD symptoms among low-income African Americans in an urban health setting. *Am J Orthopsychiatry* 2011;**81**(1):31–37.

53 Kilpatrick DG, Acierno R, Schnurr PP, Saunders B, Resnick HS, Best CL. Risk factors for adolescent substance abuse and dependence: data from a national sample. *J Consult Clin Psychol* 2000;**68**(1):19–30.

54 Kessler RC, Berglund P, Demler O, Jin R, Merikangas KR, Walters EE. Lifetime prevalence and age-of-onset distributions of DSM-IV disorders in the National Comorbidity Survey Replication. *Arch Gen Psychiatry* 2005;**62**(6):593–602.

55 Kessler RC, Berglund P, Chiu WT, et al. The US National Comorbidity Survey Replication (NCS-R): design and field procedures. *Int J Methods Psychiatr Res* 2004;**13**(2):69–92.

56 Kessler RC, Avenevoli S, Costello EJ, et al. Design and field procedures in the US National Comorbidity Survey Replication Adolescent Supplement (NCS-A). *Int J Methods Psychiatr Res* 2009;**18**(2):69–83.

57 Merikangas KR, Avenevoli S, Costello EJ, Koretz D, Kessler RC. The National Comorbidity Survey Adolescent Supplement (NCS-A): I. Background and measures. *J Am Acad Child Adolesc Psychiatry* 2009;**48**(4):367–369.

58 Breslau N, Anthony JC. Gender differences in the sensitivity to posttraumatic stress disorder: an epidemiological study of urban young adults. *J Abnorm Psychol* 2007;**116**(3):607–611.

59 Snow BR, Stellman JM, Stellman SD, Sommer JFJ. Post-traumatic stress disorder among American Legionnaires in relation to combat experience in Vietnam: associated and contributing factors. *Environ Res* 1988;**47**:175–192.

60 Kulka RA, Schlenger WE, Fairbank JA, et al. National Vietnam veterans readjustment study (NVVRS): Description, current status, and initial PTSD prevalence estimates. Washington DC: Veterans Administration; 1988.

61 Kulka RS, Schlenger WE, Fairbank JA, et al. *Contractual report of findings from the National Vietnam Veterans Readjustment Study*, Vol. II: *Tables of findings*. Research Triangle Park, NC: Research Triangle Institute; 1988.

62 Schlenger WE, Kulka RA, Fairbank JA, et al. The prevalence of post-traumatic stress disorder in the Vietnam generation: a multimethod, multisource assessment of psychiatric disorder. *J Trauma Stress* 1992;**5**(3):333–363.

63 Weiss DS, Marmar CR, Schlenger WE, et al. The prevalence of lifetime and partial post-traumatic stress disorder in Vietnam theater veterans. *J Trauma Stress* 1992;**5**(3):365–376.

64 Kilpatrick DG, Resnick HS, Ruggiero KJ, Conoscenti LM, McCauley J. *Drug-facilitated, incapacitated, and forcible rape: a national study* (NCJ 219181—Final report). Washington DC: US Department of Justice/National Institute of Justice; 2007.

Chapter 11

Life course approach to substance use

Jennifer Ahern and Hannah H. Leslie

11.1 Introduction: life course framework applied to substance use

The life course approach has potential to enhance our understanding of the development and persistence of substance use behaviours. Overall, the life course approach considers substance use patterns as the product of choices made within the constraints of biological, social, and historical contexts as they change over time.[1,2] Research that follows this approach contains the key considerations of: (i) long term trajectories of substance use;[1,3] (ii) timing of exposures and how they shape trajectories of substance use[4]—this includes the importance of exposures during critical and sensitive periods (periods in which an exposure may affect a developmental process or may have a greater impact than at another time, respectively) as well as the sequencing and cumulative effects of exposures across the lifespan;[1-3] (iii) the role of broader contexts (e.g. social, economic) in shaping exposure and determining how exposure influences trajectories of substance use, including how contexts evolve over time, how their importance changes over the lifespan (e.g. family in early life, peers in adolescence), and how historical context influences exposure and outcome patterns.[1-3]

Several reviews have summarized research on the determinants of substance use, both broadly and within categories of exposures (e.g. social factors), or life stages (e.g. adolescence).[5] This chapter adds a review of work that takes a clear life course approach in design and/or analysis in the sense that it examines trajectories of substance use, considers time-scales and timing of exposures in shaping use or trajectories of use, or considers broader contexts in time. Our discussion of existing literature highlights the insights gleaned with a life course approach that might be missed in studies focused on substance use at one time or a single substance use transition. We focus on studies with population-representative samples when possible. We conclude by discussing challenges to conducting work that follows a life course approach, as well as potential new directions to enhance our understanding of the determinants of substance use across the life course and facilitate identification of key targets for population intervention.

11.2 Life course research on substance use

Work to date on substance use that has taken a life course approach includes studies of early life determinants, trajectories, broader contexts, and historical periods. Notable studies have integrated more than one life course element. The contributions of each of these types of studies to our understanding of substance use is now discussed.

11.2.1 **Early life determinants**

One area of research that applies a life course approach examines how early life exposures shape substance use initiation, use later in life, and trajectories of use. Gestation, infancy, and childhood are characterized by unfolding developmental processes that may be altered by exposures during critical or sensitive periods and may influence propensity toward substance use later in life.[6]

11.2.1.1 **Gestational exposure**

A set of studies has examined whether gestational exposure to substances influences substance use in the offspring. In an intergenerational study of nicotine dependence, investigators traced 1,248 adult offspring of a cohort of Rhode Island women who had been recruited as obstetric patients between 1959 and 1966.[7] Children of mothers who smoked more than one pack of cigarettes per day during pregnancy had increased odds of nicotine dependence, of progressing from smoking to nicotine dependence, and, in men only, of regular smoking. Maternal smoking was not associated with ever smoking or with marijuana use among offspring. The investigators' use of a life course perspective generated evidence that supports a physiological pathway between gestational nicotine exposure and susceptibility to nicotine dependence in adulthood. Without the linkage back to data on gestational exposures, analysis of maternal influence would likely be confined to genetics. Subsequent studies of this type would benefit from considering a range of exposures across contextual levels as well as during infancy and childhood, such as smoking in the household and smoking norms.

11.2.1.2 **Early life adversity**

A growing body of work is interested in how early life adversities may shape health broadly; a subset of this research has focused on substance use. As an example, a retrospective study of 8,613 members of the Kaiser Health Plan in California assessed the impact of adverse childhood experiences (e.g. abuse, neglect) in relation to drug use.[8] Adverse experiences tended to cluster together and demonstrated a dose–response relationship with ever using drugs, initiating early, and reporting problematic drug use, addiction, or injecting drug use. These associations were consistent across four birth cohorts spanning 1900–1978 despite changes in the prevalence of substance use across cohorts. Beyond linking exposure in early life with lifelong outcomes, this study assessed cumulative exposure to adversities, enabling estimation of a graded relationship. It further addressed historical context by assessing the stability of childhood adversity as predictors across multiple birth cohorts. However, due to the retrospective nature of the study, temporality could not be clearly established, misclassification due to recall may have increased, and characterization of use trajectories was not attempted.

11.2.2 **Trajectories**

A relatively new body of research examines trajectories of substance use over time. Substance use lends itself to consideration of trajectories because there are distinct patterns of use across the lifespan that are not well characterized by single transitions (e.g. onset or cessation). One early observation of distinct patterns was that a sizable proportion of individuals experiment with substance use during adolescence but stop in adulthood, whereas others who use in adolescence continue to use into adulthood.[9] Recent application of trajectory methods has facilitated characterization of patterns of use in more detail, as well as assessment of their determinants. A large prospective study followed a community-based cohort of injection drug users (IDUs) in Baltimore for 20 years.[10] Trajectory analysis revealed five distinct patterns of use: early, delayed, and late cessation; frequent relapse; and persistent injectors. IDUs with baseline single drug use, history of drug treatment, and less frequent injection were more likely to have an early cessation trajectory; using only cocaine at baseline was associated with persistent injection. The life course approach in this study brought into focus discrete use patterns over an extended time-period. A more typical analysis limited to use versus cessation would have failed to identify determinants of the varying patterns of cessation timing and of rapid relapse. Notably, this analysis identified factors that characterized early cessation, enabling a tailored public health response. Similarly, identification of predictors of persistent injection suggests that harm reduction strategies could be targeted to users most in need of them. Extensions of this approach, such as inclusion of time-varying covariates and measures of the broader context, would deepen our understanding of use trajectories and facilitate identification of population-level intervention targets.

11.2.3 Broader context shaping substance use in time

Several studies have considered how broader contexts shape substance use in time. Some of this research explicitly examines characteristics of different contexts over time, whereas other work parses out biological contributions from context more generally.

11.2.3.1 Characteristics of different contexts over time

Studies of contexts shaping substance use over time underscore the importance of family and peer influences, particularly family and peer use of substances, substance use norms, and supports provided. For instance, investigators constructed a sequential cohort of adolescents in the urban Northwest USA by following four groups of 11–15-year-olds for four years.[11] By modelling the eight-year patterns of alcohol, tobacco, and marijuana use, they identify a common trajectory of increasing substance use throughout adolescence. Family cohesion was associated with reduced initial use of all substances but did not affect increased use over time. Baseline peer encouragement for use was associated with initial levels of all substances and with increasing use over time; increased encouragement was associated with steeper uptake. The life course approach in this study led to a focus on the sensitive period of adolescence, an analysis of drug-using trajectories in the context of family and peer environment, and discussion of staging of substance use in the context of adolescent development. While laudable for consideration of multiple environments shaping substance use trajectories, investigators were not able to include other aspects of these environments that may be important in shaping adolescent substance use, such as substance use within the family.

11.2.3.2 Biological and contextual influences over time

A small but informative set of studies examines the roles of genetics and family environment in substance use trajectories by studying twins. In one example of this kind of research, a population-based study of 1,796 male twins in Virginia examined the roles of family environment compared with genetics in shaping alcohol, caffeine, cannabis, and nicotine use from early adolescence through middle adulthood.[12] A consistent pattern emerged: family environment was strongly influential in early adolescence but minimal by middle adulthood, whereas genetic influences gained importance in adulthood. By substance, family environment was least important for alcohol and most important for cannabis. By considering the roles of genetics and environment over time, this study revealed changing contributions of each component to substance use by age. Although the study design did not enable examination of specific aspects of the family environment, it did suggest a sensitive period for the broader environment to influence substance use during adolescence and young adulthood. The findings are consistent with hypotheses that the social environment largely determines initiation of substance use, while biology plays a larger role in progression to long term use or dependence following sufficient exposure to a substance.

11.2.4 **Historical context shaping substance use**

There has been an increasing number of studies examining the role of historical context and time in substance use, particularly attempting to disentangle age, period, and cohort effects.[9,13] Multiple studies have taken advantage of repeated cross-sectional surveys of high school seniors to describe and assess trends in youth substance use from the 1970s onwards. Taken as a whole, these studies suggest that many psychosocial and behavioural predictors of substance use have remained stable despite the changing social and historical context of substance use, and that social norms appear to play an important role in historical variations in use.[14] For example, annual cross-sectional surveys of high school seniors were combined to form seven cohort groups spanning 1976–1997 and comprising more than 180,000 individuals.[15] Predictors such as religious commitment, political beliefs, grade point average, truancy, and evenings out were consistently associated with all substances (cigarettes, alcohol, marijuana, cocaine) across all time-periods. This study examined substance use in a fixed age group across two decades of historical context and found no support for period effects in the variables identified. The authors present these findings as a baseline for further work integrating other life course constructs, including developmental time, individual and family context, and political and historical context of each type of substance. Indeed, a more recent study built upon the same historical data and incorporated follow-up data from the same respondents on heavy drinking in adulthood. As in the age-specific analysis, this longitudinal assessment identified stable correlates of heavy drinking at age 35 years (parental drinking, risk taking, use of cigarettes and marijuana) that did not vary across 11 cohorts.[16] This combination of historical and longitudinal data represents a valuable application of the life course perspective to distinguish age and period effects.

11.2.5 **Combinations of life course approaches**

The full potential of the life course approach can be realized through integration of the insights gained in each area reviewed above. The field is moving towards this goal, with several recent studies (all on youth smoking) effectively applying multiple components of the life course approach. A community-based study in France classified parents as non-smokers, declining smokers, and persistent smokers based on more than a decade of prospective observation, and identified increased odds of smoking among offspring. All associations were stronger for maternal smoking than paternal.[16] In another study, a nationally representative sample in the USA was used to categorize youth as early experimenters, early- or late-onset smokers, or non-smokers. The investigators assessed maternal smoking in terms of timing, amount, and periods of cessation before, during, and after pregnancy, enabling a detailed examination of risk of intergenerational transmission. Prenatal exposure was associated with increased odds of becoming a regular smoker, whereas only those children also exposed postnatally were more likely to be early onset than late onset smokers.[17] The combination of intergenerational analysis and categorization of smoking trajectories in these studies enables the identification of elevated risk associated with persistent parental smoking and provides support for multiple pathways of transmission: physiological, genetic, and parental—especially maternal—modelling of behaviour. These types of analyses are beginning to provide the insights required to apportion risk and to identify critical mediators and sites for intervention. Extending these integrated methods beyond tobacco is a critical next step.

11.3 **Synthesis of research on life course of substance use**

Research that takes a life course approach to the study of substance use suggests a key role for the broader context in shaping initiation and early substance use patterns.[12] Important contributions include the historical context that shapes norms around substance preferences;[14] substance availability may also be shaped by local geographical context.[18] Family and peer influences appear to be important, particularly use of substances, norms around substances, and supports provided.[11] Adversities and stressors in childhood play a role in early substance use patterns.[8] Some work hints at complex interactions among these factors in shaping progression in use (e.g. support from family may buffer effects of stressors);[19] however, these associations have not been comprehensively studied. Progression from early use to long term problematic use (e.g. misuse, dependence) appears to have a strong component of biological predisposition, but also has important influences from the broader context and early life exposures.[11,12,17,20] Among those who experience problematic use of a substance, there are suggestions that treatment and contexts that support cessation via norms or behaviours may enhance earlier cessation, but this is a relatively new area that requires further study.[10,21] Work describing use at the population level suggests wide variation across the life course by substance, with alcohol and marijuana peaking in late adolescence/early adulthood followed by a decline; whereas, to a greater extent than other substances, cigarette use tends to persist once initiated. However, there are insufficient studies on individual trajectories by substance to determine whether any substances show stable trajectories across geographical and historical context.

11.4 **Challenges in life course approaches to substance use**

Several challenges arise in conducting research using a life course approach; we highlight data requirements and measurement issues as the most pressing.

11.4.1 **Data over time**

Life course approaches to studying substance use necessitate that we examine and explain effects on different time-scales (i.e. age, period, and cohort effects). Further, we must layer on to those time-scales events and contextual characteristics that may influence substance use patterns in time. The simple description of patterns on different time-scales cannot be achieved without detailed longitudinal data from different birth cohorts followed over long time-periods. To assess the determinants of trajectories in time across contextual levels requires data on important elements of those contexts over time. It is perhaps obvious from this description that precious few studies will contain all of these elements; that scarcity is reflected in the relatively small body of literature on trajectories.

11.4.2 **Measurement**

To characterize patterns or trajectories of use in time relies on determination of times of onset, cessation, increase, and reduction in use. However, the time-frame queried, individual recall, and phrasing of the question may influence whether or not a time-period is characterized as a time of cessation or reduction.[22] Biological tests for substance use can be employed; however, they generally do not capture past use and add to study cost and respondent burden. Further validation work to identify optimal approaches to retrospective self-report measurement is necessary.

11.5 **Potential new directions**

Based on the existing research, there is great future potential in the extension of methods and full application of the life course approach.

11.5.1 **Extending life course methods**

11.5.1.1 Trajectory characterization

Methods to characterize trajectories have become more accessible.[23,24] An important element of moving research forward includes initial descriptive work characterizing trajectories of use for each substance in large population-based samples to assess whether general types can be identified and their frequencies assessed. Given the limited data sets that will facilitate this, development of instruments for retrospective self-report to characterize trajectories would expand the data resources available; recently such an instrument has been developed for smoking.[25] DSM guidelines are commonly used to identify lifetime or current dependence and misuse; working towards similar classifications with time-scales included would make trajectories more accessible and facilitate the inclusion of this element in a range of studies. In addition, use of trajectories as predictors of further behaviour has been limited.[26] Extending efforts to test the predictive power of trajectories against actual outcomes would strengthen the evidence for the construct validity of the categories.

11.5.1.2 Analytic approaches

Research would benefit from engaging more fully with analytic methods beyond latent growth analysis and logistic regression. Hierarchical modelling provides one approach to the challenge of including higher-level exposures such as school, neighborhood, or regional context along with individual factors. Particularly given the challenges of attrition and time-dependent confounding in longitudinal studies, methods from the causal inference literature such as propensity score weighting and plug-in estimation provide useful tools to estimate population parameters.[27,28]

11.5.2 **Full application of the life course approach**

All studies in the body of research reviewed included explicit life course questions. However, researchers generally did not frame their work in the context of the full life course approach. For example, studies of the trajectories rarely considered historical context. While it may pose an insurmountable challenge to quantify every element of every life course component (e.g. measurements of cost/availability of drugs, local/national drug policies, and norms), the historical context of any given study is important to discuss even if it is not analysed explicitly. Much would be gained by situating these studies in a broader life course framework to guide subsequent research priorities. For example, we know from existing work that there are elements of family and peer context that are important in shaping substance use trajectories, but because a full array of use behaviours, norms, and supports have not been considered across key environments in the same study, we do not have a sense of which elements may be the most important to guide intervention. Such a comprehensive assessment would also facilitate consideration of the interactions among these elements that may be important in shaping trajectories. Similarly, research on intergenerational transmission due to gestational substance use exposure does not typically assess environmental factors that may be highly correlated with parental use and thus cannot clearly distinguish biological from environmental effects. A broader, more explicit application of the life course framework would advance the field towards identification of optimal sites for population-level intervention.

11.6 **Summary**

The life course approach challenges us to face the complexities of patterns and effects across time and context throughout the life span. Framing work in this perspective can productively improve our understanding of substance use in a variety of ways. It alerts us to early events that may set patterns throughout life and that may be amenable to early preventive strategies. Consideration of the full range of pathways contributing to the development and transmission of substance use, from genetic to contextual, enables the identification of the optimal sites and time-frames for intervention. In particular, consideration of contextual factors makes it possible to identify determinants of substance use that hold potential for intervention at a population rather than individual level.

References

1 **Halfon N, Hochstein M.** Life course health development: an integrated framework for developing health, policy, and research. *Milbank Q* 2002;**80**(3):433–479, iii.

2 **Elder GH.** The life course as developmental theory. *Child Dev* 1998;**69**(1):1–12.

3 **Hser YI, Longshore D, Anglin MD.** The life course perspective on drug use—a conceptual framework for understanding drug use trajectories. *Evaluation Rev* 2007;**31**(6):515–547.

4 **Lynch J, Smith GD.** A life course approach to chronic disease epidemiology. *Annu Rev Public Health* 2005;**26**:1–35.

5 **Galea S, Nandi A, Vlahov D.** The social epidemiology of substance use. *Epidemiol Rev* 2004;**26**:36–52.

6 **Tarter RE.** Etiology of adolescent substance abuse: a developmental perspective. *Am J Addict* 2002;**11**(3):171–191.

7 **Buka SL, Shenassa ED, Niaura R.** Elevated risk of tobacco dependence among offspring of mothers who smoked during pregnancy: a 30-year prospective study. *Am J Psychiatry* 2003;**160**(11):1978–1984.

8 **Dube SR, Felitti VJ, Dong M, Chapman DP, Giles WH, Anda RF.** Childhood abuse, neglect, and household dysfunction and the risk of illicit drug use: the adverse childhood experiences study. *Pediatrics* 2003;**111**(3):564–572.

9 **Kandel DB, Logan JA.** Patterns of drug-use from adolescence to young adulthood. 1. Periods of risk for initiation, continued use, and discontinuation. *Am J Public Health* 1984;**74**(7):660–666.

10 **Genberg BL, Gange SJ, Go VF, Celentano DD, Kirk GD, Mehta SH.** Trajectories of injection drug use over 20 years (1988–2008) in Baltimore, Maryland. *Am J Epidemiol* 2011;**173**(7):829–836.

11 **Duncan TE, Tildesley E, Duncan SC, Hops H.** The consistency of family and peer influences on the development of substance use in adolescence. *Addiction* 1995;**90**(12):1647–1660.

12 **Kendler KS, Schmitt E, Aggen SH, Prescott CA.** Genetic and environmental influences on alcohol, caffeine, cannabis, and nicotine use from early adolescence to middle adulthood. *Arch Gen Psychiatry* 2008;**65**(6):674–682.

13 **O'Malley PM, Bachman JG, Johnston LD.** Period, age, and cohort effects on substance use among young Americans: a decade of change, 1976–86. *Am J Public Health* 1988;**78**(10):1315–1321.

14 **Bachman JG, Johnston LD, O'Malley PM.** Explaining the recent decline in cocaine use among young adults: further evidence that perceived risks and disapproval lead to reduced drug use. *J Health Social Behavior* 1990;**31**(2):173–184.

15 **Brown TN, Schulenberg J, Bachman JG, O'Malley PM, Johnston LD.** Are risk and protective factors for substance use consistent across historical time?: national data from the high school classes of 1976 through 1997. *Prev Sci* 2001;**2**(1):29–43.

16 **Merline A, Jager J, Schulenberg JE.** Adolescent risk factors for adult alcohol use and abuse: stability and change of predictive value across early and middle adulthood. *Addiction* 2008;**103**:84–99.

17 **Weden MM, Miles JNV.** Intergenerational relationships between the smoking patterns of a population-representative sample of US mothers and the smoking trajectories of their children. *Am J Public Health* 2012;**102**(4):723–731.

18 **Chilenski S, Greenberg M.** The importance of the community context in the epidemiology of early adolescent substance use and delinquency in a rural sample. *Am J Community Psychol* 2009;**44**(3):287–301.

19 **Hoffmann JP, Cerbone FG, Su SS.** A growth curve analysis of stress and adolescent drug use. *Subst Use Misuse* 2000;**35**(5):687–716.

20 **Melchior M, Chastang J-F, Mackinnon D, Galéra C, Fombonne E.** The intergenerational transmission of tobacco smoking—the role of parents' long-term smoking trajectories. *Drug Alcohol Depend* 2010;**107**(2–3):257–260.

21 **Karasek D, Ahern J, Galea S.** Social norms, collective efficacy, and smoking cessation in urban neighborhoods. *Am J Public Health* 2012;**102**(2):343–351.

22 **Richter L, Johnson PB.** Current methods of assessing substance use: a review of strengths, problems, and developments. *J Drug Issues* 2001;**31**(4):809–832.

23 **Jones BL, Nagin DS.** Advances in group-based trajectory modeling and a SAS procedure for estimating them. *Sociological Methods Res* 2007;**35**:542–571.

24 **Muthen B, Muthen LK.** Integrating person-centered and variable-centered analyses: growth mixture modeling with latent trajectory classes. *Alcohol Clin Exp Res* 2000;**24**(6):882–891.

25 **Colby SM, Clark MA, Rogers ML, et al.** Development and reliability of the Lifetime Interview on Smoking Trajectories. *Nicotine Tob Res* 2012;**14**(3):290–298.

26 **Duncan TE, Duncan SC, Hops H.** The role of parents and older siblings in predicting adolescent substance use: modeling development via structural equation latent growth methodology. *J Family Psychol* 1996;**10**(2):158–172.

27 **Ahern J, Hubbard A, Galea S.** Estimating the effects of potential public health interventions on population disease burden: a step-by-step illustration of causal inference methods. *Am J Epidemiol* 2009;**169**(9):1140–1147.

28 **Hernán MA, Robins JM.** Estimating causal effects from epidemiological data. *J Epidemiol Community Health* 2006;**60**(7):578–586.

Chapter 12

The life course perspective: a framework for autism research

Michaeline Bresnahan, Traolach Brugha, and Ezra Susser

12.1 Introduction

Life course studies change our understanding of health and disease by changing the temporal frame in which we view health outcomes. For adult onset diseases, reframing the causal window provides striking evidence of prenatal, infant, and childhood exposures affecting diseases as diverse as schizophrenia and cardiovascular disease. The frame may be extended to include exposures in previous generations causing heritable gene modifications (mutations, epigenetic alterations). Simultaneously, life course approaches transform the calculus of disease experience over a lifetime: we are persuaded to consider the trajectory of the disease expression over time, and its relation to other and subsequent health outcomes.

For childhood diseases such as autism a life course perspective is equally important but in a different way. Autism is a behaviourally defined neurodevelopmental disability characterized by social and communication deficits, and the presence of repetitive, ritualistic behaviours and restricted interests. By definition, it is expressed and diagnosed early in life, and, perhaps more than most developmental disorders, autism has been seen as a condition affecting children. Yet it is also generally a lifetime diagnosis, which means that the frame of reference for research and services should encompass the whole of life.

In this chapter we show how a life course perspective on autism leads us to pose different questions as well as to address familiar questions from a new standpoint. We first briefly mention methodological issues prominent in autism research as they provide an essential context, and then focus on the real and potential contributions of a life course approach to key areas of research in this disorder.

12.2 Methodological issues

The diagnostic criteria for autism and other autism spectrum disorders have undergone changes in successive versions of the DSM and ICD. The spectrum of disorders grouped as austism spectrum disorders (ASD) includes autistic disorder (AD), pervasive developmental disorder not otherwise specified (PDD-NOS), and Asperger syndrome.[1] Generally revisions to date have broadened the criteria for autism, although rarely to the extent adopted by the DSM-V where autism is subsumed in the broader category of autism spectrum disorder.[2]

Along with the exponential increase in autism research in the past decade, there has been significant improvement in the quality of research. Nonetheless some current as well as many past investigations have serious methodological limitations (e.g. the use of clinical or other convenience samples, the absence of comparison groups, small sample sizes). Furthermore, comparisons across studies are affected by differences over time and place in diagnostic classification and available services. It is important to keep this context in mind when interpreting results reported on autism, including many that are cited in this chapter.

12.3 **Life stages**

To illustrate how the life course perspective has the potential to shift the framework for research on autism and ASD, and enhance investigations of both aetiology and course of the disorder(s), a central issue will be presented for each stage of the life span.

12.3.1 **Pre- and perinatal period**

Many of the questions posed in pre- and perinatal research relate to the aetiology and early pathogenesis of autism and ASD. The importance of genetic causes of autism/ASD is well established and these disorders have a high heritability. It is now widely recognized, however, that this does not in any way preclude a major role for non-genetic factors. We suggest that understanding the nature and timing of non-genetic exposures that could affect the parental germline, or the parental or fetal epigenome in the preconception–perinatal period, is essential to unpacking causal mechanisms. A significant challenge to the study of this early period is to create/identify a window that allows observation of the fetal environment and fetal development.

Currently research on this early period is being transformed by large scale population-based research. The two most frequently adopted approaches involve registry linkage and birth cohort designs. In linked registry studies, birth registry data are linked to outcome registry data (patient registries, psychiatric registries, autism registries, educational systems), sometimes combining registries from many populations.[3] The ability to link families within registries adds power to these designs.[4,5] These studies have generated a number of highly replicated findings. Advancing paternal age at conception as a risk factor for autism has been reported in registries across many countries.[6,7] This risk factor is especially tractable to investigation, as it does not require specifying a window of observation for fetal development, until one initiates further investigations to determine the causal pathways that explain its relation to autism. The leading hypotheses advanced to explain the paternal age effect are de-novo mutations and epigenetic alterations. Some supportive evidence for de-novo mutations has emerged.[8,9]

The second approach is the large scale pregnancy/birth cohort study. This design expands the scope of investigation by including prospectively collected information on diet during pregnancy, and other environmental exposures, as well as prenatal and neonatal biological samples, ultrasound, clinical, and other data that is unavailable in most registry linkage studies. A good example is the Autism Birth Cohort study (ABC).[10] Thus far the ABC has reported evidence in support of a protective effect of periconceptional folate supplementation.[11] This is consistent with reports based on complementary methods.[12] Also intriguing is evidence suggesting that periconceptional maternal folate supplementation could be protective for severe language disorders in the same large birth cohort.[13]

12.3.2 **Infancy and early childhood**

Autism spectrum disorder (as well as autism alone) is generally understood as a syndrome characterized by concurrent manifestations that will ultimately be disentangled into more specific disorders. Charting the onset of a heterogeneous syndrome can offer a foothold for the identification of more homogeneous subtypes, which may facilitate the search for genetic and environmental causes. It can also initiate and inform intervention strategies. High risk designs, capitalizing on the elevated risk of autism in siblings of children affected with autism, have been brought to bear on this issue. Infant siblings are recruited for study, and through repeated observation and standardized assessments (e.g. behavioural, brain imaging) investigators are able to chart behaviour and developmental differences before the symptoms of ASD fully emerge. The granularity of timing in the assessments and sample size are limiting factors. A series of small high risk baby sib studies[14–17] form the basis of much of what is known about the onset of autism.

Thus far, these studies suggest that baby sibs who go on to have autism are not behaviourally distinctive at six months;[15,18] they engage in socially directed gaze, social smiling, and react comparably to the withdrawing of maternal attention.[19] Nonetheless, preliminary evidence reported by a baby sib imaging group[20] suggests that the neurological foundation for the disorder may be detectable at this age. Measurable behavioural differences do begin to emerge between 9 and 12 months of age, at least sufficient to differentiate children with typical versus atypical development along the lines seen in ASD. It has been difficult, however, to differentiate children who have ASD, or a specific subtype of ASD, among those with the multiplicity of patterns of onset of atypical development that have been observed between 12 and 24 months.[15,21–24]

There is a broad consensus that identifying these children at the earliest possible moment could increase the possibility of effective interventions. Efforts to uncover biomarkers of ultra-high risk for autism/ASD, or other endophenotype based on neurocognitive features, are underway. The identification of a useful endophenotype could ultimately be transformative but only represents a first step. Questions that will then need to be answered include: What is the positive predictive value for ASD? Why do some children with the endophenotype not go on to develop ASD? Is intervention indicated for all children with the endophenotype if many (or perhaps most) do not go on to develop ASD? Furthermore, if the endophenotype has a much higher positive predictive value for a broader range of neurodevelopmental disorder than for specifically ASD, is intervention indicated?

12.3.3 Childhood

Among the most marked and controversial early outcomes associated with a diagnosis of autism spectrum disorders is the loss of the diagnosis, which could be due to partial or full recovery.[25] The condition is considered a lifetime developmental disorder, yet instances of young children who pass through a diagnosis of any ASD are reported in clinical[26–28] and population-based[29] studies. There does not appear to be a necessary characteristic at intake with the potential to identify these children.[26] Predictors of losing an ASD diagnosis at an early age include diagnosis subtype (PDD-NOS > AD),[26–29] higher verbal and non-verbal IQ at first diagnosis,[27] and 'normal' motor skills.[26] Moving off the spectrum generally does not include moving on to a normal developmental trajectory; however, optimal outcomes are reported for a minority of those losing the diagnosis. Studies are beginning to address the leading alternative explanations of these reports—for example, that the children were initially misdiagnosed.[30]

Like the baby sibs studies of early development, the studies of the developmental trajectories in children with ASD through childhood and adolescence suggest great degree of heterogeneity in course. A longitudinal study of children with a recorded diagnosis of autism in California, utilizing educational assessment records, derived six trajectories each for communication and social symptoms between ages 3 and 14 years.[31] segregating by initial scores and velocity of improvement. A somewhat unexpected finding was the identification of a group of 'bloomers', whose initial functioning was low, but who showed a high rate of improvement that continued after age 10 years. Communication 'bloomers' comprised 7.5% and social 'bloomers' comprised 10.7% of the study population. Compared with their initial peers who were low-functioning, the 'bloomers' were more likely not to have intellectual disability, and more likely to have more educated mothers and non-minority mothers. Groups of ASD children exhibiting a high rate of improvement have also been reported by others.[32]

12.3.4 Childhood–adolescence: establishing diagnostic boundaries

Comorbid medical and psychiatric conditions and behaviours are frequently noted in association with ASD. Their presence is fundamental to the kind of services that persons with ASD require, can play a pivotal role in the course of illness, and may offer clues to aetiology. Prominent comorbid conditions include intellectual disability, language delay, epilepsy, and attention deficit/hyperactivity disorder. We are only beginning to understand the relationship between autism and each of these conditions. We can confidently anticipate that much insight into both ASD and these co-occurring disorders will be gained by prospective, rigorous examination of the natural history of both ASD and comorbid conditions that are now underway. Epilepsy is now discussed for illustration.

Although a wide range of prevalence estimates has been reported,[33] the elevated risk of epilepsy in autism is secure. A meta-analysis of 14 published reports (1963–2006) estimated the prevalence of epilepsy in ASD of 21.5% among individuals with intellectual disability and 8% among individuals with normal intelligence.[34] Peak ages of onset for epilepsy in children with autism are in early childhood and adolescence[35,36] although onset in adulthood also occurs.[37,38] Because the presence of epilepsy predicts poor outcomes in individuals with ASD, understanding the nature of the relationship between the two disorders holds great significance. Is early onset epilepsy causal? Are seizures an indication of a common cause or mechanism?[38–40] Is autism accompanied by later onset epilepsy a subtype of autism (and epilepsy)?[36] Gaining traction on these questions necessitates longitudinal observation of both disorders.

12.3.5 Adulthood

In many respects, the most pressing outcomes for public health pertain to adulthood. Most high income countries have at least some special educational services for children with ASD, but after childhood the service structure of education falls away, and individuals with ASD must make their way for decades of life—with or without family or appropriate service support.[41] Very little is known about ASD in adulthood. In the first prevalence study of ASD in a nationally representative adult population, Brugha et al.[42] reported that nearly 1% of the adult population living outside of institutions met criteria for ASD. These individuals were largely under the radar of psychiatric services. They were more likely to be male and unmarried, with little or no educational qualifications, often reliant on social support for housing.

Long term follow-up studies of individuals coming to the attention of specialist services and diagnosed in childhood report that a vast majority do not achieve independence in adulthood.[43–45] Childhood IQ and early language development are the main predictors of better outcomes in these clinically recognized cases; however, the 'better' outcomes elude even those in the higher functioning range. The most optimistic report by far is from a study in Utah that comes closer to being population-based.[46] A follow-up study focused on cases of ASD identified 20 years prior in a prevalence study[47] including only those with IQ >70 without a major medical condition that would interfere with independent living. Half were in independent employment, 16% had been married or were in long term relationships, 11% lived in their own homes or apartment, and 85% regularly attended church services. The better outcomes reported—even by comparison with studies also reporting outcome for individuals with IQ > 70 (e.g. Cedurland et al.,[45] Engstrom et al.[4])—may be in part due to community support, as well as the potential inclusion of less severe cases due to sampling methodology.

There is reason to hope that the 'better' outcomes will be more frequent for newer cohorts of adults, many of whom have received early intervention and specialized education for ASD. The adult health and human services systems will nonetheless be called upon to facilitate positive outcomes for all of those affected with ASD. Adult services research is crucial to advance the agenda.[41]

Furthermore, follow-up studies do not directly address the issue of ageing during adulthood. Adults are, by and large, treated as one group of 'not children'. The complexity of examining age effects in a heterogeneous population, with heterogeneous early life experience and heterogeneous disease, must also be confronted with meaningful research and analysis.[49,50] Age-related changes in phenotype are vital for service planning. Understanding these changes later in the life course may also, however, illuminate the nature of ASD and perhaps other disorders. This possibility is underscored by studies of Down syndrome, in which (among other things) early onset of Alzheimer disease has been documented.

12.5 **Summary**

Perhaps more than most developmental disorders, autism has been seen as a condition affecting children. In this brief review we have illustrated the potential for a life course framework to greatly accelerate understanding of autism/ASD. The essence of this perspective is to shift in frame of reference for research and services so as to encompass the whole of life and all of those affected.

References

1 **American Psychiatric Association.** *Diagnostic and statistical manual of mental disorders.* 4th ed. text revision (DSM-IV-TR). Washington DC; APA; 2000.

2 **American Psychiatric Association.** *Diagnostic and statistical manual of mental disorders.* 5th edition (DMS-V). Washington DC; APA; 2013.

3 **Schendel D, Bresnahan M, Carter K, et al.** The International Collaboration for Autism Registry Epidemiology (iCARE): multinational registry-based investigations of autism risk factors and trends. *J Autism Dev Disord* 2013 Apr 7 [Epub ahead of print].

4 **Cheslack-Postava K, Liu K, Bearman PS.** Closely spaced pregnancies are associated with increased odds of autism in California sibling births. *Pediatrics* 2011;**127**(2):246–253.

5 **Frans EM, McGrath JJ, Sandin S, et al.** Advanced paternal and grandpaternal age and schizophrenia: a three-generation perspective. *Schizophr Res* 2011;**133**(1–3):120–124.

6 **Croen LA, Najjar DV, Fireman B, Grether JK.** Maternal and paternal age and risk of autism spectrum disorders. *Arch Pediatr Adolesc Med* 2007;**161**(4):334–340.

7 **Hultman CM, Sandin S, Levine SZ, Lichtenstein P, Reichenberg A.** Advancing paternal age and risk of autism: new evidence from a population-based study and a meta-analysis of epidemiologic studies. *Mol Psychiatry* 2011;**16**(12):1203–1212.

8 **Kong A, Frigge ML, Masson G, et al.** Rate of de novo mutations and the importance of father's age to disease risk. *Nature* 2012; **488**(7412):471–475.

9 **Sanders SJ, Murtha MT, Gupta AR, et al.** De novo mutations revealed by whole-exome sequencing are strongly associated with autism. *Nature* 2012;**485**(7397):237–241.

10 Stoltenberg C, Schjølberg S, Bresnahan M, et al. ABC Study Group. The Autism Birth Cohort: a paradigm for gene–environment–timing research. *Mol Psychiatry* 2010;**15**(7):676–680.

11 Surén P, Roth C, Bresnahan M, et al. Folic acid supplements in pregnancy and autism in children. *JAMA* 2013;**309**(6):570–577.

12 Schmidt RJ, Hansen R, Hartiala J, et al. Prenatal vitamins, one-carbon metabolism gene variants and risk for autism. *Epidemiology* 2011;**22**(4):476–485.

13 Roth C, Magnus P, Schjolberg S, et al. Folic acid supplements in pregnancy and severe language delay in children. *JAMA* 2011;**306**(14):1566–1573.

14 Landa RJ, Holman KC, Garrett-Mayer E. Social and communication development in toddlers with early and later diagnosis of autism spectrum disorders. *Arch Gen Psychiatry* 2007;**64**(7):853–64.

15 Ozonoff S, Iosif AM, Baguio F, et al. A prospective study of the emergence of early behavioral signs of autism. *Am Acad Child Adolesc Psychiatry* 2010;**49**(3):256–266.e1–2.

16 Zwaigenbaum L, Thurm A, Stone W, et al. Studying the emergence of autism spectrum disorders in high risk infants: methodological and practical issues. *J Autism Dev Disord* 2007;**37**(3):466–480.

17 Tager Flusberg H. The origins of social impairments in autism spectrum disorder: studies of infants at risk. *Neural Netw* 2010;**23**(9):1072–1076.

18 Rogers SJ. What are infant siblings teaching us about autism in infancy? *Autism Res* 2009;**2**(3):125–137.

19 Rozga A, Hutman T, Young GS, et al. Behavioral profiles of affected and unaffected siblings of children with autism: contribution of measures of mother–infant interaction and nonverbal communication. *J Autism Dev Disord* 2011;**41**(3):287–301.

20 Wolff JJ, Gu H, Gerig G, et al. Differences in white matter fiber tract development present from 6 to 24 months in infants with autism. *Am J Psychiatry* 2012;**169**(6):589–600.

21 Macari S, Campbell D, Gengoux GW, Saulnier CA, Klin AJ, Chawarska K. Predicting developmental status from 12 to 24 months in infants at risk for autism spectrum disorder: a preliminary report. *J Autism Dev Disord* 2012;**42**(12):2636–2647.

22 Werner E, Dawson G. Validation of the phenomenon of autistic regression using home videotapes. *Arch Gen Psychiatry* 2005;**62**(8):889–895.

23 Landa RJ, Gross AL, Stuart EA, Bauman M. Latent class analysis of early developmental trajectory in baby siblings of children with autism. *J Child Psychol Psychiatry* 2012;**53**(9):986–996.

24 Lord C, Luyster R, Guthrie W, Pickles A. Patterns of developmental trajectories in toddlers with autism spectrum disorders. *J Consult Clin Psychol* 2012;**80**(3):477–489.

25 Helt M, Kelley E, Kinsbourne M, et al. Can children with autism recover? If so, how? *Neuropsychol Rev* 2008;**18**(4):339–366.

26 Sutera S, Pandly J, Essser EI, et al. Predictors of optimal outcome in toddlers diagnosed with autism spectrum disorders. *J Autism Dev Disord* 2007;**37**(1):98–107.

27 Turner L, Stone WL. Variability in outcome for children with an ASD diagnosis at age 2. *J Child Psychol Psychiatry* 2007;**48**(8):793–802.

28 Lord C, Risi S, diLavore PS, Shulman C, Thurm A, Pickles A. Autism from 2 to 9 years of age. *Arch Gen Psychiatry* 2006;**63**(6):694–701.

29 van Daalen E, Kemner C, Dietz C, Swinkels S, Buitelaar J, van Engeland H. Inter-rater reliability and stability of diagnoses of autism spectrum disorder in children identified through screening at a very young age. *Eur Child Adolesc Psychiatry* 2009;**18**(11):663–674.

30 Fein D, Barton M, Eigsti IM, et al. Optimal outcome in individuals with a history of autism. *J Child Psychol Psychiatry* 2013;**54**(2):195–205.

31 Fountain C, Winter AS, Bearman PS. Six developmental trajectories characterize children with autism. *Pediatrics* 2012;**129**(5):e1112–e1120.

32 Anderson DK, Oti RS, Lord C, Welch K. Patterns of growth in adaptive social abilities among children with autism spectrum disorders. *J Abnorm Child Psychol* 2009;**37**(7):1019–1034.

33 Tuchman R, Cuccaro M, Alessandri M. Autism and epilepsy: historical perspective. *Brain Dev* 2010;**32**(9):709–718.

34 Amiet C, Gourfinkel-An I, Bouzamondo A, et al. Epilepsy in autism is associated with intellectual disability and gender: evidence from a meta-analysis. *Biol Psychiatry* 2008;**64**(7):577–582.

35 Volkmar FR, Nelson DS. Seizure disorders in autism. *J Am Acad Child Adolesc Psychiatry* 1990;**29**(1):127–129.

36 Hara H. Autism in epilepsy: a retrospective follow-up study. *Brain Dev* 2007;**29**(8):486–490.

37 Bolton PF, Carcani-Rathwell I, Hutton J, Goode S, Howlin P, Rutter M. Epilepsy in autism: features and correlates. *Br J Psychiatry* 2011;**198**(4):289–294.

38 Saemundsen E, Ludvigsson P, Rafnsson V. Risk of autism spectrum disorders after infantile spasms: a population-based study nested in a cohort with seizures in the first year of life. *Epilepsia* 2008;**49**(11):1865–1870.

39 Brooks-Kayal A. Epilepsy and autism spectrum disorders: are there common developmental mechanisms? *Brain Dev* 2010;**32**(9):731–738.

40 Simonoff E, Pickles A, Charman T, Chandler S, Loucas T, Baird G. Psychiatric disorders in children with autism spectrum disorders: prevalence, comorbidity and associated factors in a population-derived sample. *J Am Acad Child Adolesc Psychiatry* 2008;**47**(8):921–929.

41 Bresnahan M, Li G, Susser E. Hidden in plain sight. *Int J Epidemiol* 2009; **38**(5):1172–1174.

42 Brugha TS, McManus S, Bankart J, et al. Epidemiology of autism spectrum disorders in adults in the community in England. *Arch Gen Psychiatry* 2011;**68**(5):459–466.

43 Howlin P, Goode S, Hutton J, Rutter M. Adult outcome for children with autism. *J Child Psychol Psychiatry* 2004;**45**(2):561–578.

44 Billstedt E, Gillberg C, Gillberg C. Autism after adolescence: population based 13–22 year follow-up study of 120 individuals with autism diagnosed in childhood. *J Autism Dev Disord* 2005;**35**(3):351–260.

45 Cedurland M, Hagberg B, Billstedt E, Gillberg IC, Gillberg C. Asperger syndrome and autism: a comparative longitudinal follow-up study more than 5 years after original diagnosis. *J Autism Dev Disord* 2008;**38**(1):72–85.

46 Farley MA, McMahon WM, Fombonne E, et al. Twenty-year outcome for individuals with autism and average or near-average cognitive abilities. *Autism Res* 2009;**2**(2):109–118.

47 Ritov ER, Freeman BJ, Pingree C, et al. The UCLA-University of Utah epidemiologic survey of autism prevalence. *Am J Psychiatry* 1989;**146**(2):194–199.

48 Engstrom I, Ekstrom L, Emilsson B. Psychosocial functioning in a group of Swedish adults with Asperger syndrome or high-functioning autism. *Autism* 2003;**7**(1):99–110.

49 Happe F, Charlton RA. Aging in autism spectrum disorders: a mini-review. *Gerontology* 2012;**58**(1): 70–77.

50 Mukaetova-Landinska EB, Perry E, Baron M, Povey C; Autism Ageing Writing Group. Ageing in people with autistic spectrum disorder. *Int J Geriatr Psychiatry* 2012;**27**(2):109–118.

Chapter 13

Life course epidemiology of eating disorders

Karen S. Mitchell and Cynthia M. Bulik

13.1 Introduction

Eating disorders (EDs) are pernicious conditions with among the highest mortality rates of any psychiatric disorder.[1] The EDs included in DSM-IV-TR[2] are anorexia nervosa (AN), characterized by extremely low weight and fear of gaining weight; bulimia nervosa (BN), characterized by binge eating episodes followed by use of inappropriate compensatory behaviours; binge eating disorder (BED; as a criteria set for further study), the key feature of which is binge eating episodes that are not accompanied by compensatory behaviours; and eating disorder not otherwise specified (EDNOS), which encompasses a variety of clinical presentations that do not fit the criteria for the three aforementioned disorders. Population-based studies have shown that EDs affect approximately 0.9–3.5% of women, and 0.3–2.0% of men, in their lifetimes.[3] However, men as well as ethnic minorities remain relatively understudied in this field, due to longstanding beliefs that EDs primarily affect Caucasian, middle- and upper-class young women. Not only have many of our investigations not included men and ethnic minorities, but our basic definitions of illness may preclude detection of gender-based and culturally influenced variants in clinical presentation. Further, the current epidemiologic landscape of EDs is incomplete. For example, we have strikingly few estimates of incidence in general, no studies of incidence in women or men in their thirties or beyond, and little consensus regarding the nature and extent of differences in clinical presentation from childhood through late adulthood.

This chapter explores a life course approach to investigation of EDs. Currently, these disorders are examined most frequently in samples of adolescent and young adult women. Yet, findings about the influence of the early environment,[4–6] and the prevalence of ED symptoms in women aged >50 years,[7] emphasize the importance of studying these disorders across varying developmental periods. Only clear data from prospective epidemiological studies, and/or cross sectional studies including participants from diverse groups, will counteract stereotypes and eliminate the bias that EDs affect only young, Caucasian women.

13.2 Age of onset for eating disorders

To date, there have been two nationally representative studies in the USA that included ED assessments. The National Comorbidity Survey—Replication study (NCS-R) of adults aged ≥18 years found that the mean age of onset of AN in men and women combined was 18.9 years; age of onset for BN was 19.7 years and for BED was 25.4 years.[3] By contrast, the NCS—Adolescent Supplement (NCS-A) found that median ages of onset were 12.3 years (AN), 12.4 years (BN), and 12.6 years (BED) among the total sample of boys and girls.[8] It is possible that retrospective studies of adults overestimate ages of onset; alternatively, individuals may develop EDs later than the sampling window of the NCS-A (ages 13–17 years).

13.3 **Prevalence of eating disorders**

In the NCS-R, lifetime rates of AN, BN, and BED were 0.9%, 1.5%, and 3.5%, respectively, among women, and 0.3%, 0.5%, and 2% among men,[3] which were similar to estimates from previous US population-based studies.[9,10] The 12-month prevalence estimates of BN and BED in the NCS-R were 0.5 and 1.6 among women and 0.1 and 0.8, respectively, among men. Notably, despite previous findings that men comprise only 10% of ED cases,[2] Hudson et al.[3] found that approximately 25% of cases identified in the NCS-R interview were male.

Among adolescent participants in the NCS-A, lifetime prevalence estimates of AN, BN, and BED were 0.3%, 1.3%, and 2.3%, respectively, in girls and 0.3%, 0.5%, and 0.8% in boys.[8] Again, the female:male ratio of EDs across disorders was quite a bit lower than the 9:1 ratio reported in DSM-IV-TR,[2] underscoring the importance of population-based epidemiological studies, which include groups traditionally underrepresented in treatment-seeking samples.

13.4 **Risk factors for eating disorders**

EDs are multifactorial conditions that likely are determined through myriad interactions among biological mechanisms, genes, and psychosocial variables. Psychosocial variables which have been shown to precede the onsets of EDs include weight concerns, negative body image, and dieting.[11] It is critical to note that the study of risk factors in EDs is complicated by several issues. However, it is difficult to determine the potency of these risk factors, as many of these dimensions, such as body dissatisfaction and dieting, are nearly ubiquitous in the primarily Caucasian samples studied in ED research. In addition, these symptoms may actually be prodromal indices of these disorders and may indicate early presentations, rather than indexing risk. In many ways, identifying risk factors that are independent of the weight and shape and eating symptoms may afford earlier detection and prevention.

13.4.1 **Genetic risk factors**

There has been an increased focus on the genetic architecture of EDs, although there is much left to be discovered. Twin studies have demonstrated that 40–50% of the variance of AN, BN, and BED is due to genetic factors.[12] Molecular genetic studies of EDs have trailed the path of psychiatric genetics in general. The majority of early investigations applied candidate-gene methods, which attempt statistically to associate specific genes or single nucleotide polymorphisms (SNPs) with a given trait. Unfortunately, the typical pattern of these investigations has been early identification of association followed by a parade of mixed replication and non-replication.[13]

Significant findings have implicated genes in the serotonin system,[14,15] brain-derived neurotophic factor,[16] ovarian hormone,[17] dopamine system genes,[18] and the delta opiod receptor-1[19] in the aetiology of EDs. However, although these studies collectively may tell a story, they must be interpreted with extreme caution, as we do not yet have sufficiently robust and adequately statistically powered investigations needed to draw any clear conclusions.

Given the issues of lack of power and replicability in candidate gene association studies, more innovative approaches, including genome-wide association studies (GWAS) and sequencing, are currently being explored. However, due to the very large number of statistical comparisons in GWAS, a strict correction for multiple testing is required. In the case of psychiatric phenotypes with low prevalences, such as EDs, it can be quite difficult to achieve the large sample sizes necessary to provide adequate power. Two GWAS have been published, including one investigation of AN[20] and another of ED-related phenotypes, including drive for thinness, body dissatisfaction, bulimia symptoms, childhood obsessive-compulsive personality disorder traits, breakfast-skipping, and weight fluctuation.[21] No SNPs reached genome-wide significance in either study. Another, larger global GWAS is currently underway as part of the Wellcome Trust Case Control Consortium 3.

Next generation sequencing, including whole exome (protein-coding region) and whole genome, potentially may be useful for psychiatric phenotypes. Exome sequencing is best suited for the discovery of rare variants (i.e. <5% of the population), which may be relevant to EDs.[22] In addition, investigation of copy number variations offers potentially useful approaches to the continued discovery of the genetic basis of EDs. As these methods become more powerful and less expensive, they can be more easily incorporated into large, epidemiological studies.

13.4.2 Gene–environment interactions

Given the presumed strong influence of the psychosocial environment on the development of EDs,[11] gene–environment interactions (G × E) likely play an important role in the aetiology of these conditions.[23] For example, there is some evidence that factors such as trauma (e.g. childhood sexual, physical, or emotional abuse) or dieting may trigger vulnerability to ED behaviours.[15]

In addition, epigenetic changes, which alter the expression but not the structure of DNA, are one type of G × E interaction. Prenatal and early postnatal exposures can cause changes in the offspring that initially are adaptive but later increase risk to pathology.[24] For example, there is evidence that prenatal maternal stress, maternal diet, obesity, and diabetes can impact DNA methylation and offspring health.[25] Relative to women without EDs, individuals with EDs have demonstrated differential diets during pregnancy, weight gain trajectories during and after pregnancy, caesarean section rates, and breastfeeding practices.[26] However, no studies have yet merged these epidemiological observations with epigenetic methods. Findings regarding the dynamic nature of some epigenetic patterns[27] underscore the importance of investigation of these factors across developmental periods.

13.5 Childhood and adolescence

Several early childhood factors have been associated with increased risk for EDs, although it is important to note that these are non-specific risk factors.[28] For example, a longitudinal study revealed that childhood physical neglect, sexual abuse, poverty, low parental education, and maladaptive paternal behaviours were associated with ED behaviours in adolescence and adulthood.[4] Early feeding and eating practices also have been associated with increased risk for EDs later in life.[11] For example, in a large Norwegian birth cohort, we found that mothers with BN and BED were more likely to report restrictive feeding styles and child eating problems than mothers without EDs.[29]

Adolescence may be a particularly vulnerable window for the development of EDs. Longitudinal studies in middle and high school-aged girls have demonstrated associations among low self-esteem, weight concerns, dietary restraint, body dissatisfaction, depression, negative emotionality, early maturation, and being overweight with EDs.[30] Adolescents, particularly girls, may be susceptible to social pressures to be thin, which can increase risk for EDs.[31] Finally, teasing about weight also has been associated with increased risk for EDs among girls and boys in longitudinal studies.[32]

Puberty also may represent a period of increased vulnerability to EDs due to changes in hormones and, possibly, gene expression levels. Twin studies have demonstrated that genetic factors had little to no impact on ED behaviours among pre-pubertal girls. However, in pubertal and post-pubertal females, the contributions of genetics and the environment were similar to those reported in adult samples. Moreover, there may be sex differences in the magnitude of these effects before puberty.[33] These findings suggest that specific pubertal factors, as well as socio-cultural influences, influence the development of EDs among girls. However, there is a need for future epidemiological studies in younger samples that capture incidence of both threshold and sub-threshold EDs.[34]

13.6 **Young adulthood**

The age of onset for AN and BN seems to peak by age 21 years, around the time that many women have entered college. Indeed, previous studies have found elevated rates of sub-threshold disordered eating behaviours among college students.[35] Thus, much of the aforementioned risk factor research has been conducted in this age group. There is evidence that ED symptoms and cases which begin during adolescence remain stable through at least young adulthood; however, the longitudinal course of EDs has been less frequently studied.[5]

There is a need for further study of ED onset across developmental periods. For example, Kimura et al.[36] found that women with AN onset after age 25 years had slightly lower body mass index (BMI) than did women in the 'peak' (age 15–24 years) onset group. In a multisite sample, Bueno et al.[37] found that women with onset after age 25 years reported lower rates of weekly vomiting, less drive for thinness, less impulsivity, higher BMI, and more harm avoidance than did women whose ED began earlier (mean: 17.4 years). These findings suggest that, among western but not Asian samples, late onset EDs may be associated with less pathology.

The onset of EDs has been less frequently studied among women aged >25 years; however, a growing body of literature focuses on the impact of pregnancy, the postpartum period, and the transition to motherhood on the onset and course of EDs. Symptoms may remit in pregnancy, as women seek to practice healthy eating behaviours for the sake of the developing fetus.[38] However, although pregnancy may be protective for purging and other compensatory behaviours, it is potentially a vulnerable time for binge eating, due to neuroendocrine, metabolic, mood, and appetite changes, and psychological stress.[38,39] These findings underscore the need to assess ED symptomatology among pregnant and newly postpartum women.

13.7 **Middle–late adulthood**

Eating disorders are much less frequently investigated among older samples. As high rates of relapse have been observed for EDs,[40] only 50% of EDs remit following treatment, on average,[41] and as BN symptoms may remain stable over time,[42] it is possible that EDs continue into late adulthood among some individuals. Further, evidence suggests that body dissatisfaction and thin-ideal internalization persist into middle and late adulthood,[7] and the incidence of EDs among middle-aged women may be increasing.[43] Several sociocultural factors may account for these increased rates. Emphasis on plastic surgery in the current media may result in increased pressure on middle-aged individuals to pursue unrealistically thin, and youthful, physiques.[44] In addition, concerns specific to this age group, such as one's ageing appearance, deaths of loved ones, the 'empty nest', and loss of youth, also might trigger vulnerability to ED symptoms.[45]

Some EDs among middle-aged and elderly individuals may be a continuation of illness that begins during adolescence or young adulthood. However, there is evidence for de-novo EDs in women and men aged ≥60 years.[46] In a review of 48 case reports of EDs in men and women aged ≥50 years, Lapid et al.[47] observed that AN was the most frequent diagnosis (81%). Of the late onset cases, 58% had an onset between the ages of 45 and 62 years, and 33% had an onset after the age of 65 years. Of these cases, 42% reported successful outcomes; however, 21% of these individuals died due to the ED or related medical complications. Given cohort effects on EDs, the ageing population of baby boomers may lead to an increase in rates of EDs among the elderly. The elevated risk for medical complications secondary to EDs among older individuals[47] underscores the need for assessment and intervention among women, as well as men, of all ages.

13.8 Eating disorders among racially diverse groups

There have been inconsistent results across studies regarding the prevalence of EDs among racially and ethnically diverse groups. Findings from clinical samples have reported lower rates of EDs among minority women.[48] Notably, however, the prevalence of EDs did not differ by ethnic group in the NCS-R.[3] In the NCS-A, Hispanic adolescents had significantly higher rates of BN than did other ethnic groups.[8] Thus, African-American and Hispanic women appear to experience clinically significant levels of eating pathology. Importantly, the literature demonstrates a reduced likelihood of treatment-seeking, and treatment referrals, for minority women compared with Caucasian women,[49] possibly due to the perception that EDs are far less prevalent among other racial groups or stigmatization of EDs within their culture.

13.9 Summary

There is a strong need for prospective, longitudinal investigations of ED epidemiology and risk factors. Many extant birth cohorts have not included ED assessments, perhaps due to the misperception that these disorders are rare and to the lack of consensus in the field about how best to characterize childhood EDs. The Growing Up Today Study, Avon Longitudinal Study of Parents and Children, and Norwegian Mother and Child Cohort Study are three notable exceptions; however, they include primarily Caucasian participants. In addition, the lack of inclusion of a full spectrum of ED symptomatology in epidemiological studies may result in under-assessment of symptoms more relevant to younger as well as older individuals.[50]

In sum, epidemiological studies of EDs would benefit from a life course approach that takes into account a broad range of psychosocial, cultural, biological, and genetic factors that influence these conditions. Older adults, men, and ethnic/racial minority groups remain under-served in this area, possibly secondary to the nature of the diagnostic criteria or inaccurate stereotypes of who suffers from EDs. Further investigation is needed in order to elucidate aetiological mechanisms across stages of development and inform prevention and intervention for women and men of all ages.

References

1 **Sullivan P.** Mortality in anorexia nervosa. *Am J Psychiatry* 1995;**152**;1073–1074.
2 **American Psychiatric Association.** *Diagnostic and statistical manual of mental disorders.* 4th ed. Text revision. Washington DC: APA; 2000.
3 **Hudson JI, Hiripi E, Pope Jr HG, Kessler RC.** The prevalence and correlates of eating disorders in the National Comorbidity Survey Replication. *Biol Psychiatry* 2007;**61**:348–358.

4 **Johnson JG, Cohen P, Kasen S, Brook JS.** Childhood adversities associated with risk for eating disorders or weight problems during adolescence or early adulthood. *Am J Psychiatry* 2002;**159**:394–400.

5 **Kotler LA, Cohen P, Davies M, Pine DS, Walsh BT.** Longitudinal relationships between childhood, adolescent, and adult eating disorders. *J Am Acad Child Adolesc Psychiatry* 2001;**40**:1434–1440.

6 **Birch LL, Fisher JO.** Development of eating behaviors among children and adolescents. *Pediatrics* 1998;**101**:539–549.

7 **Gagne DA, Von Holle A, Brownley KA, et al.** Eating disorder symptoms and weight and shape concerns in a large web-based convenience sample of women ages 50 and above: results of the Gender and Body Image (GABI) study. *Int J Eat Disord* 2012;**45**:832–844.

8 **Swanson SA, Crow SJ, Le Grange D, Swendsen J, Merikangas KR.** Prevalence and correlates of eating disorders in adolescents. Results from the national comorbidity survey replication adolescent supplement. *Arch Gen Psychiatry* 2011;**68**:714–723.

9 **Kendler KS, MacLean C, Neale M, Kessler R, Heath A, Eaves L.** The genetic epidemiology of bulimia nervosa. *Am J Psychiatry* 1991;**148**:1627–1637.

10 **Walters EE, Kendler KS.** Anorexia nervosa and anorexic-like syndromes in a population-based female twin sample. *Am J Psychiatry* 1995;**152**:64–71.

11 **Jacobi C, Hayward C, de Zwaan M, Kraemer HC, Agras WS.** Coming to terms with risk factors for eating disorders: application of risk terminology and suggestions for a general taxonomy. *Psychol Bull* 2004;**130**:19–65.

12 **Mazzeo SE, Slof-Op 't Landt MCT, van Furth EF, Bulik CM.** Genetics of eating disorders. In: Wonderlich SA, Mitchell JE, De Zwaan M, Steiger H, editors. *Annual review of eating disorders—Part 2*. Oxford: Radcliffe Publishing; 2006. pp. 17–31.

13 **Pinheiro AP, Bulik CM, Thornton LM, et al.** Association study of 182 candidate genes in anorexia nervosa. *Am J Med Genet B Neuropsychiatr Genet* 2010;**53B**:1070–1080.

14 **Di Bella D, Catalano M, Cavallini MC, Riboldi C, Bellodi L.** Serotonin transporter linked polymorphic region in anorexia nervosa and bulimia nervosa. *Mol Psychiatry* 2000;**5**:233–234.

15 **Steiger H, Joober R, Israel M, et al.** The 5HTTLPR polymorphism, psychopathologic symptoms, and platelet [3H-] paroxetine binding in bulimic syndromes. *Int J Eat Disord* 2005;**37**:57–60.

16 **Ribases M, Gratacos M, Fernandez-Aranda F, et al.** Association of BDNF with anorexia, bulimia and age of onset of weight loss in six European populations. *Hum Mol Genet* 2004;**13**:1205–1212.

17 **Klump KL, Gobrogge KL.** A review and primer of molecular genetic studies of anorexia nervosa. *Int J Eat Disord* 2005;**37**(Suppl):S43–48; discussion S87–89.

18 **Bergen AW, Yeager M, Welch RA, et al.** Association of multiple DRD2 polymorphisms with anorexia nervosa. *Neuropsychopharmacology* 2005;**30**:1703–1710.

19 **Brown KM, Bujac SR, Mann ET, Campbell DA, Stubbins MJ, Blundell JE.** Further evidence of association of OPRD1 & HTR1D polymorphisms with susceptibility to anorexia nervosa. *Biol Psychiatry* 2007;**61**:367–373.

20 **Wang K, Zhang H, Bloss CS, et al.** A genome-wide association study on common SNPs and rare CNVs in anorexia nervosa. *Mol Psychiatry* 2011;**16**:949–959.

21 **Boraska V, Davis OSP, Cherkas LF, et al.** Genome wide association analysis of eating disorder-related symptoms, behaviors, and personality characteristics. *Am J Med Genet B Neuropsychiatr Genet* 2012;**159B**:803–811.

22 **Uher R.** The role of genetic variation in the causation of mental illness: an evolution-informed framework. *Mol Psychiatry* 2009;**14**:1072–1082.

23 **Bulik CM.** Exploring the gene–environment nexus in eating disorders. *J Psychiatry Neurosci* 2005;**30**:335–339.

24 **Barker DJ.** The developmental origins of adult disease. *J Am Coll Nutr* 2004;**23**:588S–595S.

25 Attig L, Gabory A, Junien C. Nutritional developmental epigenomics: immediate and long-lasting effects. *Proc Nutr Soc* 2010;**69**:221–231.

26 Micali N, Treasure J. Biological effects of a maternal ED on pregnancy and foetal development: a review. *Eur Eating Disord Rev* 2009;**17**:448–454.

27 Campbell IC, Mill J, Uher R, Schmidt U. Eating disorders, gene–environment interactions, and epigenetics. *Neurosci Biobehav Rev* 2011;**35**:784–793.

28 Bulik CM, Prescott CA, Kendler KS. Features of childhood sexual abuse and the development of psychiatric and substance use disorders. *Br J Psychiatry* 2001;**179**:444–449.

29 Reba-Harreleson L, Von Holle A, Hamer RM, Torgersen L, Reichborn-Kjennerud T, Bulik CM. Patterns of maternal feeding and child eating associated with eating disorders in the Norwegian Mother and Child Cohort Study (MoBa). *Eat Behav* 2010;**11**:54–61.

30 Shisslak CM, Crago M. Risk and protective factors in the development of eating disorders. In: Thompson JK, Smolak L editors. *Body image, eating disorders, and obesity in youth.* Washington DC: American Psychological Association; 2001. pp. 103–125.

31 McKnight Investigators. Risk factors for the onset of eating disorders in adolescent girls: results of the McKnight Longitudinal Risk Factor Survey. *Am J Psychiatry* 2003;**160**:248–254.

32 Haines J, Neumark-Sztainer D, Eisenberg ME, Hannan PJ. Weight teasing and disordered eating behaviors in adolescents: longitudinal findings from Project EAT (Eating Among Teens). *Pediatrics* 2006;**117**:e209–e215.

33 Klump KL, Culbert KM, Slane JD, Burt SA, Sisk CL, Nigg JT. The effects of puberty on genetic risk for disordered eating: evidence for a sex difference. *Psychol Med* 2012;**42**:627–637.

34 Lewinsohn PM, Striegel-Moore RH, Seeley JR. Epidemiology and natural course of eating disorders in young women from adolescence to young adulthood. *J Am Acad Child Adolesc Psychiatry* 2000;**39**:1284–1292.

35 Mitchell KS, Mazzeo SE. Binge eating and psychological distress in ethnically diverse undergraduate men and women. *Eat Behav* 2004;**5**:157–169.

36 Kimura H, Tonoike T, Muroya T, Yoshida K, Ozaki N. Age of onset has limited association with body mass index at time of presentation for anorexia nervosa: comparison of peak-onset and late-onset anorexia nervosa groups. *Psychiatry Clin Neurosci* 2007;**61**:646–650.

37 Bueno-Julia-Capmany B, Krug I, Jiménez-Murcia S, et al. Late onset eating disorders in Spain: clinical and therapeutic implications. *J Clin Psychol* (in press).

38 Morgan JF, Lacey JH, Sedgwick PM. Impact of pregnancy on bulimia nervosa. *Br J Psychiatry* 1999;**174**:135–140.

39 Bulik CM, Von Holle A, Hamer R, et al. Patterns of remission, continuation and incidence of broadly defined eating disorders during early pregnancy in the Norwegian Mother and Child Cohort Study (MoBa). *Psychol Med* 2007;**37**:1109–1118.

40 Keel PK, Dorer DJ, Franko DL, Jackson SC, Herzog DB. Postremission predictors of relapse in women with eating disorders. *Am J Psychiatry* 2005;**162**:2263–2268.

41 British Psychological Society and Royal College of Psychiatrists. *National Practice Guideline Number CG69.* London: BPS & RCP; 2004.

42 Procopio CA, Holm-Denoma JM, Gordon KH, Joiner TE, Jr. Two-three-year stability and interrelations of bulimotypic indicators and depressive and anxious symptoms in middle-aged women. *Int J Eat Disord* 2006;**39**:312–319.

43 Wiseman CV, Sunday SR, Klapper F, Harris WA, Halmi KA. Changing patterns of hospitalization in eating disorder patients. *Int J Eat Disord* 2001;**30**:69–74.

44 Midlarsky E, Nitzburg G. Eating disorders in middle-aged women. *J Gen Psychol* 2008;**135**:393–407.

45 Zerbe K, Domnitei D. Eating disorders at middle age, parts 1 and 2. *Eating Disorders Rev* 2004;**15**:1–2.

46 Beck D, Casper R, Andersen A. Truly late onset of eating disorders: a study of 11 cases averaging 60 years of age at presentation. *Int J Eat Disord* 1996;**20**:389–395.

47 Lapid MI, Prom MC, Burton MC, McAlpine DE, Sutor B, Rummans TA. Eating disorders in the elderly. *Int Psychogeriatr* 2010;**22**:523–536.

48 Striegel-Moore RH, Cachelin FM. Etiology of eating disorders in women. *Counseling Psychologist* 2001;**29**:635–661.

49 Becker AE, Franko DL, Speck A, Herzog DB. Ethnicity and differential access to care for eating disorder symptoms. *Int J Eat Disord* 2003;**33**:205–212.

50 Wade TD, Bergin JL, Tiggemann M, Bulik CM, Fairburn CG. Prevalence and long-term course of lifetime eating disorders in an adult Australian twin cohort. *Aust NZ J Psychiatry* 2006;**40**:121–128.

Chapter 14

Attention deficit/hyperactivity disorder over the life course

Jessica Agnew-Blais and Larry J. Seidman

14.1 Introduction: ADHD prevalence and diagnosis

Attention deficit/hyperactivity disorder (ADHD) affects ~3–9% of the school-age population in the USA[1,2] and accounts for up to half of the children seen for psychiatric services.[3] A diagnosis of ADHD is characterized by six or more symptoms of inattention (such as being easily distracted and forgetful) or impulsivity/hyperactivity (such as fidgeting and excessive talking). DSM criteria for ADHD require that symptoms be pervasive (occur in at least two settings) and cause impairment for at least six months. Importantly, these criteria also require that symptoms be inappropriate for the individual's developmental level,[4] (Barkley,[5] p. 99).

While ADHD was originally described as a disorder limited to childhood,[6] research now suggests that a moderate to large proportion of children with ADHD will continue to have symptoms into adolescence and adulthood.[7] In this chapter, we discuss ADHD symptom profile, gender breakdown, comorbidities and associated problems, risk factors, persistence into adolescence and adulthood, and methodological issues.

14.2 Symptoms over the life course

The age of onset for ADHD is specified in the DSM-5 as before age 12 years,[8] up from age 7 in the prior version of the manual.[4] While diagnosis appears to be valid in children as young as age 4 years,[9] it is not clear that ADHD can be accurately identified or disentangled from other disorders at younger ages.[10] Pre-school children who later develop ADHD may exhibit symptoms of hyperactivity, oppositional behaviour, and sleep disturbance.[3] Symptoms of ADHD have been found to be relatively consistent from childhood through adolescence[11,12] but may manifest somewhat differently in adulthood. Adults with ADHD tend to have more symptoms of inattention than hyperactivity,[13] and when adults do endorse symptoms of hyperactivity, they are typically described as feelings of internal restlessness, rather than gross motor hyperactivity (Barkley,[5] p. 83).

14.3 Gender differences in ADHD

Women and girls with ADHD have generally been understudied.[14] Boys are more likely to be diagnosed with ADHD, but the difference between the ratio of males to females in clinical populations (about 9:1)[4] compared with community populations (about 3:1)[15] suggests potential referral bias.[16] Core symptoms of ADHD are generally similar between boys and girls, but girls exhibit less hyperactivity and comorbid conduct disorder.[16,17] The gender ratio tends to equalize by adulthood, which could be due to a difference in recognition of ADHD based on adult self-report versus reports from teachers and parents,[18] or to the relative persistence of inattentive symptoms (more common in girls).[13,19]

14.4 **Comorbidities and associated problems**

Comorbidity with other psychiatric disorders frequently occurs with ADHD.[15] Two of the most widespread comorbidities with ADHD are oppositional defiant disorder (ODD) and conduct disorder (CD). A study following hyperactive children into adolescence found rates of ODD of 59% and of CD of 43% among those with childhood hyperactivity compared with 11% and 1.6% among controls.[20] Adolescents with persistent ADHD have been found to exhibit higher rates of CD compared with adolescents whose ADHD was childhood-limited.[21] Several studies have found increased rates of substance use among individuals with ADHD.[21,22] This association may be at least partially mediated by the presence of CD;[20,21] however, a recent study found that individuals with ADHD and no comorbid CD still had higher risk of substance use disorders than controls.[22] Several studies have also found that individuals with ADHD are at higher risk for smoking tobacco,[20,22,23] even compared with a behavior-problem control group.[23]

While elevated rates of mood disorders have also been found in clinical ADHD populations,[12] studies following ADHD children into adulthood have provided equivocal results regarding risk of mood or anxiety disorders in adulthood.[24,25] Learning disabilities (deficits in reading, mathematics or spelling), tend to be more frequent in ADHD populations,[26] and neuropsychological impairment has also been found among adults with ADHD.[27]

ADHD has been found to increase risk for problems in school. Studies indicate that hyperactive adolescents are more likely to be suspended, expelled or drop-out of school, although these outcomes may be at least partially attributed to comorbid CD.[20] In an 18-year longitudinal study, early attentional problems were associated with adverse educational outcomes, even after controlling for childhood IQ, suggesting that ADHD confers risk for school underachievement over-and-above its association with neuropsychological functioning.[28] Finally, there is some evidence that ADHD may have a negative impact on employment in adulthood, with higher rates of unemployment among adults with ADHD.[29]

14.5 **Risk factors for childhood ADHD**

The precise aetiology of ADHD is not clear, and multiple biopsychosocial risk factors may act independently or in concert to produce disorder.[30,31] However, genetic vulnerability, pre- and perinatal exposures, and psychosocial factors have been found to increase risk of the disorder and persistence (see Figure 14.1). Family history of ADHD is an important risk factor for the disorder, with an estimated heritability of 76%.[32] Low birth weight and preterm birth have been found to relate to levels of hyperactivity and inattention in childhood,[31] as has maternal depression.[30] There is mixed evidence that maternal smoking during pregnancy is related to ADHD in offspring; several studies[30,31,33] but not all[34] have found increased risk. Because ADHD is also associated with smoking, maternal smoking could be an indicator of genetic risk. Psychosocial adversity may also be related to risk of ADHD: elevated family conflict and maternal psychopathology have been found to be predictive of ADHD, even after controlling for parental ADHD and maternal smoking.[33]

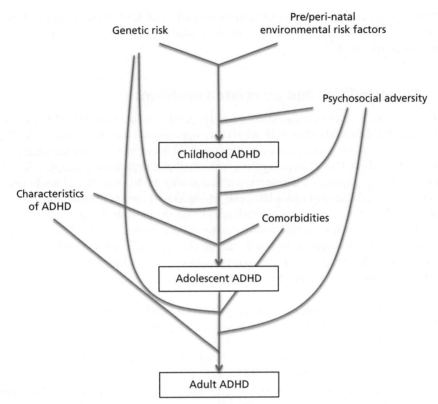

Figure 14.1 Suggested risk factors for attention deficit/hyperactivity disorder (ADHD) over development.

14.6 **Treatment**

Treatment for ADHD consists of medication, behavioural therapy, or a combination. By the mid-1990s, stimulant drugs were the most common psychotropic medication prescribed to children.[35] Concerns of overprescribing of stimulant medication have been raised,[36] although a community-based study in the mid-1990s found a combination of apparent over-and under-prescribing.[37] Behavioural treatments with some empirical support include cognitive–behavioural therapy, behaviour modification, and parent training.[38,39]

The large, multicenter Multimodal Treatment Study of Children with ADHD (MTA), found that careful medication management produced a greater improvement in symptoms than behavioural treatment and community care alone, and that the medication plus behavioural therapy arm showed improvements comparable to those in the medication-only group.[40] While all study groups showed an average reduction in the number of symptoms, there were no longer significant differences between treatment groups at 3-[41] and 8-year follow-up.[42]

14.7 **Persistence**

Longitudinal studies of ADHD have generally debunked the notion that ADHD is a disorder limited to childhood. Estimates of persistence range widely across studies, due at least in part to different definitions of ADHD used (e.g. full criteria ADHD vs partially remitted)[7] and the inclusion of study populations with different characteristics (e.g. excluding children with comorbid conduct problems).[43]

14.7.1 **Childhood**

Problems with hyperactivity among pre-schoolers are relatively non-specific, and many children who exhibit these symptoms do not go on to develop ADHD: Palfrey et al.[44] found that whereas 40% of pre-schoolers exhibited some evidence of inattention, only a minority developed ADHD. The MTA study found that on average all study arms showed decreased symptoms,[40] and studies find that some children will outgrow ADHD during childhood.[45] Children with hyperactivity in multiple settings have been found to be more likely to have continued symptoms than those with more situation-based symptoms.[46]

14.7.2 **Childhood to adolescence**

Rates of persistence of ADHD from childhood into adolescence range widely from, for example, 31%[21] up to 85%.[45] The differences in these estimates are driven by several factors, including: definition of remission, study eligibility criteria, and means of diagnosis of ADHD. However, despite variation across studies, several risk factors for persistence of ADHD into the teenage years have emerged. Family history is one risk factor: the MTA study found that children with higher levels of parental inattention were less likely to improve from study enrollment through ages 10–13 years;[41] likewise, studies suggest that individuals with a family history of ADHD are more likely to persist into adolescence.[45] Additionally, studies find that children with comorbid disorders, such as CD, are more likely to continue to experience problems with attention/hyperactivity past childhood.[45,47] Adolescent hyperactivity has also been related to lower family SES in some studies,[42] but not all.[47] Three-year follow-up of the MTA study found that children with families receiving public assistance had poorer outcomes,[41] and at 8-year follow-up, social disadvantage in childhood was related to adolescent ADHD symptom severity.[42] Parental psychopathology and conflict have also been found to be risk factors for persistence of ADHD into adolescence.[45] Finally, severity of childhood ADHD symptoms has been found to predict persistence: in the MTA trial, children with less severe clinical presentation at baseline were more likely to show symptom improvement into adolescence.[47]

14.7.3 **Adolescence into adulthood**

Fewer studies have tracked participants into midlife to assess persistence of ADHD into adulthood (see Barkley[43] for an in-depth discussion of these studies). A meta-analysis of 10 longitudinal studies found a rate persistence of full ADHD diagnosis of 15%, and partially remitted ADHD of 40-60%.[7] Some risk factors for persistence of ADHD into adulthood have been identified and are similar to those associated with persistence into adolescence. Genetic risk is one such factor, as girls with a family history of ADHD were more likely to have persistent ADHD symptoms into young adulthood.[14] Characteristics of childhood ADHD may also predict adult persistence: a retrospective study among 18–44-year-olds found that that combined-type ADHD was more likely to persist, as was ADHD that caused a higher level of impairment in role functioning.[48] A follow-up study of ADHD girls at a mean age of 22 years found that persistent individuals were more likely to have comorbid CD, more relatives with ADHD, and higher levels of family conflict compared with controls, whereas remitted individuals did not significantly differ from controls.[14]

14.8 **Methodological issues in studying ADHD over the life course**

14.8.1 **'Trait versus state' aspects of ADHD outcomes**

Studies examining ADHD over the life course may not assess whether associated problems are 'state or trait dependent'.[49] For example, some prospective studies of children with ADHD examining adult outcomes do not concurrently assess symptoms of ADHD in adulthood. Therefore, it may be difficult to disentangle whether negative adult outcomes are related to: (a) persistent ADHD symptoms in adulthood, (b) long-term consequences of problems associated with childhood ADHD (e.g. lower educational attainment), or (c) commonly co-occurring (but at least partially independent) syndromes associated with ADHD symptoms (e.g. learning disabilities). However, several follow-up studies have concurrently evaluated the persistence of ADHD symptoms, allowing better understanding of this issue. For example, one study examining cognitive functioning among young adults with childhood ADHD found no significant difference in performance between persistent and remitted ADHD groups, suggesting that cognitive deficits associated with ADHD may remain a relatively stable trait even while behavioural symptoms may abate.[49] Alternatively, when examining rates of substance use disorders in a longitudinal cohort, childhood ADHD was predictive of higher risk of substance use disorders compared with no ADHD, whereas subjects who continued to exhibit ADHD in adulthood had an even higher risk of substance use disorders, possibly suggesting that persistent ADHD symptoms may be related to substance use.[22]

14.8.2 **Problems assessing persistence of ADHD**

There is a wide range of findings as to the rate of persistence of ADHD into adulthood. One source of the inconsistent results regarding the rate of persistence of ADHD is the definition of 'remission' of ADHD. For example, Biederman et al. illustrated this issue in a study that found that while 60% of subjects no longer met full diagnostic criteria for ADHD at ages 18-20, 90% continued to experience 'partial' ADHD (some symptoms and impairment).[50] Another frequent methodological problem in assessing adult ADHD is reliance on recall of childhood symptoms, which has been shown to have limited reliability.[43,51] Additionally, unlike assessment of childhood ADHD, which relies on reports from parents and teachers, assessment of adult ADHD is based on self-report. The assumption must therefore be made that the same behaviours assessed by outside observers in childhood can be accurately self-assessed by adults with ADHD.[52] Source of report of ADHD symptoms has a significant influence on estimated rates of persistence: in one longitudinal study, when adults who were hyperactive as children were asked to self-report adult symptoms, only 5% continued to meet criteria for ADHD; however, using symptom reports from subjects' parents, this percentage increased to 46%.[43]

14.8.3 **'Outgrowing' the disorder versus the criteria**

There has been significant debate as to the appropriateness of the DSM-IV ADHD criteria, which are based on research among childhood populations, for adolescence and adulthood.[53] A central concern is that lower rates of ADHD in older populations are due to lack of applicability of the criteria for adulthood, rather than a true resolution of the disorder.[54] It has also been proposed that the number of symptoms required for diagnosis in adulthood be lowered, as a similar level of impairment could be found in adulthood with fewer symptoms. A study in a large community population of adults found that applying the DSM-IV threshold of six or more symptoms identified individuals in higher than the 99th percentile of inattentive/hyperactivity deviance, a higher percentile than is identified when this threshold is applied to childhood populations.[55] The most recent revision to the DSM, the DSM-5, has sought to address this concern by lowering the number of symptoms to meet diagnostic threshold from 6 to 5 for adults, and providing example of criterion items that apply across the life course.[8,56]

14.9 Summary and future directions

Studies have found that ADHD in childhood is related to a host of negative outcomes over the life course, including continued ADHD symptoms,[6] substance use disorders and smoking,[22] and greater risk for academic underachievement and unemployment.[28,29] Some of the risk factors for persistence of ADHD described in this chapter include family history, comorbid psychiatric disorders, psychosocial adversity, and more severe childhood ADHD symptoms.

There are many areas in the study of ADHD over the life course that require further research. The majority of prospective studies following individuals with childhood ADHD have only been able to assess persistence into young adulthood, so fewer conclusions can be made about the course of ADHD into middle and late adulthood.[7] Questions remain as to the appropriateness of the DSM criteria for ADHD for adult life, and the new DSM-5 seeks to address some of these issues. Additionally, females tend to remain underrepresented in studies of ADHD. Finally, future research should address which forms of treatment for ADHD are most effective over the long term in reducing symptoms and minimizing the negative outcomes associated with ADHD.

References

1 **Goldman LS, Genel M, Bezman RJ, Slanetz PJ.** Diagnosis and treatment of attention-deficit/ hyperactivity disorder in children and adults. *JAMA* 1998;**279**:1100–1107.

2 **Froehlich TE, Lanphear BP, Epstein JL, et al.** Prevalence, recognition, and treatment of attention-deficit/hyperactivity disorder in a national sample of US children. *Arch Pediatr Adolesc Med* 2007;**161**(9):857–864.

3 **Cantwell DP.** Attention deficit disorder: a review of the past 10 years. *J Am Acad Child Adolesc Psychiatry* 1996;**35**(8):978–987.

4 **American Psychiatric Association.** *Diagnostic and statistical manual of mental disorders.* 4th ed. Washington DC: APA; 2000.

5 **Barkley RA.** *Attention-deficit hyperactivity disorder: a handbook for diagnosis and treatment.* 3 ed. New York: Guilford Press; 2006.

6 **Laufer MW, Denhoff ED.** Hyperkinetic behavior syndrome in children. *J Pediatr* 1957;**50**:467–473.

7 **Faraone SV, Biederman J, Mick E.** The age-dependent decline of attention deficit hyperactivity disorder: a meta-analysis of follow-up studies. *Psychol Med* 2006;**36**:159–165.

8 **American Psychiatric Association.** *Diagnostic and statistical manual of mental disorders.* 5th ed. Washington DC: APA; 2013.

9 **Lahey BB, Pelham WE, Stein MA, et al.** Validity of DSM-IV attention-deficit/hyperactivity disorder for younger children. *J Am Acad Child Adolesc Psychiatry* 1998;**37**(7):695–702.

10 **Rappley MD, Mullan PB, Alvarez FJ, Eneli IU, Wang J, Gardiner JC.** Diagnosis of attention-deficit/ hyperactivity disorder and use of psychotropic medication in very young children. *Arch Pediatr Adolesc Med* 1999;**153**:1039–1045.

11 **Barkley RA, Anastopoulos AD, Guevremont DC, Fletcher KE.** Adolescents with ADHD: patterns of behavioral adjustment, academic functioning and treatment utilization. *J Am Acad Child Adolesc Psychiatry* 1991;**30**:752–761.

12 Faraone SV, Biederman J, Monuteaux MC. Further evidence for diagnostic continuity between child and adolescent ADHD. *J Atten Disord* 2002;**6**(1):5–13.

13 Wilens TE, Biederman J, Faraone SV, Martelon M, Westerberg D, Spencer TJ. Presenting ADHD symptoms, subtypes, and comorbid disorders in clinically referred adults with ADHD. *J Clin Psychiatry* 2009;**70**(11):1557–1562.

14 Biederman J, Petty CR, O'Connor KB, Hyder LL, Faraone SV. Predictors of persistence in girls with attention deficit hyperactivity disorder: results from an 11-year controlled follow-up study. *Acta Psychiatr Scand* 2012;**125**:147–156.

15 Szatmari P, Offord DR, Boyle MH. Ontario Child Health Study: prevalence of attention deficit disorder with hyperactivity. *J Child Psychol Psychiatry* 1989;**30**(2):219–30.

16 Biederman J, Faraone SV, Mick E, et al. Clinical correlates of ADHD in females: findings for a large group of girls ascertained from pediatric and psychiatric referral sources. *J Am Acad Child Adolesc Psychiatry* 1999;**38**(8):966–975.

17 Gaub M, Carlson CL. Gender differences in ADHD: a meta-analysis and critical review. *J Am Acad Child Adolesc Psychiatry* 1997;**36**(8):1036–1045.

18 Biederman J, Faraone SV, Monuteaux MC, Bober M, Cadogen E. Gender effects on attention-deficit/ hyperactivity disorders in adults, revised. *Biol Psychiatry* 2004;**55**:692–700.

19 Biederman J, Mick E, Faraone SV, et al. Influence of gender on attention deficit hyperactivity disorder in children referred to a psychatric clinic. *Am J Psychiatry* 2002;**159**:36–42.

20 Barkley RA, Fischer M, Edelbrock CS, Smallish L. The adolescent outcome of hyperactive children diagnosed by research criteria: I. An 8-year prospective follow-up study. *J Am Acad Child Adolesc Psychiatry* 1990;**29**:546–557.

21 Gittelman R, Mannuzza S, Shenker R, Bonagura N. Hyperactive boys almost grown up: I. Psychiatric status. *Arch Gen Psychiatry* 1985;**42**:937–947.

22 Wilens TE, Martelon M, Joshi G, et al. Does ADHD predict substance-use disorders? A 10-year follow-up study of young adults with ADHD. *J Am Acad Child Adolesc Psychiatry* 2011;**50**(6):543–553.

23 Lambert NM, Hartsough CS. Prospective study of tobacco smoking and substance dependencies among samples of ADHD and non-ADHD participants. *J Learn Disabil* 1998;**31**:533–544.

24 Biederman J, Monuteaux MC, Mick E, et al. Young adult outcome of attention deficit hyperactivity disorder: a controlled 10-year follow-up study. *Psychol Med* 2006;**36**:167–179.

25 Klein RG, Mannuzza S. Long-term outcome of hyperactive children: a review. *J Am Acad Child Adolesc Psychiatry* 1991;**30**(3):383–387.

26 Seidman LJ. Neuropsychological functioning in people with ADHD across the lifespan. *Clin Psychol Rev* 2006;**26**:466–485.

27 Seidman LJ, Biederman J, Weber W, Hatch M, Faraone SV. Neuropsychological funtion in adults with attention-deficit hyperactivity disorder. *Biol Psychiatry* 1998;**44**:260–268.

28 Fergusson DM, Lynskey MT, Horwood LJ. Attentional difficulties in middle childhood and psychosocial outcomes in young adulthood. *J Child Psychol Psychiatry* 1997;**38**:633–644.

29 Kessler RC, Adler L, Barkley R, et al. The prevalence and correlates of adult ADHD in the United States: results from the National Comorbidity Survey Replication. *Am J Psychiatry* 2006; **163**:716.

30 Sagiv SK, Epstein JN, Bellinger CD, Korrick SA. Pre- and postnatal risk factors for ADHD in a nonclinical pediatric population. *J Atten Disord* 2013;**17**(1):47–57.

31 Galera C, Cote SM, Bouvard MO, et al. Early risk factors for hyperactivity–impulsivity and inattention trajectories from age 17 months to 8 years. *Arch Gen Psychiatry* 2012;**68**(12):1267–1275.

32 Faraone SV, Perlis RH, Doyle AE, et al. Molecular genetics of attention-deficit/hyperactivity disorder. *Biol Psychiatry* 2005;**57**:1313–1323.

33 **Biederman J, Faraone SV, Monuteaux MC.** Differential effect of environmental adversity by gender: Rutter's index of adversity in a group of boys and girls with and without ADHD. *Am J Psychiatry* 2002;**159**(9):1556–1562.

34 **Ball SW, Gilman SE, Mick E, et al.** Revisiting the association between maternal smoking during pregnancy and ADHD. *J Psychiatr Res* 2010;**44**:1058–1062.

35 **Olfson M, Marcus SC, Weissman MM, Jensen PS.** National trends in the use of psychotropic medications by children. *J Am Acad Child Adolesc Psychiatry* 2002;**41**(5):514–521.

36 **Jensen PS, Kettle L, Roper MT, et al.** Are stimulants overprescribed? Treatment of ADHD in four US communities. *J Am Acad Child Adolesc Psychiatry* 1999 **38**(7): 797–804.

37 **Angold A, Erkanli A, Egger HL, Costello EJ.** Stimulant treatment for children: a community perspective. *J Am Acad Child Adolesc Psychiatry* 2000;**39**(8):975–984; discussion 84–94.

38 **Biederman J, Faraone SV.** Attention-deficit hyperactivity disorder. *Lancet* 2005;**366**:237–248.

39 **Sonuga-Barke EJS, Daley D, Thompson M, Laver-Bradbury CAW.** Parent-based therapies for school attention-deficit/hyperactivity disorder: a randomized controlled trial with a community sample. *J Am Acad Child Adolesc Psychiatry* 2001;**40**(4):402–408.

40 **MTA Cooperative Group.** A 14-month randomized clinical trial of treatment strategies for attention-deficit/hyperactivity disorder. *Arch Gen Psychiatry* 1999;**56**(12):1073–1086.

41 **Jensen PS, Arnold LE, Swanson JM, et al.** 3-year follow-up of the NIMH MTA study. *J Am Acad Child Adolesc Psychiatry* 2007;**46**(8):989–1002.

42 **Molina BSG, Hinshaw SP, Swanson JM, et al.** The MTA at 8 years: prospective follow-up of children treated for combined type ADHD in a multisite study. *J Am Acad Child Adolesc Psychiatry* 2009;**48**(5):484–500.

43 **Barkley RA, Fischer M, Smallish L, Fletcher K.** The persistence of attention-deficit/hyperactivity disorder into young adulthood as a function of reporting source and definition of disorder. *J Abnorm Psychol* 2002;**111**(2):279–89.

44 **Palfrey JS, Levine MD, Walker DK, Sullivan M.** The emergence of attention deficits in early childhood: a prospective study. *Dev Behav Pediatr* 1985;**6**(6):339–348.

45 **Biederman J, Faraone SV, Milberger S, et al.** Predictors of persistence and remission of ADHD into adolescence: results from a four-year prospective follow-up study. *J Am Acad Child Adolesc Psychiatry* 1996;**35**(3):343–351.

46 **Campbell SB, Endman MW, Bernfeld G.** A three-year follow-up of hyperactive preschoolers into elementary school. *J Child Adolesc Psychiatry* 1977;**18**:239–249.

47 **Hart EL, Lahey BB, Loeber R, Applegate B, Frick PJ.** Developmental change in attention-deficit hyperactivity disorder in boys: a four-year longitudinal study. *J Abnorm Child Psychol* 1995;**23**(6): 729–749.

48 **Kessler RC, Adler LA, Barkley R, et al.** Patterns and predictors of attention-deficit/hyperactivity disorders persistence into adulthood: results from the National Comorbidity Survey Replication. *Biol Psychiatry* 2005;**57**:1442–1451.

49 **Biederman J, Petty CR, Ball SW, et al.** Are cognitive deficits in ADHD related to the course of the disorder? A prospective controlled follow-up study of grown up boys with persistent and remitting couse. *Psychiatry Res* 2009;**170**(2–3):177–182.

50 **Biederman J, Mick E, Faraone SV.** Age-dependent decline of symptoms of attention deficit hyperactivity disorder: impact of remission defintion and symptom type. *Am J Psychiatry* 2000;**157**(5):816–818.

51 **Henry HB, Caspi A, Langley K, Silva PA.** On the "remembrance of things past": a longitudinal evaluation of retrospective method. *Psychol Assess* 1994;**6**:92–101.

52 **Murphy P, Schacher R.** Use of self-ratings in the assessment of symptoms of attention deficit hyperactivity disorder in adults. *Am J Psychiatry* 2000;**157**:1156–1159.

53 **McGough JJ, Barkley RA.** Diagnostic controversies in adult attention deficit hyperactivity disorder. *Am J Psychiatry* 2004;**161**:1948–1956.

54 **Biederman J, Petty CR, Evans M, et al.** How persistent is ADHD? a controlled 10-year follow-up of boys with ADHD. *Psychiatry Res* 2010;**177**:299–304.

55 **Murphy K, Barkley RA.** Prevalence of DSM-IV symptms of ADHD in adult licensed drivers: Implications for clinical diagnosis. *J Atten Disord* 1996;**1**(3):147–161.

56 **American Psychiatric Association.** 2013. *Highlights of Changes from DSM-IV-TR to DSM-5.* http://www.dsm5.org/Documents/changes%20from%20dsm-iv-tr%20to%20dsm-5.pdf

Chapter 15

Conduct disorder across the life course

Sara R. Jaffee and Candice L. Odgers

15.1 Introduction

This chapter synthesizes the literature with regard to a life course perspective on conduct disorder. First, the disorder is defined and its prevalence and comorbidity with other disorders is described. The developmental course of conduct disorder is then charted, with attention to taxonomic issues as well as predictors and sequelae of different trajectories of conduct problems. The literature on individual and contextual risk factors for conduct disorder is summarized and the implications for public health discussed.

15.1.1 Definitions and prevalence

According to DSM-IV-TR,[1] conduct disorder is characterized by 'a repetitive and persistent pattern of behaviour in which the basic rights of others or major age-appropriate societal norms or rules are violated' (p. 93). Symptoms include aggression towards people or animals (e.g. bullying, using a weapon), destructive behaviour (e.g. fire setting), deceitfulness or theft, and rule violations (e.g. truancy, running away from home). In population studies the prevalence rate of conduct disorder ranges from <1% to 10%.[1] Conduct disorder is more frequent among boys than in girls throughout childhood and adolescence at a rate of about 2:1, although this sex difference narrows in adolescence.[2] In community samples in the USA, some studies have identified high rates of conduct disorder among African-American (10%) compared with Hispanic (6%) or non-Hispanic, non-African-American (5%) youth,[3] but others have not identified differences between African-American and Caucasian-American youth.[4]

Conduct disorder is related to oppositional defiant disorder (ODD), which is characterized by 'a recurrent pattern of negativistic, defiant, disobedient, and hostile behaviour toward authority figures' (p. 100).[1] In a community sample, the past-year prevalence rate of ODD ranged from 8% to 9% and did not vary by race or ethnicity.[3] The genetic influences on ODD and conduct disorder are substantially overlapping.[5,6] ODD is typically viewed as a developmental precursor to conduct disorder and is not diagnosed if criteria for conduct disorder are met. There is some empirical support for this developmental sequence, particularly in boys.[7]

In general population surveys, there are high rates of comorbidity between conduct disorder and other disorders, particularly attention deficit/hyperactivity disorder (ADHD) and depression.[8,9] Approximately one-third of pre-schoolers with severe ADHD go on to develop conduct disorder later in childhood,[10] and children with combined conduct disorder and ADHD have a particularly poor prognosis.[11]

15.2 **Taxonomic issues and developmental course**

Conduct problem symptoms exhibit an age-graded relationship. At the population level, the base rate of serious conduct problems tends to be relatively low in childhood, increases during adolescence, and then decreases rapidly during the transition to adulthood.[12,13] Longitudinal studies that track conduct problem symptoms within the same individuals over time have shown that the 'age–crime' curve comprises a mixture of developmental pathways.

Several theories have been proposed to explain the course and substantial heterogeneity in the development of antisocial behaviour.[14-16] Moffitt's[17] often-cited taxonomic theory of antisocial behaviour proposed that at least two prototypical subtypes underlie the observed age-by-crime distribution: a life-course-persistent (LCP) pathway that onsets in early childhood, is characterized by social, familial, and neurodevelopmental deficits, and that characterizes a relatively small, yet persistent and pathological, subgroup of individuals; and an adolescence-limited pathway that is hypothesized to be more frequent and relatively transient. Adolescence-limited involvement in antisocial behaviour is believed to emerge alongside puberty as a relatively normative response to the 'maturity gap', wherein adolescents—who are biologically mature, but not yet treated by society as adults—mimic the antisocial behaviour of their LCP peers who, for example, drink alcohol, father children, possess expensive material goods, and do not adhere to curfews. By contrast with those on the LCP pathway, Moffitt[17] predicted that individuals following the adolescence-limited pathway would not be characterized by any significant early childhood vulnerability or familial risk. Whereas those on the LCP pathway are expected to experience multiple problems in adulthood (including violence), adolescence-limited individuals, given the normative nature of their pre-teen development and their growing access to adult rights and privileges, are hypothesized to be more successful in their transition to adulthood provided they do not encounter snares, such as substance dependency or a criminal record.

15.2.1 **Developmental course: pathways and predictors**

Longitudinal studies using group-based trajectory models (e.g. the Christchurch Health and Development Longitudinal Study, the Dunedin Multidisciplinary Health and Development Study, the National Longitudinal Survey of Youth, the Quebec Longitudinal Study of Kindergarten Children) have identified four or five prototypical conduct problem pathways (four of which are displayed in Figure 15.1). The early-onset-persistent or life-course persistent pathway typically captures between 5% and 10% of children and is characterized by symptoms that onset in childhood and continue across adolescence and into young adulthood. The adolescence-limited (or onset) pathway is characterized by the emergence of conduct problems during adolescence and (for the most part) desistance thereafter. A childhood-limited pathway has also surfaced in some studies; this subgroup captures a relatively large percentage of the population (up to 25% in some studies) who surpass the criteria for conduct disorder in childhood but who desist rapidly as they move through the elementary school years,[18] and by late adolescence/young adulthood these individuals cannot be distinguished from those on the low/no-conduct problem pathway.[19] The childhood-limited group may reflect a normative developmental phenomenon, whereby many children exhibit conduct-problem-like behaviours during early childhood before they have acquired the necessary skills to obtain their goals through more prosocial means. This general pattern of decline in antisocial behaviour is also consistent with Robins'[20] early observations that 'adult antisocial behaviour virtually requires childhood antisocial behaviour . . . [but that] most antisocial children do not become antisocial adults' (p. 611). Finally, the majority of children, an

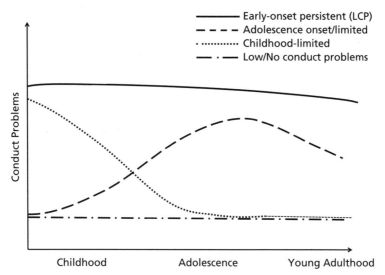

Figure 15.1 Prototypical developmental pathways of conduct problems identified within prospective cohort studies using group based-trajectory modelling.

estimated 50–60% depending on the measures that are used, never reach the clinically elevated range (three or more symptoms) of conduct disorder.[21]

Children following the LCP pathway have repeatedly been shown to suffer from a wide range of neurodevelopmental, familial and social risks.[22,23] For example, children following the LCP pathway from the Dunedin Study scored worse on virtually every marker of childhood risk (e.g. maltreatment, inconsistent discipline, mother's mental health, child IQ) when compared with their counterparts on the adolescence-limited and low conduct problem pathways. By contrast, children in this study who followed the adolescence-limited pathway were found to resemble the cohort norm across the majority of childhood risk measures. Less is known about the predictors of the childhood limited pathway. Although there has been limited success in identifying childhood risk factors that distinguish children on the LCP versus childhood-limited pathways, there is some evidence that a family history of psychiatric illness and family violence is more characteristic of the former than the latter.[24,25]

15.2.2 Developmental course: consequences

Although conduct problems in childhood are widespread, only a fraction of children (between 5% and 10%) continue to exhibit clinically elevated levels of conduct problem symptoms into adolescence and adulthood.[21] Approximately 45–75% of youth with conduct disorder meet criteria for antisocial personality disorder in adulthood.[26–28] Individuals following a life-course persistent pathway of antisocial behaviour are responsible for 50–70% of officially sanctioned violent crime,[29–31] and are also more likely than those within the other conduct problem subgroups to engage in violence towards themselves, exhibit controlling and abusive behaviour towards their spouses, and act aggressively towards their children in adulthood.[19,30,32,33]

Like their male counterparts, women following the LCP pathway are at an increased risk for violence towards their partners and their children. For example, in the Dunedin Study, more than 75% of women on the LCP pathway had engaged in at least one form of physical violence over the past 6 months.[19] Although antisocial personality disorder often follows from a childhood history of conduct disorder in girls,[26,28] other personality disorders—particularly borderline personality disorder—are also frequently reported among women with a childhood history of conduct disorder.[34] Moreover, girls with a history of conduct disorder are at elevated risk for substance use disorder diagnoses, even accounting for concurrent comorbidity.[28,35]

The evidence is mixed as to whether youth on the adolescent-onset pathway exit a life of crime as they assume adult roles. In general, rates of antisocial behaviour and involvement in official crime among this subgroup have been significantly lower than those documented among individuals on the LCP pathway, but complete desistance from involvement in antisocial behaviour and related problems among this group has not always been observed.[19,36,37] Although some researchers have hypothesized that adolescent onset antisocial behaviour among girls is analogous to the LCP pathway with respect to the presence of early risk and the increased risk for poor prognosis,[38] the 17% of women following the adolescence-limited pathway in the Dunedin study resembled the cohort norm on childhood risk factors and demonstrated very little continuity in their antisocial behaviour into adulthood.[19]

As implied by the name, individuals following the childhood-limited pathway have not been found to be at an increased risk for involvement in antisocial and closely related behaviours as they move through adolescence and young adulthood. In fact, the cardinal feature of this trajectory group appears to be the presence of a complete desistance from involvement in externalizing behaviours and an increase in prosocial behaviours,[39] although there is some evidence that males following this pathway experience some difficulties with internalizing disorders and tobacco use later in life.[19] Additional research is required to determine whether individuals following this pathway represent true recoveries.

15.3 **Biosocial perspective**

Both individual and contextual risk factors for conduct disorder have been identified. Individual risk factors include low heart rate,[40,41] deficits in executive function,[42,43] an inability to learn from punishment,[44,45] and difficulties recognizing expressions of sadness and fearfulness.[44,46–49] Although many of these individual risk factors were hypothesized to differentiate individuals with life course persistent versus adolescent onset antisocial behaviour, recent studies have suggested that the groups may differ in degree rather than in kind.[43,49,46]

A recent review of studies that used quasi-experimental and statistical matching methods to test for associations between contextual risk factors and youth antisocial behaviour supported a causal role for some, but not others.[50] Specifically, there was evidence that maltreatment and harsh, inconsistent discipline, parental divorce, parental depression and antisocial behaviour, adolescent motherhood, poverty, and peer delinquency played a causal role in the development of antisocial behaviour. By contrast, support was not found for the hypothesis that smoking during pregnancy, parental drug use, or neighbourhood disadvantage were causally related to youth antisocial behaviour—though the set of studies related to neighbourhood disadvantage was small—and, more recently, results from a quasi-experimental study of cousins supported the hypothesis that neighbourhood disadvantage is a cause of youth antisocial behaviour.[51]

A biosocial perspective proposes that individual risk factors are exacerbated in the context of environmental risk, increasing the likelihood that conduct problems will emerge and persist across the life course.[52,53] Deficits in the ability to inhibit behaviour, to recognize fear and to respond to punishment may be potentiated in criminogenic environments characterized by suboptimal caregiving, high levels of threat, and abundant opportunities for antisocial behaviour.

There is substantial evidence across multiple levels of individual and contextual characteristics to support the biosocial perspective. For example, quantitative behavioural genetic studies have shown that genetic effects on symptoms of externalizing disorders are amplified under conditions of various forms of contextual risk (peer delinquency, parent–child relationship problems, stressful life events).[54] Molecular genetic studies have identified specific variants that moderate the effect of environmental adversity on risk for antisocial behaviour, with the most robust finding involving an interaction between a variant of the monoamine oxidase A (MAOA) gene and childhood maltreatment.[55–57]

Several child characteristics interact with the child's environment to increase risk for conduct problems. These include child temperament,[58] hormone levels,[59] stress reactivity,[60] and pubertal status.[61] For example, prospective, longitudinal studies have shown that neuromotor impairment[62] and other indicators of neurodevelopmental impairment—such as perinatal complications and difficult temperament measured in the first 5 years of life—increase risk for persistent aggressive, antisocial outcomes in middle childhood and adolescence, but only among children who are raised under conditions of adversity.[63–65] Although framed as biologically based characteristics of the child, most of the child characteristics that are investigated in the context of biosocial interactions are likely to be influenced by genes and environments.[66]

15.4 **Implications for public health**

Conduct disorder poses a significant public health burden with real psychological and financial costs for victims, for conduct-disordered youth and their families, and for society. One study in the UK of conduct-disordered youth followed into adulthood found that the cost of providing services to this group (including, among others, foster care, education services, benefits, juvenile justice services) was 10-fold higher than for youth without conduct disorder.[67] A 2005 study in the USA found that the additional costs per child related to conduct disorder, involving education, health, mental health, and juvenile justice services, exceeded US$70,000 over a 7-year period.[68]

Although there are many evidence-based treatments for conduct disorder that are efficacious (meaning that they can work under controlled conditions), relatively few have been shown to be effective, meaning that they produce significant improvements when rolled out on a large scale.[69] Treatments that have been shown to be both efficacious and effective include multisystemic therapy[70] and multidimensional treatment foster care.[71]

15.5 **Summary**

Conduct disorder poses a significant public health burden. Youth with conduct disorder—particularly conduct disorder that emerges and persists throughout childhood—are at elevated risk for poor educational attainment and labour force participation, poor physical and mental health, and relationship difficulties with parents, peers, romantic partners, and children. These sequelae are observed well into adulthood.[72] More research is needed to better understand the aetiology of adolescent-onset conduct disorder and to determine whether early versus adolescent onset conduct disorder are qualitatively versus quantitatively distinct in terms of aetiological risk factors. Successful early interventions to prevent the emergence of clinically significant conduct problems exist (e.g. Fast Track) and are particularly effective if targeted at high risk youth.[73] Prevention and intervention programmes are likely to be best-informed by research that is designed to identify causal mechanisms in the emergence of conduct disorder and in the reduction of conduct disorder symptoms.

References

1 **American Psychiatric Association**. *Diagnostic and statistical manual of mental disorders*: 4th ed. Text revision. Washington, DC: American Psychiatric Association; 2000.

2 **Moffitt TE, Caspi A, Rutter M, Silva PA**. *Sex differences in antisocial behaviour: conduct disorder, delinquency, and violence in the Dunedin Longitudinal Study*. Cambridge: Cambridge University Press; 2001.

3 **Buka SL, Stichick TL, Birdthistle I, Earls FJ**. Youth exposure to violence: prevalence, risks, and consequences. *Am J Orthopsychiatry* 2001;**71**:298–310.

4 **Angold A, Erkanli A, Farmer EMZ, et al**. Psychiatric disorder, impairment, and service use in rural African American and white youth. *Arch Gen Psychiatry* 2002;**59**:893–901.

5 **Dick DM, Viken RJ, Kaprio J, Pulkkinen L, Rose RJ**. Understanding the covariation among childhood externalizing symptoms: genetic and environmental influences on conduct disorder, attention deficit hyperactivity disorder, and oppositional defiant disorder symptoms. *J Abnormal Child Psychol* 2005;**33**:219–229.

6 **Meyer JM, Rutter M, Silberg JL, et al**. Familial aggregation for conduct disorder symptomatology: the role of genes, marital discord and family adaptability. *Psychol Med* 2000;**30**:759–774.

7 **Rowe R, Costello EJ, Angold A, Copeland WE, Maughan B**. Developmental pathways in oppositional defiant disorder and conduct disorder. *J Abnormal Psychol* 2010;**119**:726–738.

8 **Angold A, Costello EJ, Erkanli A**. Comorbidity. *J Child Psychol Psychiatry* 1999;**40**:57–87.

9 **Maughan B, Rowe R, Messer J, Goodman R, Meltzer H**. Conduct disorder and oppositional defiant disorder in a national sample: developmental epidemiology. *J Child Psychol Psychiatry* 2004;**45**:609–621.

10 **Beauchaine TP, Hinshaw SP, Pang KL**. Comorbidity of attention-deficit/hyperactivity disorder and early-onset conduct disorder: biological, environmental, and developmental mechanisms. *Clin Psychol Sci Pract* 2010;**17**:327–336.

11 **Waschbusch DA**. A meta-analytic examination of comorbid hyperactive–impulsive–attention problems and conduct problems. *Psychol Bull* 2002;**128**:118–150.

12 **Hirschi T, Gottfredson M**. Age and the explanation of crime. *Am J Sociol* 1983;**89**:552–584.

13 **Sampson RJ, Laub JH**. Crime and deviance in the life course. *Annu Rev Sociol* 1992;**18**:63–84.

14 **Dodge KA, Pettit GS**. A biopsychosocial model of the development of chronic conduct problems in adolescence. *Dev Psychol* 2003;**39**:349–371.

15 **Loeber R**. Development and risk factors of juvenile antisocial behavior and delinquency. *Clin Psychol Rev* 1990;**10**:1–41.

16 **Patterson GR, DeBaryshe BD, Ramsey E**. A developmental perspective on antisocial behavior. *Am Psychologist* 1989;**44**:329–335.

17 **Moffitt TE**. Adolescence-limited and life-course-persistent antisocial behavior: a developmental taxonomy. *Psychol Rev* 1993;**100**:674–701.

18 **Veenstra R, Lindenberg S, Verhulst FC, Ormel J**. Childhood-limited versus persistent antisocial behavior why do some recover and others do not? The TRAILS study. *J Early Adolescence* 2009;**29**:718–742.

19 **Odgers CL, Moffitt TE, Broadbent JM, et al**. Female and male antisocial trajectories: from childhood origins to adult outcomes. *Dev Psychopathol* 2008;**20**:673–716.

20 **Robins LN**. Sturdy childhood predictors of adult antisocial behavior: Replications from longitudinal studies. *Psychol Med* 1978;**8**:611–622.

21 **Broidy LM, Nagin DS, Tremblay RE, et al**. Developmental trajectories of childhood disruptive behaviors and adolescent delinquency: a six-site, cross-national study. *Dev Psychol* 2003;**39**:222–245.

22 **Moffitt TE, Caspi A**. Childhood predictors differentiate life-course persistent and adolescence-limited antisocial pathways among males and females. *Dev Psychopathol* 2001;**13**:355–375.

23 **Nagin DS, Tremblay RE**. Parental and early childhood predictors of persistent physical aggression in boys from kindergarten to high school. *Arch Gen Psychiatry* 2001;**58**:389–394.

24 **Odgers CL, Milne BJ, Caspi A, Crump R, Poulton R, Moffitt TE.** Predicting prognosis for the conduct-problem boy: can family history help? *J Am Acad Child Adolescent Psychiatry* 2007;**46**:1240–1249.

25 **Barker ED, Maughan B.** Differentiating early-onset persistent versus childhood-limited conduct problem youth. *Am J Psychiatry* 2009;**166**:900–908.

26 **Gelhorn HL, Sakai JT, Price RK, Crowley TJ.** DSM-IV conduct disorder criteria as predictors of antisocial personality disorder. *Comprehensive Psychiatry* 2007;**48**:529–538.

27 **Kim-Cohen J, Caspi A, Moffitt TE, Harrington H, Milne BJ, Poulton R.** Prior juvenile diagnoses in adults with mental disorder. *Arch Gen Psychiatry* 2003;**60**:709–717.

28 **Morcillo C, Duarte CS, Sala R, et al.** Conduct disorder and adult psychiatric diagnoses: associations and gender differences in the U.S. adult population. *J Psychiat Res* 2012;**46**:323–330.

29 **Hodgins S.** Status at age 30 of children with conduct problems. *Stud Crime Crime Prev* 1994;**3**:41–62.

30 **Moffitt TE, Caspi A, Harrington H, Milne BJ.** Males on the life-course-persistent and adolescence-limited antisocial pathways: follow-up at age 26 years. *Dev Psychopathol* 2002;**14**:179–207.

31 **Odgers CL, Caspi A, Broadbent JM, et al.** Prediction of differential adult health burden by conduct problem subtypes in males. *Arch Gen Psychiatry* 2007;**64**:476–484.

32 **Fergusson DM, Horwood JL, Ridder EM.** Show me the child at seven: the consequences of conduct problems in childhood for psychosocial functioning in adulthood. *J Child Psychol Psychiatry* 2004;**45**:1–13.

33 **Woodward LJ, Fergusson DM, Horwood LJ.** Romantic relationships of young people with childhood and adolescent onset antisocial behavior problems. *J Abnormal Child Psychol* 2002;**30**:231–243.

34 **Beauchaine TP, Klein DN, Crowell SE, Derbidge C, Gatzke-Kopp L.** Multifinality in the development of personality disorders: a biology × sex × environment interaction model of antisocial and borderline traits. *Dev Psychopathol* 2009;**21**:735–770.

35 **Costello EJ, Mustillo S, Erkanli A, Keeler G, Angold A.** Prevalence and development of psychiatric disorders in childhood and adolescence. *Archives of General Psychiatry* 2003;**60**:837–844.

36 **Marmorstein NR, Iacono WG.** Longitudinal follow-up of adolescents with late-onset antisocial behavior: a pathological yet overlooked group. *J Am Acad Child Adolescent Psychiatry* 2005;**44**:1284–1291.

37 **Roisman GI, Aguilar B, Egeland B.** Antisocial behavior in the transition to adulthood: the independent and interactive roles of developmental history and emerging developmental tasks. *Dev Psychopathol* 2004;**16**:857–871.

38 **Silverthorn P, Frick PJ.** Developmental pathways to antisocial behavior: the delayed-onset pathway in girls. *Dev Psychopathol* 1999;**11**:101–126.

39 **Barker ED, Oliver BR, Maughan B.** Co-occurring problems of early onset persistent, childhood limited, and adolescent onset conduct problem youth. *J Child Psychol Psychiatry* 2010;**51**:1217–1226.

40 **Lorber MF.** Psychophysiology of aggression, psychopathy, and conduct problems: a meta-analysis. *Psychol Bull* 2004;**130**:531–552.

41 **Ortiz J, Raine A.** Heart rate level and antisocial behavior in children and adolescents: a meta-analysis. *J Am Acad Child Adolescent Psychiatry* 2004;**43**:154–162.

42 **Morgan AB, Lilienfeld SO.** A meta-analytic review of the relation between antisocial behavior and neuropsychological measures of executive function. *Clin Psychol Review* 2000;**20**:113–136.

43 **Fairchild G, Van Goozen SH, Stollery SJ, et al.** Decision making and executive function in male adolescents with early-onset or adolescence-onset conduct disorder and control subjects. *Biol Psychiatry* 2009;**66**:162–168.

44 **Fairchild G, Stobbe Y, Van Goozen SHM, Calder AJ, Goodyer IM.** Facial expression recognition, fear conditioning, and startle modulation in female subjects with conduct disorder. *Biol Psychiatry* 2010;**68**:272–279.

45 **Raine A.** *The psychopathology of crime.* San Diego: Academic Press; 1993.

46 Fairchild G, Van Goozen SH, Calder AJ, Stollery SJ, Goodyer IM. Deficits in facial expression recognition in male adolescents with early-onset or adolescence-onset conduct disorder. *J Child Psychol Psychiatry* 2009;**50**:627–636.

47 Jones AP, Laurens KR, Herba CM, Barker GJ, Viding E. Amygdala hypoactivity to fearful faces in boys with conduct problems and callous-unemotional traits. *Am J Psychiatry* 2009;**166**:95–102.

48 Marsh AA, Finger EC, Mitchell DG, et al. Reduced amygdala response to fearful expressions in children and adolescents with callous-unemotional traits and disruptive behavior disorders. *Am J Psychiatry* 2008;**165**, 712–720.

49 Passamonti L, Fairchild G, Goodyer IM, et al. Neural abnormalities in early-onset and adolescence-onset conduct disorder. *Arch Gen Psychiatry* 2010;**67**, 729–738.

50 Jaffee SR, Strait LB, Odgers CL. From correlates to causes: can quasi-experimental studies and statistical innovations bring us closer to identifying the causes of antisocial behavior? *Psychol Bull* 2012;**138**:272–295.

51 Goodnight JA, Lahey BB, Van Hulle CA, et al. A quasi-experimental analysis of the influence of neighborhood disadvantage on child and adolescent conduct problems. *J Abnormal Psychol* 2012;**121**:95–108.

52 Moffitt TE. Adolescence-limited and life-course-persistent antisocial behavior: a developmental taxonomy. *Psychol Rev* 1993;**100**:674–701.

53 Raine A. Biosocial studies of antisocial and violent behavior in children and adults: a review. *J Abnormal Child Psychol* 2002;**30**:311–326.

54 Hicks BM, South SC, DiRago AC, Iacono WG, McGue M. Environmental adversity and increasing genetic risk for externalizing disorders. *Arch Gen Psychiatry* 2009;**66**:640–648.

55 Caspi A, McClay J, Moffitt TE, et al. Role of genotype in the cycle of violence in maltreated children. *Science* 2002;**297**:851–854.

56 Kim-Cohen J, Caspi A, Taylor A, et al. MAOA, maltreatment, and gene–environment interaction predicting children's mental health: new evidence and a meta-analysis. *Mol Psychiatry* 2006;**11**:903–913.

57 Jaffee SR. Teasing out the role of genotype in the development of psychopathology in maltreated children. In: Widom CS, ed. *Trauma, psychopathology, and violence: causes, consequences, or correlates?* New York: Oxford University Press; 2012. pp. 49–75.

58 Lynam DR, Caspi A, Moffitt TE, Wikstrom POH, Loeber R, Novak S. The interaction between impulsivity and neighborhood context on offending: The effects of impulsivity are stronger in poorer neighborhoods. *J Abnormal Psychol* 2000;**109**:563–574.

59 Rowe R, Maughan B, Worthman CM, Costello EJ, Angold A. Testosterone, antisocial behavior, and social dominance in boys: pubertal development and biosocial interaction. *Biol Psychiatry* 2004;**55**:546–552.

60 Erath SA, El-Sheikh M, Hinnant JB, Cummings EM. Skin conductance level reactivity moderates the association between harsh parenting and growth in child externalizing behavior. *Dev Psychol* 2011;**47**:693–706.

61 Harden KP, Mendle J. Gene–environment interplay in the association between pubertal timing and delinquency in adolescent girls. *J Abnormal Psychol* 2012;**121**:73–87.

62 Raine A, Brennan P, Mednick B, Mednick SA. High rates of violence, crime, academic problems, and behavioral problems in males with both early neuromotor deficits and unstable family environments. *Arch Gen Psychiatry* 1996;**53**:544–549.

63 Arseneault L, Tremblay R, Boulerice B, Saucier J-F. Obstetrical complications and violent delinquency: testing two developmental pathways. *Child Dev* 2002;**73**:496–508.

64 Beck JE, Shaw DS. The influence of perinatal complications and environmental adversity on boys' antisocial behavior. *J Child Psychol Psychiatry* 2005;**46**:35–46.

65 Brennan PA, Hall J, Bor W, Najman JM, Williams G. Integrating biological and social processes in relation to early-onset persistent aggression in boys and girls. *Dev Psychol* 2003;**39**:309–323.

66 **Boyce WT, Ellis BJ.** Biological sensitivity to context: I. An evolutionary–developmental theory of origins and functions of stress reactivity. *Dev Psychopathol* 2005;**17**:271–301.

67 **Scott S, Knapp M, Henderson J, Maughan B.** Financial cost of social exclusion: follow-up study of antisocial children into adulthood. *BMJ* 2001;**232**:1–5.

68 **Foster EM, Jones DE.** The high costs of aggression: public expenditures resulting from conduct disorder. *Am J Public Health* 2005;**95**:1767–1772.

69 **Weisz JR, Kazdin AE.** *Evidence-based psychotherapies for children and adolescents*. New York: Guilford Press; 2010.

70 **Henggeler SW, Schoenwalk SK, Borduin CM, Rowland MD, Cunningham PB.** *Multisystemic therapy for antisocial behavior in children and adolescents*. 2nd ed. New York: Guilford Press; 2009.

71 **Chamberlain P.** *Treating chronic juvenile offenders: advances made through the Oregon multidimensional treatment foster care model*. Washington DC: American Psychological Association; 2003.

72 **Farrington DP.** The development of offending and antisocial behaviour from childhood: key findings from the Cambridge Study of Delinquent Development. *J Child Psychol Psychiatry* 1995;**36**:929–964.

73 **Conduct Problems Prevention Research Group.** The effects of the Fast Track preventive intervention on the development of conduct disorder across childhood. *Child Dev* 2011;**82**:331–345.

Chapter 16

Borderline, schizotypal, avoidant, obsessive–compulsive, and other personality disorders

Andrew E. Skodol

16.1 Introduction

A personality disorder (PD) is defined in DSM-IV-TR[1] as 'an enduring pattern of inner experience and behaviour that deviates markedly from the expectations of the individual's culture, is pervasive and inflexible, has an onset in adolescence or early adulthood, is stable over time, and leads to distress or impairment' (p. 685). This definition reflects a traditional view of these disorders as enduring and stable over time.

Although the onset of PDs is believed to occur in adolescence or early adulthood, temperamental antecedents can be observed in childhood.[2] PDs typically present when a young person is faced with a challenging adaptive milestone, such as leaving home or school to begin a life of greater self-sufficiency or attempting to develop close intimate relationships with people outside of his or her immediate family. And although the DSM-IV-TR definition of a PD implies an onset no later than early adulthood, there are individuals who may not come to clinical attention until later in life, as a result of a major life change in their support systems or life circumstances[3] or the onset of a medical condition.

The notion of PDs as stable disorders to be distinguished from more episodic mental disorders, such as mood disorders, has persisted despite a large number of one-time follow-up studies in DSM-III and DSM-III-R eras that showed that fewer than 50% of patients diagnosed with PDs retained these diagnoses over time.[4] Because of the substantial methodological limitations of these studies, however, a new generation of more rigorous follow-along studies was spawned.

16.2 Three naturalistic studies of clinical course in personality disorder

The results of three large-scale studies of the naturalistic course of PDs are informative for describing their life course: the Collaborative Longitudinal Personality Disorders Study (CLPS),[5] the McLean Study of Adult Development (MSAD),[6] and the Children in the Community Study (CICS).[7] Course and outcome in these studies has been examined in several different ways: in this chapter, results on diagnoses; criteria, symptoms, or traits; and psychosocial functioning are described. The studies were conducted on both patient (CLPS and MSAD) and community (CICS) populations.

16.2.1 **Collaborative Longitudinal Personality Disorders Study**

The CLPS[5] is a multi-site, National Institute of Mental Health (NIMH)-funded longitudinal study of the natural course of PDs. Participating sites are at Brown, Columbia (now in collaboration with the University of Arizona), Harvard, Yale, and Texas A&M Universities. The aims of the CLPS have been to determine the stability of PD diagnoses and criteria, personality traits, and functional impairment, and to determine predictors of clinical course. The CLPS recruited 668 treatment-seeking or recently treated patients who were diagnosed with one of four DSM-IV PDs—schizotypal (STPD), borderline (BPD), avoidant (AVPD), or obsessive–compulsive (OCPD)—or with major depressive disorder (MDD) and no PD and were followed annually for 10 years. The age range of the sample was from 18 to 45 years—the ages during which traditional views hold that PDs first become evident and are most stable.

16.2.2 **McLean Study of Adult Development**

The MSAD[6] was the first NIMH-funded prospective study of the course and outcome of border-line personality disorder (BPD). The MSAD sample consists of 290 inpatients at McLean Hospital who were diagnosed with BPD and 72 with other PDs. The comparison group included ~4% with cluster A PDs, 18% with other non-borderline cluster B PDs, 33% with cluster C PDs, and 53% with personality disorder not otherwise specified (PD-NOS). All patients in the MSAD were between the ages of 18 and 35 years when they entered the study and have been followed every 2 years for 16 years.

16.2.3 **Children in the Community Study (CICS)**

The CICS[7] is a longitudinal study of a sample of ~800 children, who were originally recruited (with their mothers) in upstate New York, when they were between 1 and 10 years of age. They have been followed periodically for 30 years. PDs have been assessed four times, when the subjects were at mean ages 14, 16, 22 and 33. This study provides a unique perspective on the development and course of personality pathology in adolescents aged <18 years.

16.3 **Course of personality disorder diagnoses, criteria, symptoms, and traits**

16.3.1 **CLPS**

In the CLPS, two definitions of remission have been used to allow contrasts between the courses of PDs and the comparison group of MDD without PD.[8] One definition requires at least two consecutive months with no more than two criteria present. The other requires 12 consecutive months. The 2-month definition allows for a direct comparison of PD remission with the widely accepted definition used for MDD, and the 12-month definition provides a more clinically sig-nificant indicator of improvement.

The CLPS study has found surprising rates of improvement in patients diagnosed with PDs.[8] Within the first 2 years of follow-up, between 33% (schizotypal) and 55% (obsessive–compulsive) of patients with PDs experienced a period of remission according to the 2-month standard. Between 23% (schizotypal) and 38% (obsessive–compulsive) experienced a 12-month remission. In addition, on blind retest at 2 years, 50–60% were below the threshold for a PD diagnosis. The mean proportion of criteria met declined significantly for each of the PDs. By 10 years, 85% of patients with BPD in the CLPS had remitted according to the 12-month remission definition and

91% according to the 2-month definition.[9] Remission from BPD was slower than from MDD and minimally slower than from AVPD and OCPD. Despite significant changes, PDs have been consistently more stable than MDD in the CLPS.

Ten per cent of patients with BPD remitted in the first 6 months of follow-up, most often in association with situational changes, such as leaving stressful relationships or stopping use of substances of abuse, raising immediate questions about whether at least certain PDs are more temporally fluctuating than previously assumed.[10] More severe baseline psychopathology and a history of childhood trauma predicted poorer outcomes in BPD over 2 years.[11] Criteria referring to unstable relationships and to suicidality and self-injury were most predictive of a BPD diagnosis 2 years later.[12] Criteria for preoccupation with details, rigidity and stubbornness, and reluctance to delegate were most predictive of an OCPD diagnosis at 2 years.[13] Positive experiences during childhood and adolescence, including achievements and positive interpersonal relationships, were associated with remission from both AVPD and STPD over 4 years of follow-up.[14] There has been no evidence in the CLPS that older age was associated with remission from BPD, as is commonly believed.[15]

Relapses of PDs in the CLPS have also occurred. Relapse rates vary by PD diagnosis: STPD has had the lowest relapse rates and AVPD has had the highest relapse rates within the first 6 years.[4] By 10 years, 12% of patients with BPD who had a 12-month remission have relapsed and 21% who had a 2-month remission—rates less frequent and slower than for patients with MDD or other PDs.[9]

Viewed as dimensions, PDs showed considerably more stability than as categories. Although the mean number of criteria decreased over time for each group, a continuous measure of number of criteria met was highly correlated across assessments during the first two years of follow-up[8] and very similar to correlations of personality traits across the age groups represented in the CLPS (18–45 years) as reported in a meta-analysis of 152 longitudinal studies by Roberts and Del Vecchio.[16] These findings suggest that PDs may be characterized by maladaptive trait constellations that are stable in their structure (individual differences) but can change in severity or expression over time.

Furthermore, some diagnostic criteria for PDs appear to be more stable than others—findings that are important in the search for phenotypes. For example, 'affective instability' was the most stable of the BPD criteria over the first 2 years of follow-up, followed by 'inappropriate, intense anger'.[17] The least stable BPD criteria were 'frantic efforts to avoid abandonment' and 'self-injury'. For AVPD, the most stable criteria were 'feels socially inept' and 'feels inadequate' and the least stable was 'avoids jobs with interpersonal contact'. These findings have led CLPS investigators to hypothesize that PDs may be reconceptualized as hybrids of more stable personality traits that may have normal variants, but that in PDs are pathologically skewed or exaggerated, and dysfunctional behaviours that are attempts at adapting to, defending against, coping with, or compensating for these pathological traits.

The CLPS has also demonstrated that traits of general personality functioning tend to be stable, with stability estimates in the $r = 0.70$ to 0.80 range over 2 years.[18] However, when study patients change on these traits, the changes are followed by lagged changes in PD psychopathology, across the spectrum of PDs. Importantly, these relationships are non-reciprocal, in that changes in PD features are not predictive of subsequent changes in personality traits. In BPD, traits of neuroticism and conscientiousness showed more change than in patients with other PDs, with mean-level neuroticism declining faster and conscientiousness increasing faster.[19] In addition, BPD was characterized by greater individual level instability for these two traits. These results point to the possible importance of personality trait instability underlying the instability of BPD itself. Trait and disorder models of personality pathology have been compared to each other with respect to stability over time in the CLPS. Dimensional trait models, both of normal personality and abnormal personality, have been found to be more stable than PD categories and even 'dimensionalized' (i.e. criteria counts) PD measures.[20]

16.3.2 MSAD

The most striking finding of the MSAD has also been the degree of improvement, especially in the patients with BPD: 93% of these patients experienced a symptomatic remission lasting at least 2 years within 10 years of follow-up.[21] and 99% within 16 years.[22] Significant predictors of earlier time to remission included younger age, absence of childhood sexual abuse, absent family history of substance use disorder, good vocational record, absence of a cluster C PD, low trait neuroticism, and high trait agreeableness.[23] Even for remissions lasting as long as 8 years, patients with BPD had high rates (78%) at 16 years. Patients with other personality disorders (OPDs) achieved similarly high rates of remission, but the time to remission was slower for the patients with BPD. Recovery rates, which required good social and vocational functioning as well as symptomatic remission, were lower in borderline patients in comparison to those with OPDs, and time to recovery was again slower. However, recovery rates over 10 years were relatively stable.[21] After 16 years, by contrast, symptomatic recurrence (36% of those with a 2-year remission compared to 7%) and loss of recovery (44% compared with 28%) occurred at substantially higher rates in patients with BPD than in patients with OPDs and also occurred more rapidly. Thus, in the MSAD, sustained symptomatic remission has been significantly more common than sustained recovery in patients with BPD and remissions and recoveries more difficult to attain and to sustain for patients with BPD than for patients with other types of PD.

Consistent with the CLPS, the MSAD found differential stability among the symptoms of BPD. Symptoms reflecting impulsivity, such as self-mutilation and suicide attempts, and activities aimed at managing interpersonal difficulties (demanding behaviour, entitlement) had the most rapid decline in frequency over time.[24] Symptoms reflecting chronic mood problems, such as anger and interpersonal symptoms reflecting abandonment and dependency issues (intolerance of being alone, counter-dependency), were more stable. The 10-year course of interpersonal disturbances thought to be at the core of BPD has been studied in detail.[25] Behaviourally oriented interpersonal features, such as recurrent break-ups, demandingness, entitlement, and boundary violations remitted quickly and were rare at the end of the follow-up. Affectively oriented interpersonal features related to intolerance of being alone and to conflicts over dependency were more persistent.

16.3.3 CICS

Too few adolescent subjects in the CICS met criteria for specific PDs to reliably obtain stability estimates. Therefore, the CICS examined the stability of PD traits and found that levels decreased by 48% between adolescence (age 14–16 years) and early adulthood (age 22 years).[26] These results have been interpreted as indicating that most children and adolescents exhibiting thoughts, feelings, and behaviours consistent with PDs will mature out of them, and that PDs in young adults may represent maturational delays.[7] Importantly, however, children and adolescents who have the highest levels of PD symptoms are at the greatest risk for having a PD in young adulthood.

The odds of PDs in young adults increased given the presence of a PD in the same cluster in adolescence.[27] Disruptive behaviour disorders, anxiety disorders, and MDD all increased the likelihood of young adult PDs independent of adolescent PDs. Major depressive disorder increased the likelihood of dependent, antisocial, passive–aggressive, and histrionic PDs.[28]

Maternal separation before age 5 years predicted elevations in BPD symptoms from early adolescence to middle adulthood independent of other significant predictors including childhood temperament, child abuse, maternal problems, and suboptimal parenting.[29] School climates focused on learning or offering opportunities for student autonomy were related to declines in PD symptoms.[30] Schools with less structure were associated with increases in symptoms.

16.4 Course of impairment in psychosocial functioning in personality disorders

16.4.1 CLPS

The diagnostic instability of PDs found in the CLPS raises the question: What is stable with respect to PD? Over the first 2 years of follow-up,[31] the CLPS found that patients with BPD or OCPD showed no improvement in any domain of functioning overall, but patients with BPD who experienced change in personality psychopathology showed some improvement in functioning. Of the different domains of functioning examined, impairment in social relationships appeared most stable in patients with PDs. Although there were significant differences in global functioning between various PDs and between PDs and MDD, the only significant change (improvement) over time occurred in the MDD group.

In a comparison of the ability of various diagnostic models of personality psychopathology to predict functioning over time, DSM-IV relationships were strongest at the baseline assessment and declined over 4 years, whereas trait-based models were less predictive at baseline, but more predictive over time.[20] These results were replicated at 6-, 8-, and 10-year follow-ups.[32] Thus, the DSM-IV representation of personality psychopathology captures important variance in functioning when patients have acute problems and are seeking treatment, but over the natural course of PD, personality traits capture variance in functioning better than DSM-IV criteria.

Which specific PD criteria or general personality traits are most associated with functional impairment over time is of interest. In an initial study from the CLPS, neuroticism was positively correlated with generally worse functioning at 2- and 5-year follow-ups.[33] Extraversion and agreeableness were negatively linked with social dysfunction and with recreational dysfunction. Openness to experience was negatively associated with recreational dysfunction and conscientiousness was negatively related to work dysfunction.

16.4.2 MSAD

Overall, the psychosocial functioning of borderline patients in the MSAD improved significantly over the first 6 years of follow-up. Compared with only 26% of the borderline sample who were rated as having good or better functioning when recruited, 56% were found to have at least good functioning 6 years later.[34] Nonetheless, borderline patients continued to function more poorly than patients with other PDs, particularly in the area of vocational achievement. Borderline patients who experienced symptomatic remission functioned significantly better socially and vocationally than those who did not remit, consistent with findings from the CLPS. At 10 years, borderline patients who did not have good psychosocial functioning at baseline continued to function with difficulty. By contrast with the CLPS, the majority of poor psychosocial functioning was in vocational performance, rather than in social performance.[35] Patients with BPD were three times more likely to have received social security disability income, at least intermittently, over the follow-up period than were patients with OPDs.[36]

16.4.3 CISC

The impact of PD psychopathology on functioning has been examined in the CICS for each DSM PD cluster. For cluster A (odd, eccentric cluster), adolescents with high symptom levels had lower education and achievement,[37] greater partner conflict, and earlier childbearing[38] in early adulthood. Adolescents with high levels of cluster B (dramatic, erratic) symptoms had lower levels of intimacy[39] and sustained conflict with partners[38] in early adulthood. Adolescents with high levels of cluster C (anxious, fearful) symptoms had greater conflict with partners, if they had a partner[38] Adolescents and young adults who qualified for a diagnosis of PD-NOS experienced significant educational failure and interpersonal difficulties.[40] Young adults at age 22 years with any PD (and each cluster) had impaired quality of life (QOL) 11 years later.[41] ASPD, BPD, and STPD had particularly strong associations with reductions in QOL.

The effects of PD stability on global functioning and impairment were also examined in the CICS.[42] Individuals with persistent PDs had markedly poorer functioning and greater impairment at mean age 33 years than did those who had never been identified as having such a disorder or who had a PD that was in remission.

16.5 Summary

In contradiction to the traditional view that PDs represent forms of psychopathology that are stable over time, three methodologically rigorous longitudinal studies in both clinical and epidemiological populations indicate that PDs improve over the life course and have a clinical course that is likely more waxing and waning than chronic. Numerous factors, both personal and environmental, have been identified that influence the likelihood of improvement from PDs. The results on the course of functional impairment in PDs suggest that impairment is more stable than personality psychopathology itself, but that when PD improves, improvement in functioning may follow.

Much more needs to be learned about the development of PDs and their course over time, so that they can be better understood, treated, and ultimately prevented. Taking a life course perspective on the development of PDs other than ASPD from childhood onwards should enhance our understanding of the developmental pathways involved in personality psychopathology, for instance the interplay over time of genetic risks and environmental adversities hypothesized in diathesis–stress models of borderline PD.[43] Understanding the links between genetic liabilities and adverse childhood experiences and specific elements of PD psychopathology, such as emotional dysregulation and self- and interpersonal functioning, should lead to more focused treatment interventions and perhaps to prevention.

References

1 **American Psychiatric Association**. *Diagnostic and statistical manual of mental disorders.* 4th ed. text revision. Washington DC: APA; 2000.
2 **Tackett JL, Balsis S, Oltmanns TF, Krueger RF**. A unifying perspective on personality pathology across the lifespan: developmental considerations for the fifth edition of the *Diagnostic and statistical manual of mental disorders. Dev Psychopathol* 2009;**21**:687–713.
3 **Oltmanns TF, Balsis S**. Personality disorders in later life: questions about the measurement, course, and impact of disorders. *Annu Rev Clin Psychol* 2011;**7**:321–349.

4 Skodol AE. Longitudinal course and outcome of personality disorders. *Psychiatr Clin North Am* 2008;**31**:495–503.

5 Gunderson JG, Shea MT, Skodol AE, et al. The Collaborative Longitudinal Personality Disorders Study: development, aims, design, and sample characteristics. *J Pers Disord* 2000;**14**:300–315.

6 Zanarini MC, Frankenburg FR, Hennen J, Reich DB, Silk KR. The McLean study of adult development (MSAD): overview and implications of the first six years of prospective follow-up. *J Pers Disord* 2005;**19**:505–523.

7 Cohen P, Crawford TN, Johnson JG, Kasen S. The children in the community study of developmental course of personality disorder. *J Pers Disord* 2005;**19**:466–486.

8 Grilo CM, Shea MT, Sanislow CA, et al. Two-year stability and change in schizotypal, borderline, avoidant and obsessive–compulsive personality disorders. *J Consult Clin Psychol* 2004;**72**:767–775.

9 Gunderson JG, Stout RL, McGlashan TH, et al. Ten year course of borderline personality disorder: psychopathology and function from the Collaborative Longitudinal Personality Disorders Study. *Arch Gen Psychiatry* 2011;**68**:827–837.

10 Gunderson JG, Bender D, Sanislow C, et al. Plausibility and possible determinants of sudden "remissions" in borderline patients. *Psychiatry* 2003;**66**:111–119.

11 Gunderson JG, Daversa MT, Grilo CM, et al. Predictors of 2-year outcome for patients with borderline personality disorder. *Am J Psychiatry* 2006;**163**:822–826.

12 Grilo CM, Sanislow CA, Skodol AE, et al. Longitudinal diagnostic efficiency of DSM-IV criteria for borderline personality disorder: a 2-year prospective study. *Can J Psychiatry* 2007;**52**:357–362.

13 Grilo CM, Skodol AE, Gunderson JG, et al. Longitudinal diagnostic efficiency of DSM-IV criteria for obsessive–compulsive personality disorder: a 2-year prospective study. *Acta Psychiatr Scand* 2004;**110**:64–68.

14 Skodol AE, Bender DS, Pagano ME, et al. Positive childhood experiences: resilience and recovery from personality disorder in early adulthood. *J Clin Psychiatry* 2007;**68**:1102–1108.

15 Shea MT, Edelen MO, Pinto A, et al. Improvement in borderline personality disorder in relationship to age. *Acta Psychiatr Scand* 2009;**119**:143–148.

16 Roberts BW, Del Vecchio WF. The rank-order consistency of personality traits from childhood to old age: a quantitative review of longitudinal studies. *Psychol Bull* 2000;**126**:3–125.

17 McGlashan TH, Grilo CM, Sanislow CA, et al. Two-year prevalence and stability of individual criteria for schizotypal, borderline, avoidant, and obsessive–compulsive personality disorders. *Am J Psychiatry* 2005;**162**:883–889.

18 Warner MB, Morey LC, Finch JF, et al. The longitudinal relationship of personality traits and disorders. *J Abnorm Psychol* 2004;**113**:217–227.

19 Hopwood CJ, Newman DA, Donnellan MB, et al. The stability of personality traits in individuals with borderline personality disorder. *J Abnorm Psychol* 2009;**118**:806–815.

20 Morey LC, Hopwood CJ, Gunderson JG, et al. Comparison of diagnostic models for personality disorders. *Psychol Med* 2007;**37**:983–994.

21 Zanarini MC, Frankenburg FR, Reich DB, Fitzmaurice G. Time to attainment of recovery from borderline personality disorder and stability of recovery: a 10-year prospective follow-up study. *Am J Psychiatry* 2010;**167**:663–667.

22 Zanarini MC, Frankenburg FR, Reich DB, Fitzmaurice G. Attainment and stability of sustained symptomatic remission and recovery among patients with borderline personality disorder and axis II comparison subjects: a 16-year prospective follow-up study. *Am J Psychiatry* 2012;**169**:476–483.

23 Zanarini MC, Frankenburg FR, Hennen J, Reich DB, Silk KR. Prediction of the 10-year course of borderline personality disorder. *Am J Psychiatry* 2006;**163**:827–832.

24 Zanarini MC, Frankenburg FR, Reich DB, Silk KR, Hudson JI, McSweeney LB. The subsyndromal phenomenology of borderline personality disorder: a 10-year follow-up study. *Am J Psychiatry* 2007;**164**:929–935.

25 Choi-Kain LW, Zanarini MC, Frankenburg FR, Fitzmaurice GM, Reich DB. A longitudinal study of the 10-year course of interpersonal features in borderline personality disorder. *J Pers Disord* 2010;**24**:365–376.

26 Johnson JG, Cohen P, Kasen S, Skodol AE, Hamagami F, Brook JS. Age-related change in personality disorder trait levels between early adolescence and adulthood: a community-based longitudinal investigation. *Acta Psychiatr Scand* 2000;**102**:265–275.

27 Kasen S, Cohen P, Skodol AE, Johnson JG, Brook JS. Influence of child and adolescent psychiatric disorders on young adult personality disorder. *Am J Psychiatry* 1999;**156**:1529–1535.

28 Kasen S, Cohen P, Skodol AE, Johnson JG, Smailes E, Brook JS. Childhood depression and adult personality disorder: alternative pathways of continuity. *Arch Gen Psychiatry* 2001;**58**:231–236.

29 Crawford TN, Cohen PR, Chen H, Anglin DM, Ehrensaft M. Early maternal separation and the trajectory of borderline personality disorder symptoms. *Dev Psychopathol* 2009;**21**:1013–1030.

30 Kasen S, Cohen P, Chen H, Johnson JG, Crawford TN. School climate and continuity of adolescent personality disorder symptoms. *J Child Psychol Psychiatry* 2009;**50**:1504–1512.

31 Skodol AE, Pagano ME, Bender DS, et al. Stability of functional impairment in patients with schizotypal, borderline, avoidant, or obsessive–compulsive personality disorder over two years. *Psychol Med* 2005;**35**:443–451.

32 Morey LC, Hopwood CJ, Markowitz JC, et al. Comparison of alternative models for personality disorders, II: 6-, 8-, and 10-year follow-up. *Psychol Med* 2012;**42**:1705–1713.

33 Hopwood CJ, Morey LC, Ansell EB, et al. The convergent, discriminant, and incremental validity of five-factor traits: current and prospective social, work, and recreational dysfunction. *J Pers Disord* 2009;**23**:466–476.

34 Zanarini MC, Frankenburg FR, Hennen J, Reich DB, Silk KR. Psychosocial functioning of borderline patients and axis II comparison subjects followed prospectively for six years. *J Pers Disord* 2005;**19**:19–29.

35 Zanarini MC, Frankenburg FR, Reich DB, Fitzmaurice G. The 10-year course of psychosocial functioning among patients with borderline personality disorder and axis II comparison subjects. *Acta Psychiatr Scand* 2010;**122**:103–109.

36 Zanarini MC, Jacoby RJ, Frankenburg FR, Reich DB, Fitzmaurice G. The 10-year course of social security disability income reported by patients with borderline personality disorder and axis II comparison subjects. *J Pers Disord* 2009;**23**:346–356.

37 Cohen P, Chen H, Kasen S, Johnson JG, Crawford TN, Gordon K. Adolescent cluster A personality disorder symptoms, role assumptions in the transition to adulthood, and resolution or persistence of symptoms. *Dev Psychopathol* 2005;**17**:549–568.

38 Chen H, Cohen P, Johnson JG, Kasen S, Sneed JR, Crawford TN. Adolescent personality disorder and conflict with romantic partners during the transition to adulthood. *J Pers Disord* 2004;**18**:507–525.

39 Crawford TN, Cohen P, Johnson JG, Sneed JR, Brook JS. The course and psychosocial correlates of personality disorder symptoms in adolescence: Erickson's developmental theory revisited. *J Youth Adolesc* 2004;**33**:373–387.

40 Johnson JG, First MB, Cohen P, Skodol AE, Kasen S, Brook JS. Adverse outcomes associated with personality disorder not otherwise specified (PDNOS) in a community sample. *Am J Psychiatry* 2005;**162**:1926–1932.

41 Chen H, Cohen P, Crawford TN, Kasen S, Johnson JG, Berenson K. Relative impact of young adult personality disorders on subsequent quality of life: findings of a community-based longitudinal study. *J Pers Disord* 2006;**20**:510–523.

42 Skodol AE, Johnson JG, Cohen P, Sneed JR, Crawford TN. Personality disorder and impaired functioning from adolescence to adulthood. *Br J Psychiatry* 2007;**190**:415–420.

43 Belsky DW, Caspi A, Arseneault L, et al. Etiologic features of borderline personality related characteristics in a birth cohort of 12-year-old children. *Dev Psychopathol* 2012;**24**:251–265.

Part 4

Understanding mechanisms

Chapter 17

Cognitive function over the life course

Marcus Richards

17.1 Introduction

Cognitive function, which involves the higher mental processes of perception, attention, learning, remembering, and reasoning, is shaped by factors operating across the whole of the life course:[1] from genes, through the uterine environment and into the highly malleable stage of infancy; through the school years and transition into the adult word of work and lifestyle choices; then finally later life, when the accumulating effects of health on brain ageing are increasingly manifest. We should first note what we mean by cognitive function. In children this is most commonly measured as general cognitive ability, often divided into two correlated factors, crystallized and fluid ability. The former refers to the acquisition and use of knowledge, whereas the latter is concerned with reasoning and problem-solving in novel situations.[2] Both sets of skills are also measured in adulthood and later life; typically fluid ability declines with age and morbidity, whereas crystallized ability is well preserved, even in the face of mild dementia, and can continue to improve in old age.[3] In the adult years other age-sensitive cognitive tests are also administered, above all those of memory, executive function, speed of processing and visuospatial function, although these can be given in childhood too.

Cognitive impairment is detectable in childhood, but can have a lifetime impact. It is also increasingly clear that risk of clinically significant cognitive decline accumulates over the life course rather than emerges purely as a phenomenon of senescence or later life morbidity.[4] Cognitive function tracks across the life course, even when the influence of educational attainment and parental and own socio-economic position are controlled;[5] and childhood[6] and early adult[7] cognition predict dementia. It therefore follows that influences on cognition in early life, childhood and adolescence can indirectly influence cognitive functioning in adulthood and later life (although see Section 17.3.2).

17.2 Widespread cognitive disorders of ageing

It is essential to distinguish cognitive problems that are detected in childhood and that persist across the life course, from cognitive impairment and decline that emerge in later life, most seriously Alzheimer disease. However, it is also important to recognize that the former may be a risk factor for the latter.[8] With regard to cognitive disorders of middle and later life, there have been various attempts to classify cognitive impairment in ageing that falls short of clinical dementia, for example 'cognitive impairment—no dementia'. Currently the most widely used is 'mild cognitive impairment' (MCI) (Box 17.1).[9]

Box 17.1: Proposed criteria for mild cognitive impairment (MCI)

- A report of cognitive impairment by the patient that represents a change.
- Evidence of preserved functional ability.
- Absence of frank dementia.
- A relevant cognitive test score performance in the mildly impaired range with respect to an appropriate norm.

Source: data from Petersen RC, Mild cognitive impairment, *New England Journal of Medicine*, Volume 364, pp. 2227–2234, Copyright © 2011 Massachusetts Medical Society. All rights reserved.

A large research effort has been devoted to establishing whether MCI is a stable entity, a risk factor for dementia, or simply an early manifestation of the latter. The 'conversion' rate to dementia is generally around 10%, but in any individual this depends on degree of cognitive impairment at presentation, the presence of the *apolipoprotein* (*APOE*) ε4 allele, and the presence of neuropathological markers on investigation.[9] With regard to dementia itself, the most common form is late onset Alzheimer's disease (AD, Box 17.2), whereas early onset AD is comparatively rare, and is mostly an autosomal dominant familiar disease. A widely quoted estimate for the prevalence of late-onset AD is ~7% at age 65 years, doubling every 5 years thereafter. Late onset AD has historically been framed as a neuropathological entity, driven by amyloidosis or other misfolded proteins, leading to neuronal death. However, a synthesis of evidence also suggests that this form of AD is a diffuse clinical syndrome representing the accumulation over the life course of multiple pathologies.[10]

Box 17.2: ICD-10 criteria for Alzheimer disease

(A) Criteria for dementia must be met:

- a decline in memory, which is most evident in the learning of new information, although in more severe cases, the recall of previously learned information may be also affected;
- a decline in other cognitive abilities characterized by deterioration in judgement and thinking, such as planning and organizing, and in the general processing of information;
- preserved awareness of the environment (i.e. absence of clouding of consciousness) during a period of time long enough to enable the unequivocal demonstration of memory decline;
- a decline in emotional control or motivation, or a change in social behaviour, manifest as at least one of: emotional lability, irritability, apathy; or coarsening of social behaviour;
- for a confident clinical diagnosis, memory decline should be present for at least six months.

> ## Box 17.2: ICD-10 criteria for Alzheimer disease *(continued)*
>
> (B) There is no evidence from the history, physical examination or special investigations for any other possible cause of dementia (e.g. cerebrovascular disease, Parkinson disease, Huntington disease, normal pressure hydrocephalus), a sysytemic disorder (e.g. hypothyroidism, vitamin B_{12} or folic acid deficiency, hypercalcaemia), or alcohol or drug misuse
> (C) At least one of the following requirements must be met:
>
> - evidence of a very slow, gradual onset and progression (the rate of the latter may be known only retrospectively after a course of ≥3 years);
>
> - predominance of memory impairment over intellectual impairment (see above general criteria for dementia);
>
> Source: adapted from *International statistical classification of diseases and related health problems*, 10th ed. (ICD-10), World Health Organization, Geneva, Switzerland, Copyright © 1992 with permission from the World Health Organization, available from <http://www.who.int/classifications/icd/en/GRNBOOK.pdf>

17.3 **A life course perspective**

17.3.1 **Genetic influence**

As O'Donovan and Owen note, 'with its role in human adaptability and survival, it would be remarkable if traits that result from variation in brain function were not influenced in part by genes.'[11] Indeed, the heritability of general cognitive ability is ~30% in early childhood, rising to as much as 80% in older adults through matching to environment, and genetic influences on neural processes of ageing.[12] Consistent with this, a large genome-wide association study (GWAS) showed that a substantial proportion of individual differences in general cognitive ability is due to genetic variation.[13] The heritability of AD has been recognized since the 1920s, but a major impetus came from the identification of a genetic locus segregating with familial AD mapped to chromosome 21, close to the *amyloid precursor protein* (*APP*) gene—the 'London mutation'.[14] GWAS has now identified a mutation in the *APP* gene that protects against late onset AD,[15] and is also associated with milder cognitive decline. This lends support to the sometimes controversial view that this more widespread form of AD represents the extreme end of the population cognitive decline distribution rather than a discreet disease entity.[16] The best-known genetic risk factor for AD, however, is the *ε4* allele of the *APOE* gene, which is also associated with normal cognitive ageing (although not development).[17] In addition to the role of the DNA sequence, genetic influence on AD also occurs through epigenetic alteration of gene expression during interaction with the environment.[18]

17.3.2 **Fetal growth**

The developmental origins theory of Barker led to increasing interest in fetal growth as a determinant of mental function. In this context there is a clear consensus that birth weight across the full population range is positively associated with cognitive ability in childhood, independently of social origins.[19] This association is biologically plausible, as almost certainly due to common physiological cause. However, effect sizes are modest;[19] there is no evidence that they have long term impact on cognitive ageing,[20] and associations may be substantially confounded by maternal cognitive ability.[21] Indeed, many apparent influences on fetal growth and pregnancy duration, such as maternal stress, maternal diet and teratogenic agents, are themselves confounded by maternal cognitive ability[22] and genetic common cause;[24] and many prenatal exposures persist into postnatal life, so estimating exposure window is difficult.[23]

17.3.3 Early childhood

Although the most rapid neural development occurs during fetal growth, this is still substantial during the first 5 years of postnatal life. Various maturational and health-related variables are associated with cognitive development, including postnatal somatic growth (independently of birth weight),[24] motor development,[25] micronutrients,[26] and physical disease.[27] As with prenatal exposures, however, confounding by maternal cognitive ability, for example in regard to putative effects of long-chain fatty acids in breast milk,[28] is a serious analytical consideration.

Shifting to the social level, the caregiver plays a role in early cognitive development. In this context, separation from a caregiver through parental divorce, one of the most widespread stressors faced by children in western cultures, is associated with lower academic achievement.[29] Consideration of the caregiver leads to the topic of parenting style. For example the authoritarian (high use of coercive discipline; low use of open dialogue; with a high control–low trust parent-centred approach) and permissive (low expectations; lack of control; and inconsistent approaches to discipline) parenting styles suggested by Baumrind hinder the development of competence and self-regulation,[30] with implications for cognitive development. Consistent with this, coercive discipline was associated with poorer cognitive development in the 1946 British birth cohort, after controlling for a wide range of confounders, including parental cognitive ability.[31]

At a wider societal level chronic poverty is associated with lower cognitive function.[32] Underlying mechanisms almost certainly involve autonomic and neuroendocrine dysregulation. There are additional effects of the neighbourhood on school achievement, independently of individual and family-level characteristics. Potential mechanisms include quality of services, control of noxious or hazardous exposures, and more subtle factors such as community responsibility for individuals.[33] Combined deprivation in all these respects may explain the striking decline in cognitive ability of urban children from age 6 to 11 years after controlling for maternal cognition and education; whereas those of suburban children in the same metropolitan area remained relatively unchanged.[34] Importantly, these two study areas are strongly segregated by race, where analysis suggests that severely disadvantaged neighbourhoods can reduce later verbal ability in African-American children to a degree equivalent to missing a year or more of schooling.[35]

17.3.4 Education

Cognition is an important determinant of educational achievement,[36] yet education is capable of augmenting cognitive skills net of this,[5,37] even allowing for genetic common cause.[38] This has been observed for adult education as well as formal schooling,[39] and effects can rapidly respond to policy changes.[40] This benefit of education should not be surprising. Schooling teaches specific knowledge, teaches practical skills for the workplace, refines other cognitive skills, socializes the individual for success, and shapes confidence and motivation.[41] Education also provides a readily identifiable credential that selects the individual into the workforce.[42] However, there are large historical racial inequalities in the provision of schooling in the USA.[43] Lower verbal and non-verbal test scores in African-Americans compared to Whites, even when matched for years of education, are largely explained by reading level, which is suggested to reflect quality rather than quantity of schooling.[44] There are racial disparities in the signalling power of a particular credential too; based on 2008 US Census Bureau statistics, mean income returns to a bachelor's degree for African-American and Hispanic males were nearly 30% lower than those for Whites.[45]

17.3.5 **Work and retirement**

Echoing the role of education, the seminal studies of Kohn and Schooler showed that, while cognitive ability is a determinant of intellectually demanding work, work complexity is also beneficial to cognitive function.[46] Importantly, this is observed when adolescent cognitive ability is controlled.[47] In regard to mechanism, a striking example of how occupational skill can directly alter brain structures supporting cognition comes from the 'taxi driver' study. Qualifying as a London cab driver requires passing a test on the layout of all 25,000 or so streets in the city. Neuroimaging revealed a shift in the hippocampus from anterior to posterior in drivers compared with controls, which favours visuo-spatial learning, the extent of which was correlated with time spent in the job.[48]

If work activities help to support cognition, it follows that loss of work through long term unemployment or retirement may be a risk factor for accelerated cognitive decline, unless compensatory activities are taken up. This is consistent with the disuse or 'use it or lose it' hypothesis.[49] Results from the UK Whitehall II study tentatively support the disuse hypothesis in regard to cognitive ageing.[50] Further such studies are urgently required now that extending working age has become a policy issue.

17.3.6 **Cognitive engagement**

The disuse hypothesis is also identified with advice to keep mentally active during ageing. Again there is evidence from Schooler of a reciprocal process between cognitive functioning and complex leisure time engagement.[51] Since then there have been attempts to estimate levels of cognitive engagement over the life course, which show an inverse association with incident AD,[52] independently of education. This leads to the topic of cognitive training. There is little question that performance specific to a cognitive training task will improve with practice; the controversial issue is whether there are subsequent 'transfer effects' to more general tests of cognitive function. A large online experiment failed to provide such evidence,[53] although criticism has arisen from sample selection and the relatively young mean age of participants. More encouraging has been a recent trial of training on a 'Space Fortress' game, given to healthy older adults. This game exercises divided attention, multi-tasking, visual scanning, working memory, long term memory, and motor control. After training, offline testing of executive control showed some modest improvement.[54]

17.3.7 **Adult health**

Just as physical health is associated with cognitive development,[27] there is little doubt that lifestyle and physical health are associated with cognitive ageing. For example, Type II diabetes is associated with cognitive impairment in ageing, to the extent that AD has been termed 'type 3 diabetes'.[55] A wide range of physiological mechanisms leading to cerebrovascular disease and amyloid deposition have been implicated, including inflammation, oxidative stress, endocrine dysregulation, and differences in gene expression.[56] Risk of cognitive impairment from midlife hypertension accumulates over decades, although hypotension becomes a risk for dementia in later life, possibly suggesting that older people need higher blood pressure to maintain cerebral perfusion.[57] Similar inversions appear with other cardiovascular risk factors.[58,59] One caution, however, is over the possibility of reverse causation, i.e. that these associations are explained by factors associated with prior cognition.[60] This does not rule out the possibility of recursive effects of physical disease on cognition, but does suggest that estimates of the latter may be inflated if such reverse causality is not controlled.

Consideration of health leads to the topic of lifestyle. Systematic reviews and meta-analyses show that physical exercise[61] and light-to-moderate alcohol consumption are associated with reduced risk of dementia,[62] whereas the opposite is true of smoking.[63] In a well-controlled prospective cohort study, adherence to a Mediterranean-type diet was associated with reduced risk of AD, particularly in those who were physically active.[64] In a comprehensive attempt to investigate the specificity of these behaviours, healthy diet was associated with slower memory decline and physical activity was associated with slower decline in processing speed, after these behaviours had been mutually adjusted as well as for other confounders.[65]

17.4 Summary

Cognitive function is modifiable across the life course, and we have attempted to trace this overall arc to gain perspective on cognitive disorders of ageing. Much is at stake if these can be prevented. In the UK alone, dementia costs the economy £23 billion (US$35 billion) per year,[10] more per patient than the median UK salary; and the impact of these disorders on individual sufferers and their families is frequently devastating. A life course approach demands joined-up thinking about prevention, suggesting ways in which change at one life stage can influence risk at subsequent stages. To take one example, early intervention in education can have wide-ranging effects that ultimately modify risk of cognitive disorders in ageing. We must also, however, ignore the ageist myth that 'the horse is out of the barn'[66] and continue to target interventions to older people themselves, for example encouraging the maintenance of physical activity. Thus the life course approach offers a holistic solution to protecting cognitive function.

Further reading

Deary IJ. *Looking down on human intelligence. From psychometrics to the brain*. Oxford: Oxford University Press; 2000.

Oakley L, Flanagan C, Banyard P. *Cognitive development*. Hove: Routledge; 2004.

Park DC, Schwartz N. *Cognitive aging: a primer*. Philadelphia: Psychology Press; 2000.

References

1 Beddington J, Cooper CL, Field J, et al. The mental wealth of nations. *Nature* 2008;**455**:1057–1060.

2 Horn JL, Cattell RB. Refinement and test of the theory of fluid and crystallised general intelligences. *J Educ Psychol* 1966;**57**:253–270.

3 Rabbitt P. Does it all go together when it goes? The nineteen Bartlett memorial Lecture. *Q J Exp Psychol* 1993;**6**:385–434.

4 Whalley LJ, Dick FD, McNeill G. A life-course approach to the aetiology of late-onset dementias. *Lancet Neurol* 2006;**5**:87–96.

5 Richards M, Sacker A. Lifetime antecedents of cognitive reserve. *J Clin Exp Neuropsychol* 2003;**25**:614–24.

6 McGurn B, Deary IJ, Starr JM. Childhood cognitive ability and risk of late-onset Alzheimer and vascular dementia. *Neurology* 2008;**71**:1051–1056.

7 **Snowdon DA, Kemper SJ, Mortimer JA, et al.** Linguistic ability in early life and cognitive function and Alzheimer's disease in late life. Findings from the Nun Study. *JAMA* 1996;**275**:528–32.

8 **Zigman WB, Lott IT.** Alzheimer's disease in Down syndrome: neurobiology and risk. *Ment Retard Dev Disabil Res Rev* 2007;**13**:237–246.

9 **Petersen RC.** Mild cognitive impairment. *N Engl J Med* 2011;**364**:2227–2234.

10 **Richards M, Brayne C.** What do we mean by Alzheimer's disease? *BMJ* 2010;**41**:865–867.

11 **O'Donovan MC, Owen MJ.** Genetics and the brain: many pathways to enlightenment. *Hum Genet* 2009;**126**:1–2.

12 **Deary IJ, Johnson W, Houlihan LM.** Genetic foundations of human intelligence. *Hum Genet* 2009;**126**:215–232.

13 **Davies G, Tenesa A, Payton A, et al.** Genome-wide association studies establish that human intelligence is highly heritable and polygenic. *Mol Psychiatry* 2011;**16**:996–1005.

14 **Goate A, Chartier-Harlin MC, Mullan M, et al.** Segregation of a missense mutation in the amyloid precursor protein gene with familial Alzheimer's disease. *Nature* 1991;**349**:704–706.

15 **Jonsson T, Atwal JK, Steinberg S, et al.** A mutation in APP protects against Alzheimer's disease and age-related cognitive decline. *Nature* 2012;**488**(7409):96–99.

16 **Brayne C.** The elephant in the room—healthy brains in later life, epidemiology and public health. *Nat Neurosci* 2007;**8**:233–239.

17 **Deary IJ, Whiteman MC, Pattie A, et al.** Cognitive change and the APOE epsilon 4 allele. *Nature* 2002;**418**:932.

18 **Chouliaras L, Rutten BP, Kenis G, et al.** Epigenetic regulation in the pathophysiology of Alzheimer's disease. *Prog Neurobiol* 2010;**90**:498–510.

19 **Shenkin SD, Starr JM, Deary IJ.** Birth weight and cognitive ability in childhood: a systematic review. *Psychol Bull* 2004;**130**:989–1013.

20 **Richards M, Hardy R, Kuh D, Wadsworth M.** Birth weight and cognitive function in the British 1946 birth cohort. *BMJ* 2001;**322**:199–202.

21 **Deary IJ, Der G, Shenkin SD.** Does mother's IQ explain the association between birth weight and cognitive ability in childhood? *Intelligence* 2005;**33**:445–454.

22 **Batty GD, Der G, Deary IJ.** Effect of maternal smoking during pregnancy on offspring's cognitive ability: empirical evidence for complete confounding in the US national longitudinal survey of youth. *Pediatrics* 2006;**118**:943–50.

23 **Thapar A, Rutter M.** Do prenatal factors cause psychiatric disorder? Be wary of causal claims. *B J Psychiatry* 2009;**195**:100–101.

24 **Richards M, Hardy R, Kuh D, Wadsworth M.** Postnatal growth and cognitive function in a national UK birth cohort. *Int J Epidemiol* 2002;**31**:342–348.

25 **Murray GK, Jones PB, Kuh D, Richards M.** Infant developmental milestones and subsequent cognitive function. *Ann Neurol* 2007;**62**:128–136.

26 **Richards M, Dangour A, Uauy R.** Infant feeding, mental development, and mental ageing. In: Wyness L, Stanner S, Buttriss J editors. *Nutrition and development: long and short term consequences for health*. A report of the British Nutrition Foundation Task Force. Chichester: Wiley–Blackwell; 2013.

27 **Eppig C, Fincher CL, Thornhill R.** Parasite prevalence and the worldwide distribution of cognitive ability. *Proc R Soc B* 2010;**277**:3801–3808.

28 **Der G, Batty GD, Deary IJ.** Effect of breast feeding on intelligence in children: prospective study, sibling pairs analysis, and meta-analysis. BMJ 2006;**333**:929–930.

29 **Amato PR.** Life-span adjustment of children to their parents' divorce. *Future Child* 1994;**4**:143–164.

30 **McLeod BD, Wood JJ, Weisz JR.** Examining the association between parenting and childhood anxiety: a meta-analysis. *Clin Psychol Rev* 2007;**27**:155–172.

31 Byford M, Kuh D, Richards M. Parenting practices and intergenerational associations in cognitive ability. Evidence from two generations of a British birth cohort. *Int J Epidemiol* 2012;**41**:263–272.

32 Lynch JW, Kaplan GA, Shame SJ. Cumulative impact of sustained economic hardship on physical, cognitive, psychological, and social functioning. *N Engl J Med* 1997;**337**:1889–1895.

33 Evans GW. Child development and the physical environment. *Annu Rev Psychol* 2006;**57**:423–451.

34 Breslau N, Chilcoat HD, Susser ES, et al. Stability and change in children's intelligence quotient scores: a comparison of two socioeconomically disparate communities. *Am J Epidemiol* 2001;**154**:711–717.

35 Sampson RJ, Sharkey P, Raudenbush SW. Durable effects of concentrated disadvantage on verbal ability among African-American children. *Proc Natl Acad Sci USA* 2008;**105**:845–852.

36 Deary IJ, Strand S, Smith P, Fernandes C. Intelligence and educational achievement. *Intelligence* 2006;**35**:13–21.

37 Lager ACJ, Modin BE, De Stavola BL, Vågerö DH. Social origin, schooling and individual change in intelligence during childhood influence long-term mortality: a 68-year follow-up study. *Int J Epidemiol* 2012;**41**:398–404.

38 Richards M, Sacker A. Is education causal? Yes. *Int J Epidemiol* 2011;**40**:516–518.

39 Hatch SL, Feinstein L, Link B, Wadsworth MEJ, Richards M. The continuing benefits of education: adult education and midlife cognitive ability in the British 1946 birth cohort. *J Gerontol B* 2007;**62**:S404–S414.

40 Richards M, Power C, Sacker A. Paths to literacy and numeracy problems: evidence from two British birth cohorts. *J Epidemiol Community Health* 2009;**63**:239–244.

41 Kohn M, Slomcznski KM. *Social structure and self-direction. A comparative analysis of the United States and Poland.* Cambridge, MA: Blackwell; 1993.

42 Collins R. *The credential society: an historical sociology of education and stratification.* New York: Academic Press; 1979.

43 Glynmour MM, Manly JJ. Lifecourse social conditions and racial and ethnic patters of cognitive aging. *Neuropsychol Rev* 2008;**18**:223–254.

44 Manly JJ, Jacobs DM, Touradji P, Small SA, Stern Y. Reading level attenuates differences in neuropsychological test performance between African American and White elders. *J Int Neuropsychol Soc* 2002;**8**:341–8.

45 Williams DR, Mohammed SA, Leavell J, Collins C. Race , socioeconomic status, and health: complexities, ongoing challenges, and research opportunities. *Ann NY Acad Sci* 2010;**1186**:69–101.

46 Kohn M, Schooler C. *Work and personality: an enquiry into the impact of social stratification.* Norwood, NJ: Ablex; 1983.

47 Hauser RM, Roan CL. Work complexity and cognitive functioning at midlife: cross-validating the Kohn–Schooler hypothesis in an American cohort (CDE Working Paper No. 2007–08). Madison: University of Wisconsin, Center for Demography and Ecology; 2007.

48 Maguire EA, Gadian DG, Johnsrude IS, et al. Navigation-related structural change in the hippocampi of taxi drivers. *Proc Natl Acad Sci USA* 2000;**97**:4398–403.

49 Hultsch DF, Hertzog C, Small BJ, et al. Use it or lose it: engaged lifestyle as a buffer of cognitive decline in aging? *Psychol Aging* 1999;**14**:245–263.

50 Roberts BA, Fuhrer R, Marmot M, Richards M. Does retirement influence cognitive performance? The Whitehall II Study. *J Epidemiol Community Health* 2011;**65**:958–963.

51 Schooler C, Mulatu MS. The reciprocal effects of leisure time activities and intellectual functioning in older people: a longitudinal analysis. *Psychol Aging* 2001;**16**:466–482.

52 Wilson RS, Mendes de Leon CF, Barnes LL, et al. Participation in cognitively stimulating activities and risk of incident Alzheimer's disease. *JAMA* 2002;**287**:742–748.

53 Owen AM, Hampshire A, Grahn JA, et al. Putting brain training to the test. *Nature* 2010;**465**:775–778.

54 Stern Y, Blumen HM, Rich LW, et al. Space Fortress game training and executive control in older adults: a pilot intervention. *Aging Neuropsychol Cogn* 2011;**18**:653–677.

55 Steen E, Terry BM, Rivera EJ, et al. Impaired insulin and insulin-like growth factor expression and signaling mechanisms in Alzheimer's disease—is this type 3 diabetes? *J Alzheimer's Dis* 2005;7:63–80.

56 Warsch JRL, Wright CB. The aging mind: vascular health in normal cognitive aging. *J Am Geriatr Soc* 2010;**58**:S319–S324.

57 Qiu C, Winblad B, Fratiglioni L. The age-dependent relation of blood pressure to cognitive function and dementia. *Lancet Neurol* 2005;4:487–499.

58 Solomon A, Kåreholt I, Ngandu T, et al. Serum cholesterol changes after midlife and late-life cognition. *Neurology* 2007;**68**:751–756.

59 Albanese E, Hardy R, Wills A, Kuh D, Guralnik J, Richards M. No association between lifecourse body mass index and midlife cognitive function and cognitive reserve—evidence from the 1946 British birth cohort study. *Alzheimer's Dementia* 2012;**8**:470–482.

60 Munang L, Starr JM, Whalley L, Deary IJ. Renal function and cognition in the 1932 Scottish mental Survey Lothian cohort. *Age Ageing* 2007;**36**:323–325.

61 Hamer M, Chida Y. Physical activity and risk of neurodegenerative disease: a systematic review of prospective evidence. *Psychol Med* 2009;**39**:3–11.

62 Anstey KJ, Mack HA, Cherbuin N. Alcohol consumption as a risk factor for dementia and cognitive decline: meta-analysis of prospective studies. *Am J Geriatr Psychiatry* 2009;**17**:542–555.

63 Peters R, Poulter R, Warner J, et al. Smoking, dementia and cognitive decline in the elderly, a systematic review. *BMC Geriatrics* 2008;**8**:36.

64 Scarmeas N, Luchsinger JA, Schupf N, et al. Physical activity, diet, and risk of Alzheimer's disease. *JAMA* 2009;**302**:627–637.

65 Cadar D, Pikhart H, Mishra G, et al. The role of lifestyle behaviours on 20 year cognitive decline. *J Ageing Res* 2012;2012:304014. doi: 10.1155/2012/304014.

66 Rowe JW, Kahn RL. Successful aging. New York: Pantheon Press; 1998.

Chapter 18

Life course approaches to the genetic epidemiology of mental illness

Elise B. Robinson, Lauren M. McGrath, and Susan L. Santangelo

18.1 Introduction

We are entering an exciting new era of psychiatric genetics research. The cost of genomic technology is decreasing rapidly, allowing researchers to ask new and important questions about the relationship between genes and mental disorders. Of the novel approaches on the horizon, the integration of life course perspectives into psychiatric genetics may be one of the most promising. To date, almost all genetic studies of major psychiatric disorders have searched exclusively for genetic differences between people that predict disease status. In other words, genetic research into diseases such as schizophrenia, bipolar disorder, and autism has concentrated on finding genetic variants found more frequently in people with the disorder (cases) than in people without the disorder (controls). This research is important, as it will provide much-needed clues to the biology of mental illness. However, the last decade of mental health research has taught us that psychiatric illness, and the manner in which it relates to genetic risk, is very complex. To fully understand the relationship between genes and major mental health problems, genetic epidemiologists will need to incorporate life-course-informed questions into their research agendas: Are chronic mental disorders influenced by the same genetic variants throughout their course? Do genetic risk factors for major mental illnesses predict different types of behaviour at different points in development (see Figure 18.1)? To date, questions such as these are largely unexplored in genetic studies of psychiatric disease. For example, to our knowledge, there are no published genome-wide association studies that examine the genetic predictors of behaviour change or other such developmentally sensitive outcomes in psychiatry.

There are many reasons to believe that genetic factors will be important when approaching mental illness from a life course perspective and, conversely, that a life course perspective will add much to the genetic investigation of behavioural disorders. Much of the research supporting these hypotheses comes from twin studies, which have been used extensively to estimate the importance of genetic variation in behavioural health outcomes, including outcomes that are measured across time. In this chapter, we introduce three questions that can be used to guide a life course approach to the genetic epidemiology of mental disorders. For each of these questions, examples are provided from the twin literature suggesting that developmentally sensitive models of genetic risk likely contribute to mental illness. We then discuss the manner in which those models may have influenced psychiatric genetic studies and ways in which a life course perspective can be productively integrated into future efforts.

Box 18.1 supplies definitions of some essential terminology.

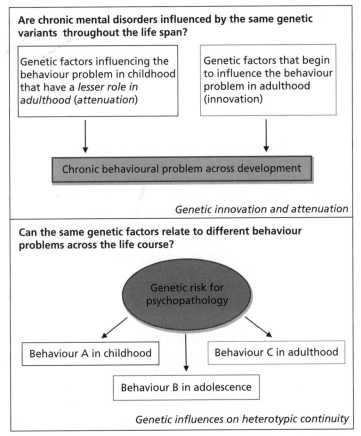

Figure 18.1 Are chronic mental disorders influenced by the same genetic variants throughout the lifespan?

Box 18.1: Terminology

Twin study: A study that uses twins to estimate the contribution of genes and the environment to a health outcome. Twin studies estimate how much genetic factors matter, but not which specific genes or genetic variants matter.

Genetic study: A study designed to identify which specific genes and genetic variants are involved in a disease.

Genetic variant: A location in the genome where the genetic code varies between individuals.

Phenotype: Observable characteristics or traits, such as hair colour, height, behaviour, or mental illness.

18.2 **Twin studies**

Twin studies are used to estimate the extent to which genetic and environmental factors influence a health outcome. They do not indicate which specific genes or genetic variants are influencing disease, but provide an estimate of 'heritability', the amount of variation in a trait that is attributable to genetic differences between people. Height, for example, is estimated to be 80% heritable. This means that ~80% of variation in height comes from genetic differences in the population. Twin studies are also used to estimate the role of the environment, but this section focuses on heritability to aid the reader's interpretation of the chapter.

Heritability is estimated by comparing the similarity of monozygotic (identical; MZ) as compared to dizygotic (fraternal; DZ) twins. MZ twins share >99% of their DNA code. DZ twins share on average 50%, the same amount as regular siblings. Unlike regular siblings, however, both MZ and DZ twins grow up at the same time in the same place. Because MZ and DZ twins are highly similar with regard to the environments that they share, greater phenotypic similarity between MZ than between DZ twins suggests that genetic variation is important to a trait. In other words, since we hypothesize that MZ and DZ twins experience 'equal environments', we believe that when MZ twins are more similar than DZ twins, it is because they are more similar genetically. There are several assumptions that underlie both this hypothesis and the statistical models that are used to estimate heritability from twin data. These assumptions are outside the scope of this chapter, but a detailed introduction to twin research is supplied by Plomin et al.[1]

Twin studies use the correlations between MZ and DZ pairs to estimate the role of genetic and environmental influences on a trait, at both a single point in time and across the life span. As an example, consider a quantitative trait that captures symptoms of depression in the population. To estimate the extent to which the genetic influences on depressive symptoms are stable over adolescence, a researcher could assess depressive symptoms in a sample of MZ and DZ twins at age 12 years and then again at age 20 years. MZ and DZ twin similarity would be estimated in part through the correlation between the depressive symptoms in twin 1 at age 12 years with depressive symptoms in twin 2 at age 20 years. Longitudinal twin designs such as these can address the extent to which genetic and environmental influences contribute to stability and change in a trait over time.

An important limitation of twin studies is that heritability estimates are always specific to the population and environment from which they have been derived. In the context of longitudinal analyses, however, this becomes an advantage. From a life course perspective, different age groups can be viewed as different populations. Twin studies are accordingly well suited to detect age-specific genetic and environmental influences that emerge over time, and can be used to inform a variety of novel questions in genetic epidemiology.

18.3 **Guiding questions for life course approaches to the genetic epidemiology of mental illness**

18.3.1 **Does the contribution of genetic differences to a trait vary over the life course?**

Genetic studies of mental illness are primarily designed to identify which specific genes and genetic variants are associated with disease. This goal is important for many reasons, one of the most significant being that genetic associations can provide clues to the biological basis of psychiatric disorders.

There are many ways to increase the chances that a genetic study will be successful. As with all other epidemiological efforts, it is important to measure the outcome (the disease or behavioural trait) and predictors (the genetic variants) well, and to account for factors that can bias a study. Genetic studies are also likely to be more powerful when the relationship between genetic variation and the outcome of interest is strong. In other words, the probability of associating genetic factors with phenotypic variation is maximized when the trait heritability is highest. In adopting a life course approach to genetic epidemiology, it is accordingly important to consider whether heritability changes over the course of development. Knowledge of when genes matter most could guide the selection of participants into genetic association studies, improving the chances of uncovering valuable genetic signals. In this section, we will introduce evidence that the heritability of behavioural phenotypes can change over time, using the specific example of substance use during adolescence and early adulthood.

There is abundant evidence from twin and family studies that the heritability of many cognitive and behavioural outcomes varies with age.[2,3] One of the most well-studied examples of this phenomenon comes from the domain of substance use research. To illustrate these findings, we focus on three frequently used substances as examples: cigarettes, alcohol, and marijuana.

Smoking is frequently initiated in adolescence. The average role of genetic factors in smoking initiation and uptake, however, appears to vary based on the age of the individual engaging in the behaviour. Specifically, many twin studies of the relationship between age and the heritability of cigarette use report that genetic factors have increasing importance through the teenage years.[3-5] In a recent research review, Maes and Neale noted that studies including young teens (aged 12 or 13 years) reported that genetic differences between people explained less than one-third of the variation in smoking initiation.[5] This means that the estimated heritability of the behaviour was <33%. Conversely, the studies including older teens and young adults (aged 17–25 years) reported that genetic differences explained 35–70% of variation in smoking initiation. A similar pattern has been noted with alcohol use among adolescents.[3] In one Finnish study, for instance, genetic factors accounted for less than one-third of the variation in intoxication frequency among teens aged ≤16 years and for more than half of the variation in teens aged ≥17 years.[6] For both smoking initiation and drinking frequency, these findings suggest that genes matter more, and the environment matters less, as adolescents age.

With an understanding that the contribution of genetic variation might change across development, one can begin to consider sources of heterogeneity in genetic epidemiology. The heritability of marijuana use provides a useful example. Many twin studies have found that genetic factors are important to marijuana use, but the estimates of heritability from these studies range from <20% to >70%.[7] There are likely many reasons why these heritability estimates vary widely. In all twin studies, the estimated contribution of genes is sensitive to study design issues such as how the behaviour is measured and how the sample is selected. In the case of marijuana use, however, there is also reason to believe that substantial heterogeneity could be introduced through mean age differences between the samples being studied.

In a developmental examination of substance use through mid-adulthood, Kendler et al. estimated the heritability of smoking, drinking, and marijuana use in a large sample of twins from the USA.[4] Consistent with the studies above, these authors found that genetic factors become relevant to smoking and drinking behaviour around age 16 years, and increase in importance through mid-adulthood. The heritability of marijuana use, however, displayed a much more dynamic pattern across development. Genetic influences did not become a strong and consistent source of variation in marijuana use until the early thirties in their sample, after which they accounted for ~60% of the variation in behaviour. Until that point, heritability estimates fluctuated substantially across development, ranging from <10% to >40%, and did not show a clear pattern with regard to age. This finding illustrates that the relationship between genetic factors and marijuana use is inconsistent until mid-adulthood, and heterogeneity in the findings from twin studies should be expected if the participants in those studies vary in age <30 years.

These patterns suggest that the strength of genetic contributions to frequently occurring substance use behaviours will vary based on the age of the participants. Since, on average, genetic factors appear to become more important as people enter adulthood, genetic studies of frequently occurring substance use behaviours may be more productively focused on post-adolescent populations. The extent to which the heritability of major psychiatric diseases such as schizophrenia and bipolar disorder may also vary with age is less clear. To our knowledge, for example, there have been no twin studies of age-based variation in the heritability of psychosis (though genetic factors do play a role in determining age of onset of psychosis in schizophrenia).[8] There will, however, be ample opportunity to address these questions when approaching genetic epidemiology from a life course perspective. As discussed below, developmental psychiatric genetics will need to be informed by considerations of: (i) the changing role of genetic risk factors across time; and (ii) the relationships between genetic risk factors at different points in time.

The next two sections of this chapter consider the dynamic, developmental relationship between genes and behaviour in two ways. First, we examine whether the same behaviours can be influenced by different genetic factors when the behaviour is measured at different periods in a person's life (Figure 18.1 upper panel). Second, we discuss whether the same genetic factors can predispose individuals to different behaviour problems across the life course (Figure 18.1, lower panel). There is evidence from twin and family studies that both of these scenarios are important to consider when adopting a developmental approach to the genetic epidemiology of mental disorders. We introduce some of this evidence, with a concentration on examples from the anxiety disorders literature, and discuss how these models of genetic risk may be influencing current research efforts.

18.3.2 Are chronic mental disorders influenced by the same genetic variants throughout their course?

Most psychiatric disorders that have been intensively investigated in genetic studies affect people for a long period of time, if not throughout their lives. Among them, schizophrenia, bipolar disorder, autism spectrum disorders, and attention deficit/hyperactivity disorder (ADHD) are all estimated to be highly heritable (~60–80%). Strong heritability, however, does not necessarily mean that the same genetic variants influence a chronic condition throughout its course. This is because heritability estimates only suggest how much of the variation in a phenotype is attributable to genetic differences between people, not which genes or genetic variants matter. In other words, it is possible that new and important genetic influences 'come online' later in the course of an illness (genetic innovation), and that the genetic factors responsible for early stages of the disease become less relevant over time (genetic attenuation).

Whereas many genetic variants have been associated with major psychiatric diseases over the last few years, little is known about the degree to which their influences are stable across the life course. For example, while more than a dozen frequently occurring genetic variants have been associated with schizophrenia in recent studies (see, for example, Ripke et al.[9]), the extent to which those variants may affect older and younger people differently is unknown. Twin studies, however, have long been used to study genetic innovation and attenuation.[10,11] In this section, we discuss evidence from some of those studies suggesting that genetic influences on behaviour are often 'developmentally dynamic', even in the case of behaviours that can be present for the majority of an individual's life.

Much of the work examining genetic influences on behaviour over time has focused on symptoms of anxiety. Anxiety disorders are particularly well suited to developmental studies given their high prevalence, early onset, and long duration. The estimated lifetime prevalence of anxiety disorders is ~30% and, very often, the behaviours typical of those disorders emerge in childhood.[12,13] Similarly, people who manifest symptoms of anxiety as children often continue to do so as they age.[14]

However, twin studies suggest that genetic influences on anxious behaviour may vary substantially over the life course.[10,11,15] For example, Kendler et al. examined the stability of genetic influences on fears in a large sample of twins at ages 8–9, 13–14, 16–17, and 19–20 years. Situational fears, one of the categories they studied, include phobias such as fear of flying or heights, and are moderately to highly heritable (50–70%). Whereas specific phobias such as these often have a chronic course,[16,17] the authors found evidence for substantial genetic innovation with age. Specifically, the genetic factors relevant to situational fears at ages 8 and 9 years accounted for only 4% of relevant genetic influences at ages 19–20 years.[10]

Twin studies such as these provide a framework for considering how genetic innovation and attenuation may be influencing genetic studies of neuropsychiatric diseases. Imagine a study designed to discover genetic variants associated with situational fears in childhood and adolescence. The cases in the study are individuals aged 8–20 years with fears; the controls are children and teens of the same age without fears. The study directors conduct a power calculation to estimate the number of individuals they will need to recruit in order to test statistically whether a genetic variant is related to situational fears. They estimate their power based on the anticipated effect size of the genetic variants and the total number of people who will be in the study. However, they do this without accounting for the observation that >90% of genetic influences on situational fears in childhood may be different from those influencing situational fears in late adolescence. Since many of the genetic variants they are interested in identifying will not be relevant to cases of all ages in their sample, the researchers will, in the case of many variants, have fewer than the number of people necessary to see a statistically significant effect. In other words, if unaccounted for, the presence of developmentally dynamic genetic influences could substantially reduce the power of the study.

To our knowledge, there has yet to be a large-scale genome-wide association study of the types of anxiety-related behaviours examined above. There is, however, evidence that similar developmentally dynamic processes may be present in behavioural disorders which have already been targeted in ambitious genetic studies.[18–22] ADHD is a frequently diagnosed, highly heritable psychiatric disorder of childhood that has already been the focus of large, well-conducted genome-wide association studies.[19,20] As with most behavioural disorders, genetic variants that consistently predict ADHD have been difficult to identify. While there are likely many reasons that studies have yet to identify replicable genetic risk factors for ADHD,[23] genetic innovation and attenuation may be contributing to the challenge.

Twin studies of traits of ADHD in the general population have suggested that genetic influences on hyperactive and inattentive behaviour may change substantially across childhood. In a twin study of parent-rated symptoms of ADHD, for example, Kuntsi et al. reported that only 10–40% of genetic influences on those traits were shared between ages 2 and 8 years.[22] A Dutch twin study of attention problems between ages 7 and 12 years described similar findings.[18] As in the studies of anxiety described above, this suggests that many of the genetic factors related to symptoms of ADHD may differ between early, mid-, and late childhood.

Although acknowledging genetic innovation and attenuation in studies of psychiatric disease may be useful in many respects, it will also present additional challenges. Specifically, the desire to identify developmental periods that maximize the homogeneity of genetic influences will need to be tempered by the realities of statistical power. That is to say, one of the great lessons of the last decade of genetic research is that the influence of any single, frequently occurring genetic variant on complex traits and diseases is likely to be small. This means that extremely large samples, often on the order of tens of thousands of individuals, will be needed to identify meaningful genetic predictors of diseases such as ADHD and anxiety disorders.[24] If researchers were to restrict their studies to some of the age ranges examined above, this would mean first collecting a very large sample of children aged 8–9 years, and then a very large sample of children aged 13–14 years, and so on. This introduces certain pragmatic obstacles.

The need for large samples will likely necessitate new ways of thinking about development in genetic studies of behaviour. We discuss one such possibility in Section 18.3.3, a framework in which genetic factors are permitted to influence different types of behaviours across development.

18.3.3 Can the same genetic factors influence different behaviour problems across the life course?

When a gene or a genetic variant influences multiple phenotypes, it is said to have 'pleiotropic effects'. In the context of psychiatric genetics, studies to date have suggested that effects of this type are widespread.[25–28] That is to say, many genetic variants that have been associated with risk for one psychiatric disorder also appear to create risk for other psychiatric disorders and cognitive/behavioural problems. For example, frequently occurring genetic variants associated with risk for schizophrenia also predict liability to bipolar disorder.[29] Similarly, many of the rare genetic variants associated with autism spectrum disorders also appear to increase risk for schizophrenia and intellectual disabilities.[26]

The investigations of pleiotropy in psychiatry to date, however, have generally lacked a developmental element. For example, very little is known about the relationship between genetic risks for adult onset psychiatric disease, such as schizophrenia and bipolar disorder, and patterns of behaviour and cognition in children. In other words, it is unclear how the risk variants that have been associated with these disorders may influence phenotypic variation in people who are not yet old enough to develop disease. Further, the limited genetic variants that have been consistently associated with childhood onset disorders, such as autism, are by and large quite rare in the general population.[30] Given the individual rarity of these risk variants, it is difficult to understand their average effect on behaviour across development in the absence of following a small cohort of individuals carrying the mutation for a long period time, or examining very large population cohorts over the life course. The latter strategy is most immediately promising for addressing developmental questions in psychiatric genetics, as large, individually genotyped general population cohorts have already been collected and followed over time. For example, the Avon Longitudinal Study of Parents and Children (ALSPAC) has collected extensive cognitive and behavioural data on a cohort of >10,000 children since birth. The cohort members are now adults, allowing their behavioural trajectories through childhood to be examined in conjunction with the genetic data that they have supplied.

Whereas genetic studies have yet to address the question of whether specific variants can predict different types of behaviour across the life course, a developing body of twin and family research suggests that, at least for some types of behaviour problems, this is likely to be the case. When behaviour is assessed at multiple points in time in the same individuals, twin studies can be used to investigate the importance of genetic factors to both homotypic continuity and heterotypic continuity in mental illness. In the context of psychiatric disease, homotypic continuity refers to the presence of one disorder predicting the presence of the same disorder later in an individual's life. Heterotypic continuity refers to the presence of one disorder at an early point in time predicting the presence of a different disorder later in life. In considering the model of genetic risk shown in the lower panel of Figure 18.1, we are interested in heterotypic continuity: to what extent is the association between different behaviour problems across development an expression of the same genetic risk factors?

As an introduction to how this question has been addressed in twin studies, we return to the anxiety disorders literature. The DSM-IV-TR includes 13 types of anxiety disorders, including specific phobias, generalized anxiety disorder, panic disorder, separation anxiety disorder, and social phobia. Anxiety disorders as a class are well suited to genetic studies of heterotypic continuity, since: (i) there is abundant evidence that different types of anxiety disorders share common genetic risk factors;[31] and (ii) the disorders show different expression patterns with age.[32,33] Specific phobias and separation anxiety, widespread problems of childhood, have the earliest average age of onset. Social phobia most often appears in early adolescence; panic disorder and generalized anxiety disorder then typically manifest themselves in late adolescence and early adulthood.[12] These differences in age of onset are consistent with shifts in the expression of anxiety across development.[32,33] In other words, some genetic and environmental factors may create risk for anxiety across the life course, but the specific behaviours associated with that risk likely change with age.

This hypothesis is beginning to be tested in twin studies of heterotypic continuity. Trzaskowski et al., for example, recently examined the stability of genetic influences on anxiety-related behaviours in twins between the ages of 7 and 9 years.[34] They considered four different types of behaviour at each time point: negative cognition, negative affect, fear, and social anxiety. Whereas the genetic contributions to homotypic continuity were strongest, the authors reported that genetic factors also played a role in the correlation between different types of anxious behaviours over time. Genetic influences explained between 28% and 66% of heterotypic continuity in the traits— the strongest genetic links were estimated between fear at age 7 years and negative cognition at age 9 years, and between negative cognition at age 7 years and negative affect at age 9 years. A recent report suggesting that childhood separation anxiety disorder and adult onset panic attacks share genetic risk factors lends further support to the hypothesis that inherited risk for anxiety may express itself differentially with age.[35]

18.4 **Summary**

Research into the genetic predictors of heterotypic continuity is in its early stages, but will play an important role in developmental approaches to psychiatric genetics. Moreover, as noted through each of the questions posed in this chapter, life course approaches require a central recognition of heterogeneity in the relationship between genetic factors and mental disorders. The relevance of genes in predicting behaviour is likely to change across development, as are the specific genetic factors related to chronic behavioural problems. Twin studies have already begun to demonstrate these possibilities; however, more work of this type is needed to inform gene-finding studies and maximize the probability of locating biologically informative genetic signals.

The technological expansion in genomics has provided opportunity to pursue large-sample genetic research more efficiently. A conceptual expansion into life course studies of behaviour, however, will be equally necessary to make meaningful gains against mental illnesses that are truly developmental in origin. Taken together, we believe that such a life course approach to genetics studies will help towards understanding the biological basis of mental disorders.

References

1 Plomin R, DeFries J, McClearn G, McGuffin P. *Behavioral genetics*, 5th ed. New York: Worth Publishers; 2008.

2 Haworth CM, Wright MJ, Luciano M, et al. The heritability of general cognitive ability increases linearly from childhood to young adulthood. *Mol Psychiatry* 2010;**15**(11):1112–1120.

3 Hopfer CJ, Crowley TJ, Hewitt JK. Review of twin and adoption studies of adolescent substance use. *J Am Acad Child Adolesc Psychiatry* 2003;**42**(6):710–719.

4 Kendler KS, Schmitt E, Aggen SH, Prescott CA. Genetic and environmental influences on alcohol, caffeine, cannabis, and nicotine use from early adolescence to middle adulthood. *Arch Gen Psychiatry* 2008;**65**(6):674–682.

5 Maes HH, Neale MC. Genetic modeling of tobacco use behavior and trajectories, In: Swan G, Baker T, Chassin L, Conti D, Lerman C, Perkins K, editors. *NCI Tobacco Control Monograph Series 20: phenotypes and endophenotypes: foundations for genetic studies of nicotine use and dependence.* Bethesda, MD: US Department of Health and Human Services, National Institutes of Health; 2009.

6 Viken RJ, Kaprio J, Koskenvuo M, Rose RJ. Longitudinal analyses of the determinants of drinking and of drinking to intoxication in adolescent twins. *Behav Genet* 1999;**29**(6):455–461.

7 Vink JM, Wolters LM, Neale MC, Boomsma DI. Heritability of cannabis initiation in Dutch adult twins. *Addict Behav* 2010;**35**(2):172–174.

8 Hare E, Glahn DC, Dassori A, et al. Heritability of age of onset of psychosis in schizophrenia. *Am J Med Genet B Neuropsychiatr Genet* 2010;**153B**(1):298–302.

9 Ripke S, Sanders AR, Kendler KS, et al. Genome-wide association study identifies five new schizophrenia loci. *Nat Genet* 2011;**43**(10):969–976.

10 Kendler KS, Gardner CO, Annas P, et al. Longitudinal twin study of fears from middle childhood to early adulthood: evidence for a developmentally dynamic genome. *Arch Gen Psychiatry* 2008;**65**(4):421–429.

11 Kendler KS, Gardner CO, Lichtenstein P. A developmental twin study of symptoms of anxiety and depression: evidence for genetic innovation and attenuation. *Psychol Med* 2008;**38**(11):1567–1575.

12 Kessler RC, Berglund P, Demler O, et al. Lifetime prevalence and age-of-onset distributions of DSM-IV disorders in the National Comorbidity Survey Replication. *Arch Gen Psychiatry* 2005;**62**(6):593–602.

13 Merikangas KR, He JP, Brody D, et al. Prevalence and treatment of mental disorders among US children in the 2001–2004 NHANES. *Pediatrics* 2010;**125**(1):75–81.

14 Hirshfeld-Becker DR, Micco JA, Simoes NA, Henin A. High risk studies and developmental antecedents of anxiety disorders. *Am J Med Genet C Semin Med Genet* 2008;**148C**(2):99–117.

15 Kendler KS, Gardner CO, Annas P, Lichtenstein P. The development of fears from early adolescence to young adulthood: a multivariate study. *Psychol Med* 2008;**38**(12):1759–1769.

16 Gregory AM, Caspi A, Moffitt TE, et al. Juvenile mental health histories of adults with anxiety disorders. *Am J Psychiatry* 2007;**164**(2):301–308.

17 Pine DS, Cohen P, Gurley D, Brook J, Ma Y. The risk for early-adulthood anxiety and depressive disorders in adolescents with anxiety and depressive disorders. *Arch Gen Psychiatry* 1998;**55**(1):56–64.

18 Rietveld MJ, Hudziak JJ, Bartels M, van Beijsterveldt CE, Boomsma DI. Heritability of attention problems in children: longitudinal results from a study of twins, age 3 to 12. *J Child Psychol Psychiatry* 2004;**45**(3):577–588.

19 Neale BM, Medland S, Ripke S, et al. Case–control genome-wide association study of attention-deficit/hyperactivity disorder. *J Am Acad Child Adolesc Psychiatry* 2010;**49**(9):906–920.

20 Neale BM, Medland SE, Ripke S, et al. Meta-analysis of genome-wide association studies of attention-deficit/hyperactivity disorder. *J Am Acad Child Adolesc Psychiatry* 2010;**49**(9):884–897.

21 Ronald A. Is the child 'father of the man'? Evaluating the stability of genetic influences across development. *Dev Sci* 2011;**14**(6):1471–1478.

22 Kuntsi J, Rijsdijk F, Ronald A, Asherson P, Plomin R. Genetic influences on the stability of attention-deficit/hyperactivity disorder symptoms from early to middle childhood. *Biol Psychiatry* 2005;**57**(6):647–654.

23 Manolio TA, Collins FS, Cox NJ, et al. Finding the missing heritability of complex diseases. *Nature* 2009;**461**(7265):747–753.

24 Sullivan P. Don't give up on GWAS. *Mol Psychiatry* 2011;**17**(1):2–3.

25 Craddock N, Owen MJ. The Kraepelinian dichotomy—going, going . . . but still not gone. *Br J Psychiatry* 2010;**196**(2):92–95.

26 Burbach JP, van der Zwaag B. Contact in the genetics of autism and schizophrenia. *Trends Neurosci* 2009;**32**(2):69–72.

27 Cook EH, Jr, Scherer SW. Copy-number variations associated with neuropsychiatric conditions. *Nature* 2008;**455**(7215):919–923.

28 O'Dushlaine C, Kenny E, Heron E, et al. Molecular pathways involved in neuronal cell adhesion and membrane scaffolding contribute to schizophrenia and bipolar disorder susceptibility. *Mol Psychiatry* 2011;**16**(3):286–292.

29 Purcell SM, Wray NR, Stone JL, et al. Common polygenic variation contributes to risk of schizophrenia and bipolar disorder. *Nature* 2009;**460**(7256):748–752.

30 Betancur C. Etiological heterogeneity in autism spectrum disorders: more than 100 genetic and genomic disorders and still counting. *Brain Res* 2011;**1380**:42–77.

31 Hettema JM, Prescott CA, Myers JM, Neale MC, Kendler KS. The structure of genetic and environmental risk factors for anxiety disorders in men and women. *Arch Gen Psychiatry* 2005;**62**(2):182–189.

32 Beesdo K, Knappe S, Pine DS. Anxiety and anxiety disorders in children and adolescents: developmental issues and implications for DSM-V. *Psychiatr Clin North Am* 2009;**32**(3):483–524.

33 Costello EJ, Egger HL, Angold A. The developmental epidemiology of anxiety disorders: phenomenology, prevalence, and comorbidity. *Child Adolesc Psychiatr Clin N Am* 2005;**14**(4):631–648, vii.

34 Trzaskowski M, Zavos HM, Haworth CM, Plomin R, Eley TC. Stable genetic influence on anxiety-related behaviours across middle childhood. *J Abnorm Child Psychol* 2011;**40**(1):85–94.

35 Roberson-Nay R, Eaves LJ, Hettema JM, Kendler KS, Silberg JL. Childhood separation anxiety disorder and adult onset panic attacks share a common genetic diathesis. *Depress Anxiety* 2012;**29**(4):320–327.

Chapter 19

Impact of early environmental exposures on mental disorders across the life course

Pam Factor-Litvak

19.1 Introduction

Emerging evidence suggests that developmental outcomes over the life course may be associated with exposures during critical times of brain development and with cumulative exposures throughout life. Developmental outcomes range from subtle deficits in cognition, behaviour, language acquisition and social functioning, to frank mental disorders such as autism, schizophrenia, and Alzheimer's disease. The range of disorders, from relatively minor to severe mental impairment, suggests that for some external exposures there is a continuum of casualty relating exposure to adverse outcomes throughout the life span. This concept, first coined by Pasamanick and Knobloch[1] refers to an exposure that is associated with various disorders over the life span;[2] the specific outcomes may depend on the timing and degree of exposure.

This chapter summarizes the adverse associations between both pre- and postnatal exposure to environmental lead and a variety of cognitive and behavioural outcomes over the life course. Environmental lead is a ubiquitous contaminant with documented exposure even in relatively pristine environments.[3] Although the ancient Greeks and Romans recognized toxicity due to lead exposure, the adverse effects of more moderate and low levels of exposure only became apparent in the past 60 years.[4] Life course outcomes include cognitive deficits, behaviour problems, deficits in academic achievement, and schizophrenia. The range of outcomes and time course of their emergence as well as hypothesized mechanisms emphasizes the importance of the life course approach. After a brief section summarizing methodological issues inherent in studying environmental exposures and developmental outcomes, the chapter focuses first on the importance of studying low levels of lead exposure, followed by an examination of the associations between lead exposure and cognitive function, behaviour problems, and schizophrenia. The biological basis for many of the associations is then discussed, followed by a summary of life course methods in relation to early lead exposure.

19.2 Methodological considerations

Studies of early environmental exposures (i.e. either in utero or during early infancy, through, for example, breastfeeding) and later life outcomes warrant special methodological considerations. These include the development of longitudinal causal models which include mediating and effect-modifying variables, the consideration of exposure timing, the estimation of the shape of dose–response relationships, and the attention to specificity in outcome definition.

To apply the life course approach to the study of the external environment and developmental outcomes, many investigators have specified longitudinal models that sequentially order exposures, background variables, and potential mediating and moderating variables.[5] For example, studies performed in the Child Health and Development Studies (CHDS), a 1960s birth cohort, specifically hypothesized that maternal thyroid hormone, which is responsible for the timely development of the brain, may be perturbed after exposure to organochlorine compounds, and thus mediate the observed associations between organochlorine exposure and decreased scores on childhood intelligence tests.[6]

Several investigators have also paid special attention to the nature and timing of exposure. Exposure can occur at a single 'critical' period during development, with consequences for the remainder of the life course. Recent examples include maternal exposure to influenza during mid-pregnancy and schizophrenia in the offspring[7] and maternal exposure to severe nutritional deficiency during early gestation, neural tube defects in newborns, and schizophrenia later in life.[8–12] Exposure can also be cumulative over the life course; for example both pre- and postnatal exposure to lead is associated with deficits in cognition which appear greater with continued exposure.[13] Attention needs to be given to the shape of the dose–response relationships, especially at low levels of exposure. This is most notable in the case of lead exposure, where deficits in scores on intelligence tests appear greater with low dose exposure.[14]

Finally, the definition of developmental and mental health outcomes has evolved over time as new technologies better define specific brain regions associated with cognitive deficits and behavioural problems. These technologies include structural and functional magnetic resonance imaging which are increasingly used in epidemiological studies.[15] However, most studies still rely on neuropsychological assessment and careful clinical histories obtained via questionnaires.

19.3 **Lead exposure**

Lead exposure is one of the most studied environmental exposures related to the outcomes of interest in this chapter. Examining the associations between blood lead (BPb) levels and broad developmental outcomes represents a moving target, as BPb levels have declined precipitously over the past three decades in the USA resulting from regulations to reduce or eliminate lead in both household paint and gasoline.[16] Thus, BPb levels in children aged 1–5 years have continued to decline, from 2.2 to 1.5 µg/dl.[17] The most recent reported data from the 2007–2008 National Health and Nutrition Survey (NHANES) indicate that the geometric mean BPb among participants aged ≥1 year is 1.3 µg/dl; only 5% of respondents had BPb ≥3.7 µg/dl. BPb levels are consistently higher in males compared with females, in Whites compared with African-Americans, and in persons with lower social circumstances compared to those with higher social circumstances.[18,19] The most recent definition of elevated BPb, effective in 2012, is tied to data from NHANES; elevated BPb is now defined as >97.5th percentile of the BPb distribution among children aged 1–5 years in the USA. The current value of the 97.5th percentile is 5 µg/dl.[20] Thus, lead exposure has significantly declined over the past 30 years, as indicated by declines in BPb levels in all age groups, particularly children. Despite the declines, lead exposure is still a concern as many health outcomes, including those described below, are associated with low level exposure.

19.4 **Lead exposure and cognitive development**

Frank encephalopathy attributable to lead was known since ancient times, but not until the 1940s did Byers and Lord[4] report a case series of children with cognitive deficits purportedly attributable to lead exposure. Following that report, cross-sectional[21–23] and longitudinal studies[13,19,24–33] collectively found adverse associations between exposure to more moderate levels of lead exposure, cognitive deficits, and behaviour problems.

Cognitive function can be divided into three major categories. First, childhood intelligence (IQ) is generally measured using standardized tests. Second, specific cognitive functions, e.g. executive function or working memory, are assessed using standardized tests. Finally, academic achievement is a recently introduced measure and is perhaps a stronger indicator of educational attainment and lifelong achievement.

19.4.1 Childhood IQ

In the 1980s a series of longitudinal birth cohort studies evaluated associations between pre- and postnatal exposure to lead, pregnancy outcomes, and childhood development. These studies took place throughout the world, including Boston,[18,24] Cincinnati,[26] Port Pirie Australia,[32] and Kosovo,[13,19,33] and included children with a range of pre- and postnatal BPb levels (from <5 to >30 μg/dl). Whereas studies used a variety of different IQ assessments at early ages, all followed similar protocols to assess IQ from age 7 years onward. The consistency of a 2–4-point decline in IQ for each 10 μg/dl increase in BPb across studies provides substantial support for the relationship between postnatal BPb and IQ. Three meta-analyses[34–36] corroborate these findings. Findings from a randomized clinical trial of chelation therapy to reduce BPb did not find reductions to be associated with improved IQ scores,[37] suggesting early damage to brain areas related to intelligence.

Recent interest focuses on the adverse effects of low dose lead. In a pooled analysis of major prospective studies,[14] associations between BPb <10 μg/dl and childhood IQ suggested that the slope of the BPb–IQ curve is steepest for very low BPb levels, that is, <5 μg/dl. Other studies corroborate this relationship.[38–41]

The analyses of the BPb–IQ relationship highlight several features of life course epidemiology. First, linear dose–response relationships cannot be assumed. Second, associations may differ by postnatal social circumstances (i.e. effect modification). Data from one study[42] suggest that the adverse effects of elevated BPb are mitigated among those with better social circumstances and among girls, compared with boys. Third, careful control of confounding is warranted especially when estimating associations at the lower end of the dose–response curve.[43] Important covariates include maternal IQ scores, maternal education, the quality of the home environment (assessed using the Home Observation for the Measurement of the Environment score[44]), and birth weight.[14] In both the Boston and Yugoslavia studies[19,24,33,38] controlling for social variables revealed the associations between BPb and IQ.

Finally, these studies highlight the importance of exposure timing. Longitudinal studies were able to obtain measures of both pre- and postnatal BPb and could address the relative importance of exposure during gestation, during early childhood or both. In several studies, including the Boston study,[38] BPb measured at age 2 years, the age of peak hand-to-mouth behaviour, had the largest association with IQ, compared with BPb either in utero or at other times in early life. Cumulative exposure using serial measures of BPb to measure 'average lifetime' exposure was also associated with decreased IQ. In Port Pirie, Australia, where there was a point source of exposure, an increase from 10 to 20 μg/dl in average lifetime BPb was associated with decreases in IQ at age 11–13 years.[32] The Yugoslavia study extended these findings to IQ measured between ages 10 and 12 years, and for bone lead measures at age 12 years. The data suggest that associations between early lead exposure and IQ are stronger for postnatal exposure.[13]

19.4.2 **Lead and specific cognitive functions**

The associations between lead exposure and specific cognitive functions largely parallel those of lead exposure and IQ. In general, the prospective studies find stronger associations between BPb and performance measures compared with verbal measures. Lead-related deficits are also found for attention, executive function, language, learning and memory, and visual–spatial function, thus suggesting various areas of brain dysfunction.[39,40,45–47]

19.4.3 **Lead and academic achievement**

Recent attention has focused on the associations between lead and academic achievement, an outcome which may more objectively measure skills and abilities with implications for later life success. Early studies found associations with scores on mathematics and vocabulary tests, teachers' assessments of academic performance and completion of high school.[48–51] Exposure was assessed early in life with either dentine lead or BPb; thus suggesting persistent effects of early life exposure. Data also suggest that associations between lead and academic achievement are independent of those with IQ.[50]

Recent studies linked BPb surveillance data in North Carolina and educational achievement scores[52,53] and found that BPb at age 2 years was associated with end-of-year academic testing for reading and arithmetic at age 6 years in several counties and the entire state. Because BPb levels were higher in African-American children than White children, the authors suggested that lead exposure may be associated with the racial achievement gap. Further, associations were strongest at the lower BPb levels.

The associations between BPb measured at age 2.5 years and academic achievement at age 7 years was studied in a subgroup of participants in the Avon Longitudinal Study of Parents and Children.[54] Mean BPb levels in this study were low (4.22 µg/dl + 3.12 (SD)) with only 6% of children having BPb >10 µg/dl. Associations were found between BPb and reading, writing, and spelling achievement. IQ did not mediate these associations. Stronger associations were found for lower BPb levels.

In summary, the associations between childhood lead exposure and academic achievement are stronger for low exposure levels, similar to the results for IQ. However, control for IQ did not change the associations, indicating no mediation. This illustrates the 'chain of events' life course model.[5]

19.5 **Behaviour**

Many of the prospective studies measured behaviour problems during childhood, and some[55–57] measured attention, delinquent behaviours, and criminality later in adolescence and early adulthood. The prospective studies found associations between BPb and features of attention deficit/hyperactivity disorder (ADHD).[48,55,56,58,59] Data from the 1999–2002 NHANES study also found that higher BPb levels were associated with parent report of ADHD diagnoses and stimulant medication use.[60] Associations were robust for BPb <5 µg/dl. Independent associations between BPb and maternal smoking during pregnancy and reported ADHD diagnoses were also reported.[61]

More recent studies have also found associations between BPb and ADHD-related behaviours. These include a cross-sectional study in Romania in children residing near a metal processing plant,[62] a case–control study in China[63] and a cross-sectional study in Chennai, India.[64] A methodological issue that arose in these studies concerns mediation by IQ. However, a series of case–control analyses found that the association between lead and ADHD was not mediated by IQ but that the association between BPb and IQ was mediated by attention problems;[65,66] this finding needs to be replicated. A 2010 review of the literature relating lead to ADHD[67] concludes that in both human and experimental animal studies exposure to lead may increase the prevalence of ADHD and ADHD-related symptoms.

Studies also find associations between lead exposure and other behaviour problems. These include conduct disorder,[68,69] oppositional defiant disorder,[65] and antisocial behaviour.[54,70,71] Most studies controlled for a wide variety of other risk factors for behaviour problems including those in the prenatal (i.e. maternal smoking, family socio-economic status) and postnatal (i.e. child IQ, family environment) periods.

In summary, the evidence strongly suggests associations between early life lead exposure and behavioural problems at least until the early adult period. These associations persist at low exposure levels.

19.6 **Schizophrenia**

Perhaps the best-studied neurodevelopmental disorder is schizophrenia.[72,73] Schizophrenia may follow a developmental trajectory, ranging from physical anomalies to prodromal symptoms,[74,75] and usually manifests in the late teenage years or in early adulthood. There is substantial evidence that prodromal symptoms, including behaviour and cognitive problems, occur years before actual symptoms develop.[76] In the 1980s a model was proposed in which an insult during early brain development predisposed to the development of schizophrenia later in life. Since that time, several studies have found abnormalities in early cognition, behaviour, and socialization among children who are later diagnosed with schizophrenia (reviewed by Cannon et al.[77]), shifting the aetiological explanation from 'psychological' to 'biological'.[78]

Interest in the possible associations between lead exposure and schizophrenia derived from the observations that the prodromal symptoms of schizophrenia are associated with lead.[49,57] Further data indicated that lead was associated with societal problems which may reflect the prevalence of psychiatric disorders. Dietrich et al.[57,79] found that prenatal BPb was associated with delinquent behaviour later in life and with criminal behaviour at ages 19–24 years. Similar associations were found using international data.[80]

Two studies examined the associations between a marker of prenatal lead exposure and schizophrenia; one within the CHDS and the second in the National Collaborative Perinatal Project.[81,82] A validated marker of lead exposure, δ-aminolevulinic acid (δ-ALA), was measured in mid-pregnancy sera and elevated δ-ALA was associated with an approximately two-fold increase in the risk of schizophrenia spectrum disorders in these studies. The major limitation of this work is the use of a marker of BPb; however, the results are compelling given corroborating evidence.

Early neuroimaging studies of children with elevated BPb (23–65 μg/dl) have found a decrease in the ratio of N-acetylaspartate (NAA) to creatinine in gray matter,[83,84] consistent with that found in the brains of schizophrenia subjects.[85,86] Studies of young adult participants from one prospective study, who had average BPb childhood concentrations of 13.3 μg/dl, found significant decreases in the volume of gray matter in several brain areas associated with executive function, mood regulation and decision-making.[87] The decrease in gray matter volume was larger in males than females, regardless of BPb.[88] Persistent effects on white matter microstructure with evidence of axonal injury and myelin damage[89] were also found; similar neuroanatomical changes are found in schizophrenic patients.[90,91]

A recent review of the literature relating early life lead exposure to schizophrenia[92] describes continuing proof-of-concept animal experiments, suggesting that lead-induced hypofunction of the N-methyl-D-aspartate (NMDA) receptor during critical periods of development may be responsible for both behaviour problems and schizophrenia. They further posit that these relationships may be attributed to gene–environment interactions. In summary, the association between early life lead exposure and schizophrenia represents an example of environmentally related brain dysfunction and long term consequences.

19.7 **Biological mechanisms**

19.7.1 **Blood–brain barrier and neurochemical perturbations**

One set of proposed biological mechanisms focuses on lead-induced perturbations of the blood–brain barrier[93] and on neurotransmitter function.[94] These result in 'synaptic noise' and inappropriate pruning of the synaptic connections, occurring late in gestation and continuing into adolescence. 'Synaptic noise' may be increased by lead-induced activation of protein kinase C, an intracellular messenger protein that plays a role in the potentiation of signals.

Studies in animals suggest that lead blocks NMDA glutamate receptor activity, a primary receptor of approximately half of brain synapses. Drugs that block this receptor are associated with deficits in learning and memory in animals.

Lead is also thought to disrupt structural components of the blood–brain barrier by injury to astrocytes and endothelial vasculature, and to preferentially damage the prefrontal cerebral cortex, hippocampus, and cerebellum, sites related to specific cognitive and behavioural deficits.

19.7.2 **Perturbation of thyroid function**

There are three hypotheses regarding the effects of lead on thyroid function, based on studies of occupational exposure and on small population samples.[95–97] The first postulated that lead impairs iodine uptake by the thyroid gland.[98] Second, lead may prevent the release of transthyretin (TTR) into the cerebrospinal fluid, preventing the transport of free thyroxine (FT4) to the brain. In both rodent and human studies, BPb is inversely associated with both TTR and FT4.[99,100] Assuming exposure during pregnancy, in both of these scenarios one would expect elevated maternal mid-pregnancy thyroid-stimulating hormone and reduced mid-pregnancy FT4. Finally, lead may affect thyroid function by triggering autoimmune thyroiditis. In the case of such a direct assault on the thyroid gland, we would expect to see elevated thyroperoxidase antibody and depressed FT4, but no effect on TSH.

Several studies have found that reductions in maternal thyroid function may result in IQ deficits in offspring. Infants and children born to mothers with frank or subclinical hypothyroidism exhibit deficits in neurodevelopment.[101–104] Maternal suboptimal thyroid function during pregnancy is associated with deficits in psychomotor development in infancy and cognition in children.[105–110] It is not known whether these deficits persist into adulthood or whether there are any early or late factors that mitigate the associations.

19.7 **Summary: environmental exposures in a life course model**

The case of in-utero and early childhood exposure to lead exemplifies many of the basic premises of a life course approach to mental illness including timing of exposure, mediation of associations by individual social circumstances, sex and other life experiences, attention to social context, the importance of proper control of confounding, and the shape of the dose–response relationships. In the case of prenatal and early childhood exposure to lead, the continuum of casualty includes minimal deficits in IQ scores, deficits on other neuropsychological functions, behaviour problems such as ADHD, and the development of schizophrenia. Remaining challenges include discriminating between the timing and degree of exposures, and identifying other contributing or mediating factors that influence outcome. These may be addressed using experimental models of exposure to inform biological mechanisms, considering genetic, epigenetic and other developmental processes, and considering the pattern of outcomes using existing data from the prospective studies.

References

1 Pasamanick B, Knobloch H. Brain damage and reproductive casualty. *Am J Orthopsychiatry* 1960;**30**:298–305.

2 Strogher CR. Minimal cerebral dysfunction: a historical overview. *Ann NY Acad Sci* 1973;**205**:6–17.

3 Piomelli S, Corash L, Corash MB, et al. Blood lead concentrations in a remote Himalayan population. *Science* 1980;**210**:1135–1137.

4 Byers RK, Lord EE. Late effects of lead poisoning on mental development. *Am J Dis Child* 1943;**66**:471–494.

5 Ben Shlomo Y, Kuh D. A life course approach to chronic disease epidemiology: conceptual models, empirical challenges and interdisciplinary perspectives. *Int J Epidemiol* 2002;**31**:285–293.

6 Factor-Litvak P, Kezios KL, Liu X, et al. Prenatal organochlorines exposure and cognition: results from the CHDS. Presented at the PPTOX III: Environmental stressors in the developmental origins of disease: evidence and mechanisms, Paris, May 2012.

7 Brown AS, Begg MD, Gravenstein S, et al. Serologic evidence of prenatal influenza in the etiology of schizophrenia. *Arch Gen Psychiatry* 2004;**61**:774–780.

8 Stein ZA, Susser M, Saenger G, Marolla F. *Famine and human development: the Dutch Hunger Winter of 1944–1945.* New York: Oxford University Press; 1975.

9 Susser E, Hoek HW, Brown A. Neurodevelopmental disorders after prenatal famine: the story of the Dutch Famine Study. *Am J Epidemiol* 1998;**147**:213–216.

10 Susser ES, Lin SP. Schizophrenia after prenatal exposure to the Dutch Hunger Winter of 1944–1945. *Arch Gen Psychiatry* 1992;**49**:983–988.

11 Susser E, Neugebauer R, Hoek HW, et al. Schizophrenia after prenatal famine. Further evidence. *Arch Gen Psychiatry* 1996;**53**:25–31.

12 St Clair D, Xu M, Wang P, et al. Rates of adult schizophrenia following prenatal exposure to the Chinese famine of 1959–1961. *JAMA* 2005;**294**:557–562.

13 Wasserman GA, Liu X, Popovac D, et al. The Yugoslavia Prospective Lead Study: contributions of prenatal and postnatal lead exposure to early intelligence. *Neurotoxicol Teratol* 2000;**22**: 811–818.

14 Lanphear BP, Horning R, Khoury J, et al. Low-level environmental lead exposure and children's intellectual function: an international pooled analysis. *Environ Health Perspect* 2005;**113**:894–899.

15 Rauh VA, Perera FP, Horton MK, et al. Brain anomalies in children exposed prenatally to a common organophosphate pesticide. *Proc Natl Acad Sci USA* 2012;**109**:7871–7876.

16 Pirkle JL, Brody DJ, Gunter EW, et al. The decline in blood lead levels in the United States. The National Health and Nutrition Examination Surveys (NHANES). *JAMA* 1994;**272**:284–291.

17 United States Environmental Protection Agency. *Report on the environment: blood lead level.* <http://cfpub.epa.gov/eroe/index.cfm?fuseaction=detail.viewInd&lv=list.listbyalpha&r=224030&subtop=208>

18 Bellinger DC. Lead neurotoxicity and socioeconomic status: conceptual and analytical issues. *Neurotoxicology* 2008;**29**:828–832.

19 Factor-Litvak P, Wasserman G, Kline JK, Graziano J. The Yugoslavia Prospective Study of environmental lead exposure. *Environ Health Perspect* 1999;**107**:9–15.

20 **CDC Response to Advisory Committee on Childhood Lead Poisoning Prevention Recommendations**. In: *Low level lead exposure harms children: a renewed call of primary prevention.* <http://www.cdc.gov/nceh/lead/acclpp/cdc_response_lead_exposure_recs.pdf>

21 **Munoz H, Romiew I, Palazuelos E, et al.** Blood lead level and neurobehavioral development among children living in Mexico City. *Arch Environ Health* 1993;**48**:132–139.

22 **Prpic-Majic D, Bobicc J, Simicc D, et al.** Lead absorption and psychological function in Zagreb (Croatia) school children. *Neurotoxicol Teratol* 2000;**22**:347–356.

23 **Surkan PJ, Zhang A, Trachtenberg F, et al.** Neuropsychological function in children with blood lead levels <10 microg/dL. *Neurotoxicology* 2007;**28**:1170–1177.

24 **Bellinger D, Leviton A, Waternaux C, et al.** Longitudinal analyses of prenatal and postnatal lead exposure and early cognitive development. *N Engl J Med* 1987;**316**:1039–1043.

25 **Canfield R, Henderson CR, Cory-Slechta DA, et al.** Intellectual impairment in children with blood lead concentrations below 10 microg/deciliter. *N Engl J Med* 2003;**348**:1517–1526.

26 **Dietrich KN, Krafft KM, Bornschein RL, et al.** Low-level fetal lead exposure effect on neurobehavioral development in early infancy. *Pediatrics* 1987;**80**:721–730.

27 **Ernhart CB, Morrow-Tlucak M, Wolf AW.** Low level lead exposure and intelligence in the preschool years. *Sci Total Environ* 1988;**71**:453–459.

28 **Hu H, Tellez-Rojo MM, Bellinger D, et al.** Fetal lead exposure at each stage of pregnancy as a predictor of infant mental development. *Environ Health Perspect* 2006;**114**:1730–1735.

29 **Schnaas L, Rothenberg SJ, Flores MF, et al.** Reduced intellectual development in children with prenatal lead exposure. *Environ Health Perspect* 2006;**114**:791–797.

30 **Tellez-Rojo MM, Bellinger DC, Arroyo-Quiroz C, et al.** Longitudinal associations between blood lead concentrations lower than 10 microg/dL and neurobehaviorial development in environmentally exposed children in Mexico City. *Pediatrics* 2006;**118**:e323–e330.

31 **Thomson GO, Raab GM, Hepburn WS, et al.** Blood lead levels and children's behavior—results from the Edinburgh Lead Study. *J Child Psychol Psychiatry* 1989;**30**:515–528.

32 **Tong S, Baghurst P, McMichael A, et al.** Lifetime exposure to environmental lead and children's intelligence at 11–13 years: the Port Pirie cohort study. *BMJ* 1996;**312**:1569–1575.

33 **Wasserman GA, Liu X, LoIacono NJ, et al.** Lead exposure and intelligence in 7-year old children: the Yugoslavia Prospective Study. *Environ Health Perspect* 1997;**105**:956–962.

34 **Schwartz J.** Low level lead exposure and children's IQ: a meta analysis and search for a threshold. *Environ Res* 1994;**65**:42–55.

35 **Pocock SJ, Smith M, Baghurst P.** Environmental lead and children's intelligence: a systematic review of the epidemiological evidence. *BMJ* 1994;**309**:1189–1197.

36 **Needleman HL, Gatonis CA.** Low-level lead exposure and the IQ of children. A meta-analysis of modern studies. *JAMA* 1990;**263**:673–678.

37 **Rogan WJ, Dietrich KN, Ware JH, et al.** The effect of chelation therapy with succimer on neuropsychological development in children exposed to lead. *N Engl J Med* 2001;**344**:1421–1426.

38 **Bellinger DC, Needleman HL.** Intellectual impairment and blood lead levels. *N Engl J Med* 2003;**349**:500–502.

39 **Chiodo LM, Jacobson SW, Jacobson JL.** Neurodevelopmental effects of postnatal lead exposure at very low levels. *Neurotoxicol Teratol* 2004;**26**:359–371.

40 **Chiodo LM, Covington C, Sokol RJ, et al.** Blood lead levels and specific attention effects in young children. *Neurotoxicol Teratol* 2007;**29**:538–546.

41 **Kim Y, Kim BN, Hong YC, et al.** Co-exposure to environmental lead and manganese affects the intelligence of school-aged children. *Neurotox* 2009;**30**:564–571.

42 **Bellinger DC.** Effect modification in epidemiologic studies of low-level neurotoxicant exposures and health outcomes. *Neurotoxicol Teratol* 2000;**22**:133–140.

43 Wasserman GA, Factor-Litvak P. Methodology , inference and causation: environmental lead exposure and childhood intelligence. *Arch Clin Neuropsychol* 2001;**16**:343–352.

44 Bradley RH, Caldwell BM. Home observation for measurement of the environment: a revision of the preschool scale. *Am J Ment Defic* 1979;**84**:235–244.

45 Walkowiak J, Altmann L, Kramer U, et al. Cognitive and sensoimotor functions in 6-year old children in relation to lead and mercury levels: adjustment for intelligence and contrast sensitivity in computerized testing. *Neurotoxicol Teratol* 1998;**20**:511–521.

46 Lanphear BP, Dietrich K, Auinger P, Cox C. Cognitive deficits associated with blood lead concentrations <10 microg/dL in US children and adolescents. *Public Health Rep* 2000;**115**:521–529.

47 Krieg EF, Butler MA, Chang MH, et al. Lead and cognitive function in VDR genotypes in the third National Health and Nutrition Examination Survey. *Neurotoxicol Teratol* 2010;**32**:262–272.

48 Needleman HL, Gunnoe C, Leviton A, et al. Deficits in psychologic and classroom performance of children with elevated dentine lead levels. *N Engl J Med* 1979;**300**:689–695.

49 Needleman HL, Schell A, Bellinger D, et al. The long-term effects of exposure to low doses of lead in childhood. An 11-year follow up report. *New Engl J Med* 1990;**322**:83–88.

50 Bellinger DC, Stiles KM, Needleman HL. Low-level lead exposure, intelligence and academic achievement: a long-term follow-up study. *Pediatrics* 1992;**90**:855–861.

51 Leviton A, Bellinger D, Allred E, et al. Pre- and postnatal low-level lead exposure and children's dysfunction in school. *Environ Res* 1993;**60**:30–43.

52 Miranda ML, Kim D, Galeano MA, et al. The relationship between early childhood blood lead levels and performance on end-of-grade tests. *Environ Health Perspect* 2007;**115**:1242–1247.

53 Miranda ML, Kim D, Reiter J, et al. Environmental contributors to the achievement gap. *Neurotoxicol* 2009;**30**:1019–1024.

54 Chandramouli K, Steer CD, Ellis M, Emond AM. Effects of early childhood lead exposure on academic performance and behavior of school age children. *Arch Dis Childh* 2009;**94**:844–848.

55 Bellinger D, Hu H, Titlebaum L, Needleman HL. Attentional correlates of dentin and bone lead levels in adolescents. *Arch Environ Health* 1994;**49**:98–105.

56 Bellinger D, Leviton A, Allred E, Rabinowitz M. Pre- and postnatal lead exposure and behavior problems in school-aged children. *Environ Res* 1994;**66**:12–30.

57 Dietrich KN, Ris MD, Succop PA, et al. Early exposure to lead and juvenile delinquency. *Neurotoxicol Teratol* 2001;**23**:511–518.

58 Wasserman GA, Liu X, Pine DS, Graziano JH. Contribution of maternal smoking during pregnancy and lead exposure to early child behavior problems. *Neurotoxicol Teratol* 2001;**23**:13–21.

59 Wasserman GA, Staghezza-Jaramillo B, Shrout P, et al. The effect of lead exposure on behavior problems in preschool children. *Am J Public Health* 1998;**88**:481–486.

60 Braun JM, Kahn RS, Froehlich T, et al. Exposures to environmental toxicants and attention deficit hyperactivity disorder in US children. *Environ Health Perspect* 2006;**114**:1904–1909.

61 Froehlich TE, Lanphear BP, Auinger P, et al. Association of tobacco and lead exposures with attention deficit/hyperactivity disorder. *Pediatrics* 2009;**124**:e1054–e1063.

62 Nicolescu R, Petcu C, Cordeanu A, et al. Environmental exposure to lead, but not other neurotoxic metals, relates to core elements of ADHD in Romanian children: performance and questionnaire data. *Environ Res* 2010;**110**:476–483.

63 Wang H-L, Chen X-T, Yang B, et al. Case–control study of blood lead levels and attention deficit activity disorder in Chinese children. *Environ Health Perspect* 2008;**116**:1401–1406.

64 Roy A, Bellinger D, Hu H, et al. Lead exposure and behavior among young children in Chennai, India. *Environ Health Perspect* 2009;**117**:1607–1611.

65 Nigg JT, Knottnerus GM, Martel MM, et al. Low blood lead levels associated with clinically diagnosed attention-deficit/hyperactivity disorder and mediated by weak cognitive control. *Biol Psychiatry* 2008;**63**:325–331.

66 Nigg JT, Nikolas M, Knottnerus GM, et al. Confirmation and extension of association of blood lead with attention-deficit/hyperactivity disorder (ADHD) and ADHD symptom domains at population-typical exposure levels. *J Child Psychol Psychiatry* 2010;**51**:58–65.

67 Eubig PA, Aguiar A, Schantz SL. Lead and PCBs as risk factors for attention deficit/hyperactivity disorder. *Environ Health Perspect* 2010;**118**:1654–1667.

68 Braun JM, Froehlich TE, Daniels JL, et al. Association of environmental toxicants and conduct disorder in US children: NHANES 2001–2004. *Environ Health Perspect* 2008;**116**:956–962.

69 Marcus DK, Fulton JJ, Clarke EJ. Lead and conduct problems: a meta analysis. *J Clin Child Adolesc Psychol* 2010;**39**:234–241.

70 Chen A, Cai B, Dietrich KN, et al. Lead exposure, IQ and behavior in urban 5- to 7- year olds: does lead affect behavior only by lowering IQ? *Pediatrics* 2007;**119**:e650–e658.

71 Burns JM, Baghurst PA, Sawyer MG, et al. Lifetime low-level exposure to environmental lead and children's emotional and behavioral development at ages 11–13. The Port Pirie Cohort Study. *Am J Epidemiol* 1999;**149**:740–749.

72 Van Os J, Kenis G, Rutten PF. The environment and schizophrenia. *Nature* 2010;**468**:203–212.

73 Murray RM, Lewis SW. Is schizophrenia a neurodevelopmental disorder? *BMJ (Clin Res Ed)* 1987;**295**(6600):681–682.

74 Kraepelin E. Dementia Praecox. In: Kraepelin E, editor. *Psychiatrie*. Leipzig: Barth, 1896. pp. 426–441.

75 Bleuler E. Die Prognose der Dementia Praecox—Schizophreniegruppe. *Allgemeine Zeitschr Psychiatrie* 1908;**65**:436–464.

76 Jones PB, Bebbington P, Foerster A, et al. Premorbid social underachievement in schizophrenia. Results from the Camberwell Collaborative Psychosis Study. *Br J Psychiatry* 1993;**162**:65–71.

77 Cannon MC, Tarrant CJ, Huttunen MO, Jones P. Childhood development and later schizophrenia: evidence from genetic high-rsk and birth cohort studies. In: Murray R, Jones P, Susser E, van OS, Cannon M, editors. *The epidemiology of schizophrenia*. Cambridge: Cambridge University Press; 2003.

78 Jones PB. Longitudinal approaches to the search for the causes of schizophrenia: past, present and future. In: Gattaz WF, Hafner H, editors. *Searches for the causes of schizophrenia*, Volume IV, *Balance of the century*. Darmstadt: Steinkopf; and Berlin: Springer; 1999. pp. 91–119.

79 Wright JP, Dietrich KN, Ris MD, et al. Association of prenatal and childhood blood lead concentrations with criminal arrests in early adulthood. *PLoS Med* 2008;**5**:e101.

80 Nevin R. Understanding international crime rates: the legacy of preschool lead exposure. *Environ Res* 2007;**104**:315–336.

81 Opler MGA, Brown AS, Graziano J, et al. Prenatal lead exposure, δ-aminolevulinic acid, and schizophrenia. *Environ Health Perspect* 2004;**112**:548–552.

82 Opler MGA, Buka SL, Groeger J, et al. Prenatal exposure to lead, δ-aminolevulinic acid, and schizophrenia: further evidence. *Environ Health Perspect* 2008;**116**:1586–1590.

83 Trope I, Lopez-Villegas D, Lenkinski RE. Magnetic resonance imaging and spectroscopy of regional brain structure in a 10-year old boy with elevated lead levels. *Pediatrics* 1998;**101**:e7.

84 Trope I, Lopez-Villegas D, Cecil KM, Lenkinski RE. Exposure to lead appears to selectively alter metabolism of cortical gray matter. *Pediatrics* 2001;**107**:1437–1442.

85 Deicken RF, Zhou L, Corwin F, et al. Decreased left frontal lobe N-acetylaspartate in schizophrenia. *Am J Psychiatry* 1997;**154**:688–690.

86 Bertolino A, Kumra S, Callicott JH, et al. Common pattern of cortical pathology in childhood-onset and adult-onset schizophrenia as identified by proton magnetic resonance spectroscopic imaging. *Am J Psychiatry* 1998;**155**:1376–1383.

87 Cecil KM, Brubaker CJ, Adler CM et al. Decreased brain volume in adults with childhood lead exposure. *PLoS Med* 2008;**5**:e112.

88 Brubaker CJ, Dietrich KN, Lanphear BP, Cecil KM. The influence of age and lead exposure on adult gray matter volume. *Neurotoxicology* 2010;**31**:259–266.

89 Brubaker CJ, Schmithorst VJ, Haynes EN, et al. Altered myelination and axonal integrity in adults with childhood lead exposure: a diffusion tensor imaging study. *Neurotoxicology* 2009;**30**:867–875.

90 Andreasen NC, Nopoulus P, Magnotta V, et al. Progressive brain changes in schizophrenia: a prospective longitudinal study of first-episode schizophrenia. *Biol Psychiatry* 2011;**70**:672–679.

91 Pearlson GD. Neurobiology of schizophrenia. *Ann Neurol* 2000;**48**:556–566.

92 Guilarte TR, Opler M, Pletnikov M. Is lead exposure in early life an environmental risk factor for schizophrenia? Neurobiological connections and testable hypotheses. *Neurotoxicology* 2012;**33**:560–574.

93 Finkelstein Y, Markowitz ME, Rosen JF. Low-level lead-induced neurotoxicity in children: an update on central nervous system effects. *Brain Res Brain Res Rev* 1998;**27**:168–176.

94 Johnston MV, Goldstein GW. Selective vulnerability of the developing brain to lead. *Curr Opin Neurol* 1998;**11**:689–693.

95 Tuppurainen M, Wagar G, Kurppa K, et al. Thyroid function as assessed by routine laboratory tests of workers with long-term lead exposure. *Scand J Work Environ Health* 1988;**14**:175–180.

96 Bledsoe M, Pinkerton L, Silver S, Deddens J, Biagini R. Thyroxine and free thyroxine levels in workers occupationally exposed to inorganic lead. *Environ Health Insights* 2011;**5**:55–61.

97 Dundar B, Oktem F, Arslan M, et al. The effect of long-term low-dose lead exposure on thyroid function in adolescents. *Environ Res* 2006;**101**:140–145.

98 Sandstead H, Stant E, Brill A, Arias L, Terry R. Lead intoxication and the thyroid. *Arch Intern Med* 1969;**123**:632–635.

99 Zheng W, Shen H, Blaner W, Zhao Q, Ren X, Graziano J. Chronic lead exposure alters transthyretin concentration in rat cerebrospinal fluid: the role of the choroid plexus. *Toxicol Appl Pharmacol* 1996;**139**(2):445–450.

100 Zheng W, Lu Y, Lu G, Zhao Q, Cheung O, Blaner W. Transthyretin, thyroxine, and retinol-binding protein in human cerebrospinal fluid: effect of lead exposure. *Toxicol Sci* 2001;**61**(1):107–114.

101 Carr E, Beierwaltes W, Raman G, et al. The effect of maternal thyroid function on fetal thyroid function and development. *J Clin Endocrinol Metab* 1959;**19**:1–18.

102 Greenman G, Gabrielson M, Howard-Flanders J, Wessel M. Thyroid dysfunction in pregnancy. *N Engl J Med* 1962;**267**:426–431.

103 Wasserstrum N, Anania CA. Perinatal consequences of maternal hypothyroidism in early pregnancy and inadequate replacement. *Clin Endocrinol (Oxf)* 1995;**42**(4):353–358.

104 Leung AS, Millar LK, Koonings PP, Montoro M, Mestman JH. Perinatal outcome in hypothyroid pregnancies. *Obstet Gynecol* 1993;**81**(3):349–353.

105 Haddow JE, Palomaki GE, Allan WC, et al. Maternal thyroid deficiency during pregnancy and subsequent neuropsychological development of the child. *N Engl J Med* 1999;**341**(8):549–555.

106 Pop VJ, Kuijpens JL, van Baar AL, et al. Low maternal free thyroxine concentrations during early pregnancy are associated with impaired psychomotor development in infancy. *Clin Endocrinol (Oxf)* 1999;**50**(2):149–155.

107 Haddow JE, Klein RZ, Mitchell M. Letter. *N Engl J Med* 1999;**341**:2017.

108 Man EB, Holden RH, Jones WS. Thyroid function in human pregnancy. VII. Development and retardation of 4-year-old progeny of euthyroid and of hypothyroxinemic women. *Am J Obstet Gynecol* 1971;**109**(1):12–19.

109 Man EB, Serunian SA. Thyroid function in human pregnancy. IX. Development or retardation of 7-year-old progeny of hypothyroxinemic women. *Am J Obstet Gynecol* 1976;**125**(7):949.

110 Man EB, Brown JF, Serunian SA. Maternal hypothyroxinemia: psychoneurological deficits of progeny. *Ann Clin Lab Sci* 1991;**21**(4):227–239.

Chapter 20

Role of the social environmental over the life course in the aetiology of psychiatric disorders

Stephen E.Gilman and Jessica R. Marden

20.1 Introduction

A hallmark of modern psychiatric epidemiology has been the search for social causes of psychiatric illness. The question of whether social environment is a cause of psychiatric disorder, posed by Alexander Leighton in 1967, remains of central interest, but even the question itself is not so straightforward. Leighton[1] humorously made the point by beginning a lecture of the same title with the following:

> As a beginning, may I apologize for the title of my talk? I see now that there are certain minor obscurities in it, such as the meaning of 'social environment', 'cause', and 'psychiatric disorder'. The 'a' and the 'of', however, are relatively clear. (p. 337)

He went on in his essay to discuss the importance of sociocultural disintegration to mental health and the need to focus on salient causes of disease—by which he meant those causes of disease that we have the capacity to change.

As early as the Midtown Manhattan study it was appreciated that comparisons of adults living under different environmental conditions provided limited traction for discerning whether such environmental conditions were causes of disease. Srole[2] noted that

> . . . such investigations are in the main static in nature, 'still photos', so to speak, of people caught in their various *current* community milieus. . . . Looked at in terms of the individual's life history, however, such a 'here-and-now' view is a grossly misleading oversimplification. (p. 456)

Environments vary systematically across the life course, in ways that profoundly influence child development and well-being,[3] and environments throughout the life course shape and constrain mental health. For this reason, attention to the life course in studies of the social and environmental determinants of mental disorders has been present since the outset of modern psychiatric epidemiology, even predating Barker's studies[4] that sparked the emergence of 'life course epidemiology' as a general discipline.

A life course perspective on the social determinants of psychiatric disorders requires simultaneous consideration of three dimensions of risk: (i) life history; (ii) disease history; and (iii) the dynamic social environment (Figure 20.1); the figure illustrates how environmental exposures across the life span provide a context for human development and ageing, and for disease aetiology.

Life history encompasses the biologically embedded patterning of human development, maturation, and ageing, and the socially embedded patterning of roles and responsibilities that adhere

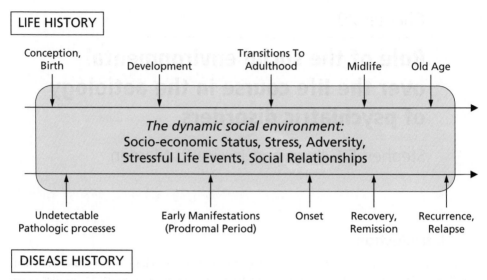

Figure 20.1 Conceptual framework for investigating social determinants of psychiatric disorders over the life course.

to life's sequential stages. Life history matters for the life course epidemiology of psychiatric disorders because life history determines what developmental processes might be perturbed by an environmental exposure, and which of life's roles and responsibilities might be interrupted. Such exposures can promote successful transitions (e.g. educational completion and entry into the work force) or delay or prevent them (e.g. financial crisis or a traumatic event leading to educational failure).[3]

Disease history refers to the 'natural history' of disease, which for the typical psychiatric disorder begins with the initiation of pathological pathways prior to manifestation of symptoms, followed by a prodromal period of subclinical symptoms, disease onset, remission of symptoms and recovery, and recurrence. Consideration of disease history in the context of life course research is critical because it may be possible to intervene among prodromal individuals to prevent disorder onset, among cases to speed recovery, and among recovered individuals to avoid recurrence. Aspects of disease history—age of onset, in particular—have been shown to vary systematically across stages of the life course, possibly indicating aetiologically distinct subtypes of disorder.[5]

Finally, we refer to the 'dynamic social environment' to underscore that environments to which individuals are exposed are patterned by stages of the life course. Intuitively, environmental exposures that impact the mental health of children—for instance, parental divorce and family disruption[6]—may be different from those that impact the mental health of older adults—for instance, spousal bereavement.[7,8] More generally, the environment provides opportunities for and constraints on human development, and these opportunities and constraints vary systematically across stages of the life course.[9]

20.2 **Systematic literature review**

We searched PubMed for published reports of the association between environmental exposures and psychiatric outcomes, within the following limits. The search was conducted among articles published from 1994 through January 2012. We included articles with the Medical Subject

Heading (MeSH) of 'mental disorders' plus any of the following MeSH terms related to environmental stressors: 'life change events', 'stress', 'psychological', 'social environment', or 'poverty'. Accordingly, the review focuses on evidence for the mental health impact of relatively widespread, and perhaps milder, forms of individual environmental stressors. We sought to identify a relatively narrow set of studies with similar design features from which we could draw general conclusions. Though the search criteria did capture some studies on more extreme forms of stress, the evidence for psychiatric consequences of traumatic events is beyond our scope.

The initial search uncovered 1,875 articles. The following restrictions were then applied : (i) English language; (ii) psychiatric disorders based on DSM-IV criteria (e.g. via structured diagnostic interviews, not symptom counts or screening scales); (iii) prospective design, with environmental exposures assessed prior to DSM-IV disorders. These inclusion criteria left 26 remaining studies, listed in Table 20.1. Using the conceptual model in Figure 20.1 as a guide, we describe the results of our review in terms of the types of environmental exposures studied, life history variations in the putative effects of environmental exposures, and disease history variations.

Table 20.1 Studies identified through systematic review

Citation	Study population	Follow-up time	Main outcome (disease history)	Main findings
Childhood				
Cheadle et al.[23]	727 North American Indigenous adolescents	7 years	Alcohol abuse or dependence (onset)	Negative events and perceived discrimination were associated with 1.1–1.4 higher odds of an alcohol use disorder
Essau et al.[34]	523 German students	15 months	Anxiety disorders (recurrence, relapse)	Each additional negative life event was associated with a 1.05 higher odds of persistent anxiety disorder
Essau et al.[33]	523 German students	15 months	Mood disorders (recurrence, relapse)	Negative life events associated with 1.09 higher odds of persistent depression
Ezpeleta et al.[41]	151 socially at-risk children	3 years	Any DSM-IV disruptive, anxiety, or depressive disorder (onset)	Being in a high risk family was associated with 11.3 higher odds of any DSM-IV disorder at ages 13–14 years, but not during other years
Fergusson et al.[14]	971 participants in a New Zealand birth cohort	25 years	Mood, anxiety, and substance disorder (onset)	Single parenthood was associated with 1.2 higher odds of an anxiety disorder
Gilman et al.[6]	1,104 offspring of mothers enrolled in a pregnancy cohort	29 years	Mood disorders (onset)	Parental divorce by age 7 years was associated with 1.79 higher odds of depression onset in adulthood

Table 20.1 (continued) Studies identified through systematic review

Citation	Study population	Follow-up time	Main outcome (disease history)	Main findings
Gilman et al.[15]	1,089 offspring of mothers enrolled in an pregnancy cohort	29 years	Mood disorders (onset)	Parental divorced by age 7 years associated with 2.39 higher odds of early onset depression; residential instability associated with 2.62 higher odds of early onset depression
Koenen et al.[18]	1037 members of the 1972–1973 New Zealand birth cohort	32 years	Anxiety disorders (onset)	Low childhood socio-economic status during childhood, parental change, and the loss of a parent before age 11 years were associated with 2-fold increased risk for PTSD
Laucht et al.[19]	309 participants in the Mannheim Study of Children at Risk	19 years	Mood and anxiety (onset)	Family adversity was associated with 1.6 higher odds of any DSM-IV depressive or anxiety disorder among those with the long form of the *5-HTTLPR* genotype
McFarlane et al.[16]	1011 adults selected based on exposure to Australian bushfire disaster as children	20 years	PTSD, mood, anxiety, and eating disorders (onset)	Children exposed to the Australian bushfire had 1.4 higher odds of an anxiety disorder other than PTSD
Mesman et al.[29]	420 children from the general population of Zuid-Holland	8 years	Any DSM-IV disorder (onset)	Stressful life events were associated with 2.55 higher odds of DSM-IV externalizing disorders
Moffitt et al.[20]	1037 participants in a New Zealand birth cohort	32 years	Mood and anxiety disorder (onset)	Child maltreatment before age 11 years was associated with 2.60 higher odds of major depression, and 4.49 higher odds of generalized anxiety disorder

Table 20.1 (continued) Studies identified through systematic review

Citation	Study population	Follow-up time	Main outcome (disease history)	Main findings
Pawlby et al.[30]	120 mother–offspring dyads from the South London Child Development Study	16 years	Mood and conduct disorders (onset)	Childhood maltreatment was associated with 11.7 higher odds of major depression or conduct disorder among those also exposed to maternal depression
Phillips et al.[21]	816 adolescents	15 years	Mood and anxiety disorders (onset)	Increasing childhood adversities associated with 1.5 higher odds of anxiety disorder
Roberts et al.[24]	3,134 youths and their parents from the Teen Health 2000 study	1 year	Mood, anxiety, and substance disorders (onset)	School and family stressors were associated with a significantly higher risk of mood, anxiety, and substance disorders
Skodol et al.[13]	520 patients with schizotypal, borderline, avoidant, or obsessive–compulsive personality disorders	4 years	Personality disorders (recovery, remission)	Positive relationships in childhood associated with 1.10 higher likelihood of remission from avoidant personality disorder and 1.27 higher likelihood of remission from schizotypal personality disorder
Wals et al.[11]	132 children of parents with bipolar disorder	14 months	Mood disorders (onset)	Severe dependent stressful life event is associated with 11.1 higher odds of depression onset; this association was reduced to 2.2 after controlling for a history of depressive symptoms
Transitions to adulthood				
Friis et al.[12]	2,389 adolescents in the Early Developmental Stages of Psychopathology Study	4–5 years	Mood disorders (onset)	Negative life events associated with 1.45 higher odds of depression onset; family-related stressful life events associated with 1.63 higher odds of depression onset

Table 20.1 (continued) Studies identified through systematic review

Citation	Study population	Follow-up time	Main outcome (disease history)	Main findings
Vriends et al.[36]	1,396 young German women in the Dresden Predictor Study	1.5 years	Anxiety disorders (recovery, remission)	Number of daily hassles was associated with 0.54 lower odds of recovery from social phobia
Zimmermann et al.[40]	1,982 German adolescents	10 years	Mood disorders (onset)	Exposure to any adverse event prior to baseline associated with 2-fold increased risk of depression
Midlife				
Beard et al.[28]	968 adult participants in a telephone survey in Australia	2 years	Any DSM-IV disorder (onset)	Adverse life events in the 12 months prior to the baseline interview were associated with a 1.5 higher odds of depression and anxiety during the follow-up period
Bromberger et al.[31]	266 women	7 years	Mood disorders (onset)	Very strong life event associated with a 2.25 higher risk of first onset depression
Gillespie et al.[45]	1,206 twins	2–4 years	Mood disorders (onset)	Personal stressful life events and network stressful life events were not associated with the onset of depression
Kersting et al.[17]	127 women in a study of pregnancy termination	14 months	Anxiety disorders (onset)	Termination of pregnancy was associated with a higher risk of any mood or anxiety disorder
Wang et al.[32]	6,008 participants in the Canadian National Population Health Survey	6 years	Mood disorders (onset)	High job strain, negative life events, chronic stress, and a history of traumatic events in childhood were associated with 1.4–1.9 higher odds of depression
Older adulthood				
Gureje et al.[22]	1,408 older adults in Nigeria	39 months	Mood disorders (onset)	Lack of regular contact with friends associated with 2.1 higher odds of depression among females

20.2.1 **Environmental stressors over the life course**

'Stressful life events', 'adverse life events', 'stress', and 'adversity' were the most frequent forms of environmental exposures investigated in the studies included in our review. The definition of these exposures varies considerably across studies, as does the strategy of relating the exposures to psychiatric outcomes, ranging from the presence of specific events to the sum total of events in a given time-period.

Table 20.1 is organized according to the time in the life course when environmental exposures were assessed. This organization makes clear that social exposures vary systematically over the life course. For example, during childhood, environmental exposures in families are most common; exposures such as job stress become important following the transition to adulthood.

Many studies included in this review analysed responses to checklist measures of stressful life events in relation to subsequent mental health. Fewer studies used a more intensive assessment method of assessing the presence of specific types of events or stressors, and then adjudicating qualitative aspects of the stressor. For example, Wals et al. used Brown and Harris's Life Events and Difficulties Schedule[10] to determine the presence of dependent or independent life events, that is, events that arose either from the respondent's own behaviour (dependent) or that could not have been caused by the respondent (independent).[11] Friis et al. distinguished controllable from uncontrollable events.[12] Other studies focused on the presence of negative events, e.g., 'physical abuse, unwanted pregnancy, abortion or miscarriage, major financial difficulties and serious problems at work or in school'[11] or, less frequently, positive experience, e.g. children's academic achievements.[13]

Studies in our review focused on specific types of environmental exposures, e.g. single parenthood and familial disruption,[6,14,15] exposure to a natural disaster,[16] or early termination of pregnancy,[17] as well as the presence of multiple environmental exposures during childhood.[18–21] Finally, several studies in our review investigated social relationships and subsequent psychopathology, including social networks,[22] social support,[23] and social resources.[24]

The general pattern that emerges across studies is that researchers asked participants in their studies one or more of the following questions: (i) Did specific things happen in your life?; (ii) When did they happen?; and (iii) What brought them about? Researchers then related participants' responses to their subsequent risk of a psychiatric disorder. Inherent in this approach is the reliance on participants to accurately report events.

Environmental risk factors for psychiatric disorders are often correlated with one another;[25] this poses a challenge for studies that aim to determine the causal influences of any individual factor. For instance, in the studies we reviewed, Fergusson et al. found that the association between exposure to single parenthood and the subsequent risk of anxiety disorders was due in large part to familial factors that cluster in single-parent households.[14] In part this is an issue of simple confounding. More broadly, and of specific relevance to life course epidemiology, it is important to consider how environmental risk factors co-occur with one another at a single point in time and prospectively over time. At a single point in time, children exposed to one type of adversity are likely to be exposed to multiple types of adversity;[25] across time, living conditions in childhood significantly predict living conditions in adulthood.[26] For life course epidemiology, a central implication is that understanding what gives rise to the clustering of risk factors within individuals may be critical for discerning the putative causal effects of any single factor.

20.2.2 **Environmental exposures and subsequent psychiatric disorders over the life course**

Anxiety and mood disorders, primarily major depressive disorder, were the most frequently occurring disorders investigated in relation to environmental exposures over the life course, perhaps owing to the fact that these are the most common disorders. Several additional studies focused on alcohol and substance use disorders, and one study focused on personality disorder.

Many of the studies investigated environmental risk factors for 'aggregate' disorders, e.g. any anxiety disorder, or any mood or anxiety disorder. The implicit assumption of this methodology is that disorders that are aggregated together arise from common aetiological pathways. This approach is also consistent with the principle of multi-finality as articulated in the field of developmental psychopathology—that individual risk factors give rise to a range of adverse outcomes.[27] If the assumption of shared aetiological pathways is correct, then aggregating disorders into a single outcome can increase the power to detect associations with hypothesized risk factors. In this case, individual variation in the specific type of disorder expressed may be less important than the presence of an increased risk for a broad category of disorders. On the other hand, if the assumption of shared aetiology pathways is incorrect, aggregating multiple disorders into a single outcome will obscure any underlying specificity in risk factor–disorder associations.

In the realm of anxiety disorders, 'any anxiety disorder' uniformly included generalized anxiety disorder as well as some combination of panic disorder and phobic disorders; there is less consistency across studies of 'any anxiety disorder' in the inclusion of post-traumatic stress disorder and obsessive–compulsive disorder. The environmental exposures investigated in these three studies were: recent adverse life events,[28] single parenthood during childhood,[14] and exposure to a natural disaster.[16]

These examples concern the aggregation of disorders within the broad domain of anxiety pathology. Many other studies in our review aggregated disorders across domains, most commonly mood and anxiety disorders.[19,29,30] These studies provide evidence for generalized effects of environmental exposures on multiple forms of psychopathology.

There was considerable variation across studies in the analysis of incident disorders, incident episodes, and episode recurrence. An incident disorder refers to the first lifetime onset of a disorder, whereas an incident episode refers to the occurrence of a new episode of a disorder over a period time, and episode recurrence refers to the development of a new episode of a disorder among individuals with a prior history of the disorder. Gilman et al. and Bromberger et al. analysed risk factors for the first lifetime onset of major depression (incident disorders).[6,31] Wang and Schmitz analysed risks for new onset depressive episodes in a sample without depression during the first several waves of follow-up; as they did not exclude from their analysis individuals with depression prior to study enrolment, theirs was an analysis of incident episodes.[32] Other studies analysed risks for recurrent episodes (and also recovery) among lifetime cases.[33–36] In general, these studies reported more similarities than differences in the predictors of onset and the predictors of recurrence.

Theoretical arguments have been made for disaggregating risks associated with the initial onset of a disorder from risks associated with disorder recurrence.[37,38] It is conceivable that certain exposures would be uniquely associated with disorder onset, and have no relation with persistence, or alternatively that certain factors would precipitate a recurrent episode but not increase the risk for initial onset. Yet the studies in our review do not provide strong support for the theory of distinct aetiologies of the incidence and recurrence of psychiatric disorders. At the same time there is moderate support in the studies reviewed that some risk factors have stronger associations with disorder onset than disorder persistence,[11] which could be due in part to the tendency of risk factor effects to decay over time.[15,39] If that is the case, then continued exposure to adverse conditions would be expected to confer ongoing excess risk for subsequent episodes.

20.2.3 **Magnitude of associations between environmental exposures and psychiatric disorders**

The majority of effect sizes relating environmental exposures to psychiatric disorders, in relative risk terms, ranged between just over 1.0 to 2.5. On the face of it, scanning the 'Main findings' column in Table 20.1, effect sizes were generally similar across studies, with the exception of studies detecting statistically significant but small relative risks in the range of 1.1–1.2. The caveat to this impression is that there are important differences across studies in the analytical procedures used to determine relative risks of psychiatric disorders associated with environmental exposures. The most directly comparable effect sizes are those involving specific environmental exposures, e.g. single parenthood (1.2),[14] a natural disaster (1.4),[16] or parental divorce (1.8).[6] Other comparable studies reported associations between 'any adversity' and a psychiatric disorder: two studies reported that exposure to any serious life event was associated with a two-fold increased risk of depression.[31,40]

Effect sizes that are least comparable across studies are those that relate the number of environmental exposures to psychiatric outcomes, where effect sizes are given in terms of 'each additional life event'. In other words, these studies relate unit differences in life events to differences in the relative risk or odds of a psychiatric disorder. Even assuming linearity, the challenge is obvious: is a unit difference in one study comparable to a unit difference in another? For example, Phillips et al. reported that the number of adversities is associated with 1.5 higher odds of an anxiety disorder,[21] and Essau reported that the number of negative life events was associated with 1.05 times higher odds of anxiety persistence.[34] One cannot directly compare the 1.5 and 1.05 odds ratios without also comparing the composition and number of items included in the original scales. Essau et al.'s measure of life events was based on a checklist of 55 events, each of which is categorized as positive or negative (they do not indicate how many negative events were among the 55 queried). Phillips et al. recorded the number of adversities across five domains, but did not give the exact number of adversities included in their sum score. It is unclear whether a point on Essau et al.'s scale is qualitatively similar to a point on Phillips et al.'s scale.

From the studies we reviewed, negative environmental exposures conferred excess risks for psychiatric disorders in the range of 50–250%. Since population prevalences of widespread mental disorders range from 10% to 20%, these excess risks lead to the following conclusions. First, environmental exposures are related to meaningful increases in the risk of psychiatric disorders, and if these relationships represent causal associations, preventing or reducing them could lead to a substantial reduction in the burden of mental illness. Second, most individuals exposed to environmental adversity do not go on to develop a psychiatric disorder. It is therefore essential to determine who, among those exposed, is most vulnerable to the adverse psychiatric consequences of environmental adversity.

20.2.4 **Specificity of associations between environmental exposures and psychiatric outcomes**

To what extent do the studies in our review support the proposition that the environmental risk factors differ across psychiatric disorders? Several studies in our review assessed associations between environmental exposures and more than one disorder.[14,16,17,19,24,28,41] However, only two studies made the comparisons needed to assess the specificity of risk factor associations across psychiatric diagnoses. Moffitt et al. compared risk factors for major depressive disorder alone, generalized anxiety disorder alone, and both conditions together.[20] Their study found that environmental risk factors were most highly concentrated among individuals with generalized anxiety disorder occurring together with major depressive disorder, and, to a somewhat lesser degree, among those with generalized anxiety disorder alone. They found few childhood risk factors for depression in the absence of anxiety. Similarly, Philips et al. reported that childhood adversities predicted an anxiety disorder (either generalized anxiety disorder, obsessive–compulsive disorder, panic disorder, post-traumatic stress disorder, social phobia, or specific phobia) more strongly than a depressive disorder (depression or dysthymia), in analyses comparing risks for anxiety versus depressive disorders.[21] These analyses highlight the importance of directly comparing risks for different psychiatric diagnoses in order to assess the specificity of associations, and by implication the presence of unique risk factor profiles across disorder categories. On the basis of these two studies alone, evidence would suggest that environmental exposures have their strongest effects on anxiety disorders, and that associations with mood disorders are either smaller in magnitude or secondary to their effects on anxiety.

20.4 Summary

Substantial work remains to determine the aetiological significance of environmental exposures over the life course to mood, anxiety, substance, and other forms of psychiatric disorders. Moreover, research is needed to evaluate whether environmental exposures can be targeted by interventions, at what stage in the life course those interventions would be most effective, and if such interventions can lead to reductions in the risk of psychopathology. Quasi-experimental designs, and a small number of randomized controlled trials, support the development of such interventions.[42,43]

The studies included in our review that focus on the persistence of psychopathology among those with a history of a disorder suggest that environmental exposures significantly predict episode recovery. The DSM has for decades contemplated incorporating such knowledge into treatment planning. Since the revision of the DSM in 1980, the multi-axial diagnostic system has held a place for including the presence of psychosocial and environmental stressors into the diagnostic evaluation—Axis IV. Evidence directly assessing the clinical utility of Axis IV suggests that recent and past exposure to environmental adversity predicts the recurrence risk of multiple forms of psychopathology.[44] Significant work is needed both to further evaluate the prognostic value of environmental exposures in the recovery and relapse of psychiatric disorders, and to evaluate whether incorporating this information into treatment planning can enhance treatment effectiveness.

Acknowledgement

This work was supported in part by grant RO1087544 from the National Institute of Mental Health.

References

1 Leighton A. Is social environment a cause of psychiatric disorder? *Psychiatr Res Rep Am Psychiatr Assoc* 1967;**22**:337–345.

2 Srole L. Urbanization and mental health: a reformulation. *Psychiatr Q* 1972;**46**(4):449–460.

3 Elder GH, Rockwell RC. The life-course and human development: an ecological perspective. *Int J Behav Dev* 1979;2(1):1–21.

4 Barker DJ, Winter PD, Osmond C, et al. Weight in infancy and death from ischaemic heart disease. *Lancet* 1989;2(8663):577–580.

5 Buka SL, Gilman SE. Psychopathology and the life course. In: Helzer JE, Hudziak JJ, editors. *Defining psychopathology in the 21st century: DSM-V and beyond.* Washington DC: American Psychiatric Press; 2002. pp. 129–141.

6 Gilman SE, Kawachi I, Fitzmaurice GM, et al. Family disruption in childhood and risk of adult depression. *Am J Psychiatry* 2003;**160**(5):939–946.

7 Gilman SE, Breslau J, Trinh NH, et al. Bereavement and the diagnosis of major depressive episode in the National Epidemiologic Survey on Alcohol and Related Conditions. *J Clin Psychiatry* 2012;**73**(2):208–215.

8 Gilman SE, Carliner H, Cohen A. The social determinants of depression in older adulthood. In: Reynolds CF, Sajatovic M, Lavretsky H, editors. *Late-life mood disorders*: New York: Oxford University Press (in press).

9 Baltes PB. On the incomplete architecture of human ontogeny. Selection, optimization, and compensation as foundation of developmental theory. *Am Psychol* 1997;**52**(4):366–380.

10 Brown GW, Harris TO. *Social origins of depression: a study of psychiatric disorder in women.* London: Tavistock; 1978.

11 Wals M, Hillegers MH, Reichart CG, et al. Stressful life events and onset of mood disorders in children of bipolar parents during 14-month follow-up. *J Affect Disord* 2005;**87**(2–3):253–263.

12 Friis RH, Wittchen HU, Pfister H, et al. Life events and changes in the course of depression in young adults. *Eur Psychiatry* 2002;**17**(5):241–253.

13 Skodol AE, Bender DS, Pagano ME, et al. Positive childhood experiences: resilience and recovery from personality disorder in early adulthood. *J Clin Psychiatry* 2007;**68**(7):1102–1108.

14 Fergusson DM, Boden JM, Horwood LJ. Exposure to single parenthood in childhood and later mental health, educational, economic, and criminal behavior outcomes. *Arch Gen Psychiatry* 2007;**64**(9):1089–1095.

15 Gilman SE, Kawachi I, Fitzmaurice GM, et al. Socio-economic status, family disruption and residential stability in childhood: relation to onset, recurrence and remission of major depression. *Psychol Med* 2003;**33**(8):1341–1355.

16 McFarlane AC, Van Hooff M. Impact of childhood exposure to a natural disaster on adult mental health: 20-year longitudinal follow-up study. *Br J Psychiatry* 2009;**195**(2):142–148.

17 Kersting A, Kroker K, Steinhard J, et al. Complicated grief after traumatic loss: a 14-month follow up study. *Eur Arch Psychiatry Clin Neurosci* 2007;**257**(8):437–443.

18 Koenen KC, Moffitt TE, Poulton R, et al. Early childhood factors associated with the development of post-traumatic stress disorder: results from a longitudinal birth cohort. *Psychol Med* 2007;**37**(2): 181–192.

19 Laucht M, Treutlein J, Blomeyer D, et al. Interaction between the 5-HTTLPR serotonin transporter polymorphism and environmental adversity for mood and anxiety psychopathology: evidence from a high-risk community sample of young adults. *Int J Neuropsychopharmacol* 2009;**12**(6):737–747.

20 Moffitt TE, Caspi A, Harrington H, et al. Generalized anxiety disorder and depression: childhood risk factors in a birth cohort followed to age 32. *Psychol Med* 2007;**37**(3):1–12.

21 Phillips NK, Hammen CL, Brennan PA, et al. Early adversity and the prospective prediction of depressive and anxiety disorders in adolescents. *J Abnorm Child Psychol* 2005;**33**(1):13–24.

22 Gureje O, Oladeji B, Abiona T. Incidence and risk factors for late-life depression in the Ibadan Study of Ageing. *Psychol Med* 2011;**41**(9):1897–1906.

23 Cheadle JE, Whitbeck LB. Alcohol use trajectories and problem drinking over the course of adolescence: a study of North American indigenous youth and their caretakers. *J Health Soc Behav* 2011;**52**(2):228–245.

24 Roberts RE, Roberts CR, Chan W. One-year incidence of psychiatric disorders and associated risk factors among adolescents in the community. *J Child Psychol Psychiatry* 2009;**50**(4):405–415.

25 **Slopen N, Fitzmaurice GM, Williams DR, et al.** Common patterns of violence experiences and depression and anxiety among adolescents. *Soc Psychiatry Psychiatr Epidemiol* 2012;**47**(10):1591–1605.

26 **Power C, Matthews S.** Origins of health inequalities in a national population sample. *Lancet* 1997;**350**(9091):1584–1589.

27 **Cicchetti D, Rogosch F.** Equifinality and multifinality in developmental psychopathology. *Dev Psychopathol* 1996;**8**:597–600.

28 **Beard JR, Heathcote K, Brooks R, et al.** Predictors of mental disorders and their outcome in a community based cohort. *Soc Psychiatry Psychiatr Epidemiol* 2007;**42**(8):623–630.

29 **Mesman J, Koot HM.** Early preschool predictors of preadolescent internalizing and externalizing DSM-IV diagnoses. *J Am Acad Child Adolesc Psychiatry* 2001;**40**(9):1029–1036.

30 **Pawlby S, Hay D, Sharp D, et al.** Antenatal depression and offspring psychopathology: the influence of childhood maltreatment. *Br J Psychiatry* 2011;**199**(2):106–112.

31 **Bromberger JT, Kravitz HM, Matthews K, et al.** Predictors of first lifetime episodes of major depression in midlife women. *Psychol Med* 2009;**39**(1):55–64.

32 **Wang J, Schmitz N.** Does job strain interact with psychosocial factors outside of the workplace in relation to the risk of major depression? The Canadian National Population Health Survey. *Soc Psychiatry Psychiatr Epidemiol* 2011;**46**(7):577–584.

33 **Essau CA.** Course and outcome of major depressive disorder in non-referred adolescents. *J Affect Disord* 2007;**99**(1–3):191–201.

34 **Essau CA, Conradt J, Petermann F.** Course and outcome of anxiety disorders in adolescents. *J Anxiety Disord* 2002;**16**(1):67–81.

35 **Leskela U, Rytsala H, Komulainen E, et al.** The influence of adversity and perceived social support on the outcome of major depressive disorder in subjects with different levels of depressive symptoms. *Psychol Med* 2006;**36**(6):779–788.

36 **Vriends N, Becker ES, Meyer A, et al.** Recovery from social phobia in the community and its predictors: data from a longitudinal epidemiological study. *J Anxiety Disord* 2007;**21**(3):320–337.

37 **Kessler RC.** The effects of stressful life events on depression. *Annu Rev Psychol* 1997;**48**:191–214.

38 **Post RM.** Transduction of psychosocial stress into the neurobiology of recurrent affective disorder. *Am J Psychiatry* 1992;**149**(8):999–1010.

39 **Surtees PG, Wainwright NW.** Surviving adversity: event decay, vulnerability and the onset of anxiety and depressive disorder. *Eur Arch Psychiatry Clin Neurosci* 1999;**249**(2):86–95.

40 **Zimmermann P, Bruckl T, Lieb R, et al.** The interplay of familial depression liability and adverse events in predicting the first onset of depression during a 10-year follow-up. *Biol Psychiatry* 2008;**63**(4):406–414.

41 **Ezpeleta L, Granero R, de la Osa N, et al.** Risk factor clustering for psychopathology in socially at-risk Spanish children. *Soc Psychiatry Psychiatr Epidemiol* 2008;**43**(7):559–568.

42 **Jackson L, Langille L, Lyons R, et al.** Does moving from a high-poverty to lower-poverty neighborhood improve mental health? A realist review of 'Moving to Opportunity'. *Health Place* 2009;**15**(4):961–970.

43 **Costello EJ, Compton SN, Keeler G, et al.** Relationships between poverty and psychopathology: a natural experiment. *JAMA* 2003;**290**(15):2023–2029.

44 **Gilman SE, Trinh NH, Smoller JW, et al.** Psychosocial stressors and the prognosis of major depression: a test of Axis IV. *Psychol Med* 2013;**43**(2):303–316.

45 **Gillespie NA, Whitfield JB, Williams B, et al.** The relationship between stressful life events, the serotonin transporter (5-HTTLPR) genotype and major depression. *Psychol Med* 2005;**35**(1):101–111.

Chapter 21

Social context and mental health over the life course

Arijit Nandi and Lauren Welsh

21.1 Introduction

The life course perspective, in addition to other frameworks for investigating social determinants of health,[1,2] has the potential to provide important insights concerning the relevance of social, behavioural, and biological factors, including their independent, cumulative, and interactive effects across the life span, as well as how experiences in one period of the life course might influence illness in another.[3,4] The aims of this chapter are to address three key questions that have helped define this burgeoning literature. First, what are the theoretical mechanisms hypothesized to link social context to mental health outcomes? Second, what is the evidence for 'independent' effects of social contextual factors on mental health at various stages of the life course, in general, and for social context at one stage of the life course influencing health at a later stage, in particular? Third, what are the main challenges to causal inference with respect to estimating contextual mental health effects over the life course? In all of these aims, we have chosen to focus on salient aspects of social context in three phases of life: childhood and adolescence, adulthood, and older age. In the next section, we briefly introduce a model to help structure our discussions of empirical findings.

21.2 Mechanisms hypothesized to link social context to mental illness

Life course and social epidemiological theories are useful for discussing the plausibility of societal influences on population mental health.[5] For the purposes of this chapter, we adapt the modified stream of causation metaphor developed by Glass and McAtee for the multilevel study of health behaviours and outcomes,[1] primarily because it focuses on articulating how 'mezzo-level' contextual characteristics, which have been the principal targets of empirical research concerning social context and mental health, shape health behaviours and population health. These intermediate contextual conditions include the social, material, and physical features of the school, workplace, neighbourhood, and other environments that we occupy over the life course. The material environment includes objective components, such as the quality of schools and the institutional and teaching resources available to students, as well as the accessibility of mental health and supportive social services in our workplaces and neighbourhoods. The social environment refers to subjective features that arise out of social interactions between individuals, including social resources (e.g. social cohesiveness), risks (e.g. neighbourhood exposure to violence and crime), and norms.[6] Finally, the physical environment encompasses features of our built environment, including housing quality and exposure to noise and air pollution, although these have been sparsely studied in

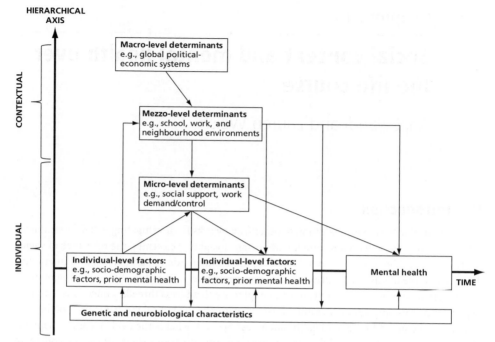

Figure 21.1 Conceptual model for how multilevel factors influence mental health over the life course.

the context of mental health outcomes. As seen in Figure 21.1, the social, material, and physical conditions of our family, school, workplace, and neighbourhood environments are nested within a hierarchy of factors, ranging from individual-level genetic, neurobiological, and psychological determinants to macro-level characteristics, including global political–economic systems and attendant government policies.

21.3 Summary of empirical evidence

21.3.1 Family and school environments in early life

The family social environment is an important aspect of social context in early life that is hypothesized to influence mental health over the life course.[7] There is substantial evidence to suggest that 'risky' family social environments characterized by interpersonal conflicts, aggression, and minimal warmth and affection are associated with poorer mental health, including increased internalizing and externalizing problems, and self-harm.[8–11] Maternal parenting styles, in particular, appear to have a stronger effect on childhood mental disorders than paternal parenting.[12,13] A family history of mental disorder remains the single most predictive risk factor for developing a mental disorder oneself,[14,15] and genetic predispositions for mental illness may both confound and modify the effects of the family environment on mental health in early life.

The life course effect of early life exposure to adverse family environments on mental health in adulthood is unclear. Some work suggests that a stressful early family environment was associated with depression in early adulthood.[16] Exposure to adverse family environments may interfere with or dysregulate children's emotional development and increase risks for substance abuse, both of which are associated with subsequent mental illness in adulthood. However, few studies have examined these effects over the life course.

In addition to family context, the school environment may play an important role in shaping cognitive experience and development during childhood and adolescence. School material and social context are associated with the propensity to exhibit internalizing problems, externalizing problems, and learning problems in early life. In particular, a lack of material resources in the classroom, school disrepair, low school income, and certain school population compositions are correlated with poorer mental health.[17–19]

Individual-level social inclusion, social support, and group dynamics have profound implications for individual's self-esteem and identity formation during adolescence, suggesting that friendships and social dynamics may mediate the effects of the school environment on mental health, although these pathways have not been explicitly tested. Involvement in bullying, as both the bully and the victim, has been linked to increased symptoms of mental disorder; victims of frequent bullying are also more likely to self-harm and attempt suicide.[20]

21.3.2 **Work environment and mental health during adulthood**

Time-use surveys indicate that the greatest proportion of waking hours for the average adult are spent working. Interventions to the psychosocial work environment are constantly occurring and studies evaluating the effects of these 'natural experiments' offer insights regarding the contextual effects of the work environment on mental health. This includes, for example, interventions to enhance employee control, such as the integration of participatory employee committees, as well as changes to the organization of work. A review of the quasi-experimental evidence suggested that increasing employee participation and control through workplace reorganization was associated with better mental health, although many of these studies were uncontrolled.[21] Changes to organizational structure, including patterns of shift work and restructuring induced by privatization, may also influence mental health.[22] Few studies have examined whether the effects of work interventions vary by individual-level socio-demographic or occupational characteristics. Similarly, there are few empirical data on the pathways linking the work environment to mental health. There is substantial evidence in support of the demand control model proposed by Karasek;[23] in particular, high demands in combination with low decisional latitude and high efforts in combination with low rewards may be associated with increased risk for common mental disorders.[24] Therefore, the association between the psychosocial work environment and mental health may be mediated by changes to individuals' levels of decisional latitude relative to their work demands. Future work should examine whether these factors mediate associations between the psychosocial work environment and mental health.

21.3.3 **Neighbourhood context and mental health over the life course**

Individuals often describe places with the same language used to characterize general affect. For example, blighted urban areas may be labelled 'depressing'. Is this an implicit recognition that certain contexts elicit a psychological response, and, if so, what specific qualities of these contexts matter for mental health? Answering these questions has long been an objective of empirical research in the social sciences[25,26] and these seminal studies established a foundation for contemporary observational research on neighbourhood effects and mental health. In this section, we briefly summarize selected work examining neighbourhood effects on mental health from early to later life.

21.3.3.1 Neighbourhood context in early life and mental health

The effects of structural features of neighbourhoods, including neighbourhood socio-economic disadvantage, racial composition, and mental health in early life have been investigated in relation to suicidal behaviours, internalizing and externalizing problems, anxiety, and depressed mood.[27–31] Several studies have assessed whether aspects of the social environment, including both the resources (e.g. social capital) and risks (e.g. exposure to violence and crime) that arise out of social interactions between residents[6] are associated with mental health outcomes among children and adolescents. A positive association between perceptions of neighbourhood disorder and adolescent alcohol and/or drug use and dependence has been consistently reported.[32,33] Comparatively few studies have assessed the association between neighbourhood disorder and mood and anxiety disorders in early life. Using methods for measuring neighbourhood social processes akin to systematic social observation,[34] both Schaefer-McDaniel[35] and Natsuaki et al.[36] found insubstantial evidence for an effect of neighbourhood disorder or stressors on depressive symptoms among adolescents. By contrast, greater perceived 'ambient hazards', a subjective measure of social disorder based on respondents' ratings of potential dangers in their neighbourhoods, was associated with more symptoms of anxiety and depression, as well as oppositional defiant and conduct disorders, among adolescents in Los Angeles County.[30]

Neighbourhood social resources, by contrast with the potentially destabilizing effects of neighbourhood disorder, are posited to benefit mental health.[29,30,33] There is divergent evidence concerning the effect of neighbourhood social capital in early life on mental health. For example, a UK study showed that children's ratings of neighbourhood trust and safety were associated with decreased odds of emotional and conduct disorders.[37] By contrast, Harpham et al. found that dimensions of social capital were not consistently associated with mental health among youth aged 15–25 years living in a low income community in Cali, Columbia, after accounting for individual-level socio-demographic characteristics and ratings of community violence.[38]

21.3.3.2 Neighbourhood context and mental health in adulthood and older age

The association between neighbourhood disadvantage in adulthood and mental health, particularly depression, has been widely studied and the subject of recent reviews.[39,40] In their assessment of the literature up to 2007, Mair et al.[39] found that roughly one-half of studies supported an association between neighbourhood socio-economic conditions and depression or depressive symptoms, after controlling for individual-level characteristics. For example, in one of the few longitudinal studies, Galea et al.[41] found that the relative odds of incident depression were more than twice as high for participants living in low socio-economic status (SES) compared with high SES neighbourhoods in multivariable models adjusting for individual covariates; research from other contexts informs similar inference.[42] However, other work suggests that there is insubstantial variation in the levels of, and changes in, common mental disorders at the neighbourhood level,[43,44] no evidence of a crude association between deprivation and mental health,[45] or rather that contextual effects of neighbourhood disadvantage on anxiety and depression are explained by individual-level compositional characteristics.[46] Outcomes besides mood and anxiety disorders have rarely been investigated.

Research concerning neighbourhood racial composition or segregation and mental health has been notably mixed, both in terms of methods (e.g. methods for exposure assessment) and results. Residential segregation, measured by the isolation index, was positively associated with symptoms of depression and anxiety among Mexican-Americans in Chicago, but not among Puerto Rican-Americans, after controlling for individual-level socio-demographic characteristics and neighbourhood income.[47] However, segregation, measured by the neighbourhood percentage of Mexican-Americans, was associated with fewer depressive symptoms among Mexican-Americans aged ≥65 years from the south-western USA.[48] Other work suggests that individual-level characteristics may confound contextual effects of neighbourhood racial composition on mental health; for example, cross-sectional analyses from the CARDIA study showed that the percentages of White and Black residents were not associated with depressive symptoms among Whites or Blacks after adjusting for individual and neighbourhood socio-economic variables.[49]

Relatively consistent associations have been reported between social disorder, or alternatively measures of supportive social interactions among neighbourhood residents (e.g. collective efficacy), and mental health outcomes, with depression again being the most frequently assessed outcome.[50] Research also suggests that higher levels of social cohesion and collective efficacy are associated with lower levels of depressive symptoms.[51,52]

There is growing interest in whether physical features of urban areas, including our internal and external built environments, the availability of green spaces, and characteristics such as urban density, are associated with mental health. A study of adult residents of a South Wales district found that respondents' with more positive ratings of their built environments, based on perceptions of the presence of litter, graffiti, green areas, as well as other indicators of neighbourhood quality, experienced better psychological well-being.[53] Other work has relied on administrative data or objective assessments of neighbourhoods to characterize the built environment.[54]

21.3.3.3 Neighbourhood conditions and mental health over the life course

Generalizing from the broader literature on life course SES and health,[55] there are at least three distinct hypotheses for explaining effects of early life neighbourhood circumstances on adult mental health. First, according to the latent effects model, early life neighbourhood conditions have an independent effect on adult mental illness. Second, according to the pathway or social trajectories model, early life neighbourhood context is associated with adult mental health only through its effect on adult neighbourhood conditions. Third, according to the cumulative exposure model, neighbourhood conditions in both early life and adulthood directly influence mental health in later life. Due to the need for cohorts with extended follow-up, research testing whether neighbourhood context in early life is associated with mental health in adulthood is especially scant. Using three waves of data from the National Survey of Children (1976–1987), Wheaton and Clarke found that early life, but not current, neighbourhood disadvantage was associated with externalizing and internalizing problems in early adulthood after controlling for individual and family-level risk factors, and that these associations were strongest for respondents of parents with lower educational attainment.[56] This work provides provisional support for an independent effect of early life neighbourhood disadvantage on mental health in early adulthood. Additionally, Stafford et al., using data from the Whitehall II cohort, provided longitudinal evidence of cumulative effects by showing that longer exposure to deprived or fragmented neighbourhood environments had incremental effects on poorer mental health.[57] Further work assessing the effects of early life neighbourhood conditions on adult mental health, in addition to mediation analyses testing whether these effects are independent of adult neighbourhood conditions, is needed.

21.3.4 Macro-level effects

There is growing evidence that 'macro-level' determinants, including global economic systems and macro-economic conditions, as well as legal frameworks and policies, are associated with population mental health. With respect to legal frameworks, several studies have examined the population health effects of regulatory policies concerning the use of substances. Research from the USA, for example, suggests that increases in state tobacco control programme expenditures and US state cigarette taxes have resulted in a significant reduction in smoking participation and frequency among youth, as well adults.[58,59] State policies governing the minimum legal drinking age have been associated with the reduced consumption of alcohol and related problems.[60] There has also been growing interest in assessing the impacts of economic downturns on population mental health, including suicide. Zivin et al. recently reviewed empirical work concerning the population mental health effects of economic conditions and concluded that there was a consistently negative association between economic crises and population mental health.[61]

21.4 Challenges to causal inference in the study of social context and mental health

As highlighted by our review, observational research has, in some cases, produced consistent evidence for an association between social context and mental health. Do these associations represent contextual influences and, if so, are they causal? Alternatively, do associations reflect compositional variations between individuals in different contexts? If so, are these compositional variations the result of the non-random residential selection of individuals into various contexts (i.e. social selection), or, conversely, the true aetiologic effect of social processes (i.e. social causation)?

21.4.1 Contextual causal effects

Within the potential outcomes framework that has guided causal inference in public health research,[62] average causal effects are identifiable when two outcomes, one in which a treatment (or exposure) is given and another in which the same treatment is withheld, are simultaneously compared. Because only potential outcomes for the treatment actually received are observed in real-life settings, the other must be inferred. Randomized experiments, considered the gold standard for evaluating causal hypotheses in epidemiology and public health, allow estimation of the average causal effect of a treatment by comparing the outcomes of treatment and control groups that have comparable or 'exchangeable' distributions of measured and unmeasured characteristics.

Estimates of the influence of contextual factors on health are seldom characterized as causal, primarily because group-level exposures are not easily articulated with the potential outcomes model. Say, for example, that we are interested in estimating the effect of living in a racially segregated neighbourhood on individual-level depressive symptoms. Within the potential outcomes framework, this effect is only identifiable if we can compare the outcomes of residents of segregated neighbourhoods with those of another neighbourhood in which all neighbourhood and individual-level conditions are identical, with the exception of neighbourhood segregation. Whether such a comparison is feasible given the inextricability of neighbourhood exposures and shifting of neighbourhood residents is questionable. Further complicating identification of causal contextual effects is the challenge of manipulating environments using randomized experiments. Readers may point to randomized controlled trials, such as the Moving to Opportunities (MTO) programme, which randomly offered families living in public housing in high poverty neighbourhoods a voucher to move to a near-poor or non-poor neighbourhood, showing that such moves had beneficial mental health effects for younger boys and adolescent girls.[63,64] However, these do not represent the contextual effects of neighbourhood income on mental health because rather than intervening to change one feature of the neighbourhood environment, the intervention of moving individuals to different neighbourhoods inevitably changes many things (e.g. the disruption of social networks). While debate continues concerning contextual causal effects, we suggest that it is constructive to underline the challenges to extant observational work and to point toward new approaches and methodologies for addressing them.

21.4.2 Confounding by non-random selection into social contexts

As both epidemiologists and sociologists have noted, the selection issue (i.e. the non-random migration of individuals into particular contexts based on individual-level characteristics that may be related to health) is the largest challenge to causal inference in observational studies of contextual effects.[65,66] Failing to account for these compositional differences threatens the exchangeability of contexts, an issue that would not exist had we been able to easily randomize group-level treatments.

How can we account for potential confounding due to compositional differences between contexts? The modus operandi is to estimate the effect of social context on individual mental health after multivariable adjustment for individual-level characteristics. Alternative strategies for estimating the effects of social context on mental health, including marginal structural models using inverse probability weights, are emerging[67-70] and gradually being incorporated into the literature.[71,72]

21.5 Summary

Advances in the application of multi-level analysis during the past decades have allowed investigators to tease out compositional influences from potential contextual effects and test longstanding hypotheses concerning the associations between social context and mental health. The empirical literature reveals substantial heterogeneity, both in terms of methods and findings. Inconsistent findings either suggest this relation is context specific (true heterogeneity) or perhaps confounded. Consistent findings cannot be inferred as causal, as even multi-level longitudinal study designs are insufficient to address the challenges of selection into social contexts using standard regression methods. Innovative approaches to analysis, including inverse probability weighting marginal structural models (to overcome time-varying confounding), utilization of natural experiments (instruments), and group-randomized trials represent promising directions for further research with the potential to inform policies and interventions for improving population mental health.

References

1 **Glass TA, McAtee MJ.** Behavioral science at the crossroads in public health: extending horizons, envisioning the future. *Soc Sci Med* 2006;**62**(7):1650–1671.

2 **Susser M, Susser E.** Choosing a future for epidemiology: II. From black box to Chinese boxes and eco-epidemiology. *Am J Public Health* 1996;**86**(5):674–677.

3 **Ben-Shlomo Y, Kuh D.** A life course approach to chronic disease epidemiology: conceptual models, empirical challenges and interdisciplinary perspectives. *Int J Epidemiol* 2002;**31**(2):285–293.

4 **Halfon N, Hochstein M.** Life course health development: an integrated framework for developing health, policy, and research. *Milbank Q* 2002;**80**(3):433–479, iii.

5 **Krieger N.** *Epidemiology and the people's health: theory and context.* New York: Oxford University Press; 2011.

6 Coutts A, Kawachi I. The urban social environment and its impact on health. In: Freudenberg N, Galea S, Vlahov D, editors. *Cities and the health of the public*. Nashville: Vanderbilt University Press; 2006. pp. 49–60.

7 Repetti RL, Taylor SE, Seeman TE. Risky families: family social environments and the mental and physical health of offspring. *Psychol Bull* 2002;**128**(2):330–366.

8 Bayer JK, Hiscock H, Ukoumunne OC, Price A, Wake M. Early childhood aetiology of mental health problems: a longitudinal population-based study. *J Child Psychol Psychiatry* 2008;**49**(11):1166–1174.

9 Bayer JK, Sanson AV, Hemphill SA. Parent influences on early childhood internalizing difficulties. *J Appl Dev Psychol* 2006;**27**(6):542–559.

10 Michelson D, Bhugra D. Family environment, expressed emotion and adolescent self-harm: a review of conceptual, empirical, cross-cultural and clinical perspectives. *Int Rev Psychiatry* 2012;**24**(2):106–114.

11 Bakker MP, Ormel J, Verhulst FC, Oldehinkel AJ. Childhood family instability and mental health problems during late adolescence: a test of two mediation models—the TRAILS study. *J Clin Child Adolesc Psychol* 2012;**41**(2):166–176.

12 Connell AMAM, Goodman SHSH. The association between psychopathology in fathers versus mothers and children's internalizing and externalizing behavior problems: a meta-analysis. *Psychol Bull* 2002;**128**(5):746–773.

13 Leve LD, Kerr DC, Shaw D, et al. Infant pathways to externalizing behavior: evidence of genotype × environment interaction. *Child Dev* 2010;**81**(1):340–356.

14 Rice F, Harold G, Thapar A. The link between depression in mothers and offspring: an extended twin analysis. *Behav Genet* 2005;**35**(5):565–577.

15 Thapar A, McGuffin P. A twin study of depressive symptoms in childhood. *Br J Psychiatry* 1994;**165**(2):259–265.

16 Taylor SE, Way BM, Welch WT, Hilmert CJ, Lehman BJ, Eisenberger NI. Early family environment, current adversity, the serotonin transporter promoter polymorphism, and depressive symptomatology. *Biol Psychiatry* 2006;**60**(7):671–676.

17 Goodman E, Huang B, Wade TJ, Kahn RS. A multilevel analysis of the relation of socioeconomic status to adolescent depressive symptoms: does school context matter? *J Pediatrics* 2003;**143**(4):451–456.

18 Grana RA, Black D, Sun P, Rohrbach LA, Gunning M, Sussman S. School disrepair and substance use among regular and alternative high school students. *J Sch Health* 2010;**80**(8):387–393.

19 Milkie MA, Warner CH. Classroom learning environments and the mental health of first grade children. *J Health Soc Behav* 2011;**52**(1):4–22.

20 Fisher HL, Moffitt TE, Houts RM, Belsky DW, Arseneault L, Caspi A. Bullying victimisation and risk of self harm in early adolescence: longitudinal cohort study. *BMJ* 2012;**344**:e2683.

21 Egan M, Bambra C, Thomas S, Petticrew M, Whitehead M, Thomson H. The psychosocial and health effects of workplace reorganisation. 1. A systematic review of organisational-level interventions that aim to increase employee control. *J Epidemiol Community Health* 2007;**61**(11):945–954.

22 Egan M, Petticrew M, Ogilvie D, Hamilton V, Drever F. "Profits before people"? A systematic review of the health and safety impacts of privatising public utilities and industries in developed countries. *J Epidemiol Community Health* 2007;**61**(10):862–870.

23 Karasek RA. Job demands, job decision latitude, and mental strain: implications for job redesign. *Adm Sci Q* 1979;**24**:285–309.

24 Stansfeld S, Candy B. Psychosocial work environment and mental health—a meta-analytic review. *Scand J Work Environ Health* 2006;**32**(6):443–462.

25 Faris RE, Dunham HW. *Mental disorders in urban areas: an ecological study of schizophrenia and other psychoses*. Chicago: University of Chiacgo; 1939.

26 White W. The geographic distribution of insanity in the United States. *J Nerv Ment Dis* 1902;**30**: 257–279.

27 **Dupere V, Leventhal T, Lacourse E.** Neighborhood poverty and suicidal thoughts and attempts in late adolescence. *Psychol Med* 2009;**39**(8):1295–1306.

28 **Schneiders J, Drukker M, van der Ende J, Verhulst FC, van Os J, Nicolson NA.** Neighbourhood socioeconomic disadvantage and behavioural problems from late childhood into early adolescence. *J Epidemiol Community Health* 2003;**57**(9):699–703.

29 **Xue Y, Leventhal T, Brooks-Gunn J, Earls FJ.** Neighborhood residence and mental health problems of 5- to 11-year-olds. *Arch Gen Psychiatry* 2005;**62**(5):554–563.

30 **Aneshensel CS, Sucoff CA.** The neighborhood context of adolescent mental health. *J Health Soc Behav* 1996;**37**(4):293–310.

31 **Kalff AC, Kroes M, Vles JS, et al.** Neighbourhood level and individual level SES effects on child problem behaviour: a multilevel analysis. *J Epidemiol Community Health* 2001;**55**(4):246–250.

32 **Jang SJ, Johnson BR.** Neighborhood disorder, individual religiosity, and adolescent use of illicit drugs: a test of multilevel hypotheses. *Criminology* 2001;**39**:109–144.

33 **Winstanley EL, Steinwachs DM, Ensminger ME, Latkin CA, Stitzer ML, Olsen Y.** The association of self-reported neighborhood disorganization and social capital with adolescent alcohol and drug use, dependence, and access to treatment. *Drug Alcohol Depend* 2008;**92**(1–3):173–182.

34 **Sampson RJ, Raudenbush SW.** Systematic social observation of public spaces: a new look at disorder in urban neighborhoods. *Am J Sociol* 1999;**105**(3):603–651.

35 **Schaefer-McDaniel N.** Neighborhood stressors, perceived neighborhood quality, and child mental health in New York City. *Health Place* 2009;**15**(1):148–155.

36 **Natsuaki MN, Ge X, Brody GH, Simons RL, Gibbons FX, Cutrona CE.** African American children's depressive symptoms: the prospective effects of neighborhood disorder, stressful life events, and parenting. *Am J Community Psychol* 2007;**39**(1–2):163–176.

37 **Meltzer H, Vostanis P, Goodman R, Ford T.** Children's perceptions of neighbourhood trustworthiness and safety and their mental health. *J Child Psychol Psychiatry* 2007;**48**(12):1208–1213.

38 **Harpham T, Grant E, Rodriguez C.** Mental health and social capital in Cali, Colombia. *Soc Sci Med* 2004;**58**(11):2267–2277.

39 **Mair C, Diez Roux AV, Galea S.** Are neighbourhood characteristics associated with depressive symptoms? A review of evidence. *J Epidemiol Community Health* 2008;**62**(11):940–946.

40 **Truong KD, Ma S.** A systematic review of relations between neighborhoods and mental health. *J Mental Health Policy Econ* 2006;**9**(3):137–154.

41 **Galea S, Ahern J, Nandi A, Tracy M, Beard J, Vlahov D.** Urban neighborhood poverty and the incidence of depression in a population based cohort study. *Ann Epidemiol* 2007;**17**(3):171–179.

42 **Sundquist K, Ahlen H.** Neighbourhood income and mental health: a multilevel follow-up study of psychiatric hospital admissions among 4.5 million women and men. *Health Place* 2006;**12**(4):594–602.

43 **Drukker M, Krabbendam L, Driessen G, van Os J.** Social disadvantage and schizophrenia—a combined neighbourhood and individual-level analysis. *Soc Psychiatry Psychiatr Epidemiol* 2006;**41**(8):595–604.

44 **Drukker M, Kaplan C, Schneiders J, Feron FJM, van Os J.** The wider social environment and changes in self-reported quality of life in the transition from late childhood to early adolescence: a cohort study. *BMC Public Health* 2006;**6**:133.

45 **Schootman M, Andresen EM, Wolinsky FD, Malmstrom TK, Miller JP, Miller DK.** Neighbourhood environment and the incidence of depressive symptoms among middle-aged African Americans. *J Epidemiol Community Health* 2007;**61**(6):527–532.

46 **Pikhartova J, Chandola T, Kubinova R, Bobak M, Nicholson A, Pikhart H.** Neighbourhood socioeconomic indicators and depressive symptoms in the Czech Republic: a population based study. *Int J Public Health* 2009;**54**(4):283–293.

47 **Lee M-A.** Neighborhood residential segregation and mental health: a multilevel analysis on Hispanic Americans in Chicago. *Soc Sci Med* 2009;**68**(11):1975–1984.

48 Ostir GV, Eschbach K, Markides KS, Goodwin JS. Neighbourhood composition and depressive symptoms among older Mexican Americans. *J Epidemiol Community Health* 2003;**57**(12):987–992.

49 Henderson C, Roux AVD, Jacobs DR, Kiefe CI, West D, Williams DR. Neighbourhood characteristics, individual level socioeconomic factors, and depressive symptoms in young adults: the CARDIA study. *J Epidemiol Community Health* 2005;**59**(4):322–328.

50 Mair C, Diez Roux AV, Morenoff JD. Neighborhood stressors and social support as predictors of depressive symptoms in the Chicago Community Adult Health Study. *Health Place* 2010;**16**(5):811–819.

51 Mair C, Diez Roux AV, Shen M, et al. Cross-sectional and longitudinal associations of neighborhood cohesion and stressors with depressive symptoms in the multiethnic study of atherosclerosis. *Ann Epidemiol* 2009;**19**(1):49–57.

52 Ahern J, Galea S. Collective efficacy and major depression in urban neighborhoods. *Am J Epidemiol* 2011;**173**(12):1453–1462.

53 Araya R, Dunstan F, Playle R, Thomas H, Palmer S, Lewis G. Perceptions of social capital and the built environment and mental health. *Social Sci Med* 2006;**62**(12):3072–3083.

54 Araya R, Montgomery A, Rojas G, et al. Common mental disorders and the built environment in Santiago, Chile. *Br J Psychiatry* 2007;**190**:394–401.

55 Lynch J, Smith GD. A life course approach to chronic disease epidemiology. *Annu Rev Public Health* 2005;**26**:1–35.

56 Wheaton B, Clarke P. Space meets time: integrating temporal and contextual influences on mental health in early adulthood. *Am Sociol Rev* 2003;**68**(5):680–706.

57 Stafford M, Gimeno D, Marmot MG. Neighbourhood characteristics and trajectories of health functioning: a multilevel prospective analysis. *Eur J Public Health* 2008;**18**(6):604–610.

58 Farrelly MC, Pechacek TF, Thomas KY, Nelson D. The impact of tobacco control programs on adult smoking. *Am J Public Health* 2008;**98**(2):304–309.

59 Ciecierski CC, Chatterji P, Chaloupka FJ, Wechsler H. Do state expenditures on tobacco control programs decrease use of tobacco products among college students? *Health Econ* 2011;**20**(3):253–272.

60 Yoruk BK, Yoruk CE. The impact of minimum legal drinking age laws on alcohol consumption, smoking, and marijuana use: evidence from a regression discontinuity design using exact date of birth. *J Health Econ* 2011;**30**(4):740–752.

61 Zivin K, Paczkowski M, Galea S. Economic downturns and population mental health: research findings, gaps, challenges and priorities. *Psychol Med* 2011;**41**(7):1343–1348.

62 Little RJ, Rubin DB. Causal effects in clinical and epidemiological studies via potential outcomes: concepts and analytical approaches. *Annu Rev Public Health* 2000;**21**:121–145.

63 Leventhal T, Brooks-Gunn J. Moving to opportunity: an experimental study of neighborhood effects on mental health. *Am J Public Health* 2003;**93**(9):1576–1582.

64 Jackson L, Langille L, Lyons R, Hughes J, Martin D, Winstanley V. Does moving from a high-poverty to lower-poverty neighborhood improve mental health? A realist review of 'Moving to Opportunity'. *Health Place* 2009;**15**(4):961–970.

65 Diez Roux AV. Estimating neighborhood health effects: the challenges of causal inference in a complex world. *Soc Sci Med* 2004;**58**(10):1953–1960.

66 Harding DJ. Counterfactual models of neighborhood effects: the effect of neighborhood poverty on dropping out and teenage pregnancy. *Am J Sociol* 2003;**109**(3):676–719.

67 Cole SR, Hernan MA, Robins JM, et al. Effect of highly active antiretroviral therapy on time to acquired immunodeficiency syndrome or death using marginal structural models. *Am J Epidemiol* 2003;**158**(7):687–694.

68 Hernan MA, Brumback B, Robins JM. Marginal structural models to estimate the causal effect of zidovudine on the survival of HIV-positive men. *Epidemiology* 2000;**11**(5):561–570.

69 **Hernan MA, Robins JM.** Estimating causal effects from epidemiological data. *J Epidemiol Community Health* 2006;**60**(7):578–586.

70 **Robins JM, Hernan MA, Brumback B.** Marginal structural models and causal inference in epidemiology. *Epidemiology* 2000;**11**(5):550–560.

71 **Nandi A, Glass TA, Cole SR, et al.** Neighborhood poverty and injection cessation in a sample of injection drug users. *Am J Epidemiol* 2010;**171**(4):391–398.

72 **Cerda M, Diez-Roux AV, Tchetgen ET, Gordon-Larsen P, Kiefe C.** The relationship between neighborhood poverty and alcohol use: estimation by marginal structural models. *Epidemiology* 2010;**21**(4):482–489.

Chapter 22

Epigenetic influences on mental illness over the life course

Monica Uddin and Levent Sipahi

22.1 Introduction

The influence of lifetime experiences, including early life experiences, on mental health has been recognized for some time. Foundational research[1,2] provided evidence of the importance of early life experiences (principally maternal care) to physical and mental health. Decades of research since have further elucidated the effects of lifetime experiences on mental health, demonstrating, for example, that birth weight, maternal mental health, and home and neighbourhood environments during development are associated with emotional and mental effects in later childhood.[3] Despite the longstanding recognition of such influences, the underlying biological mechanisms by which they are translated into psychological effects have remained, until recently, largely unknown. In this chapter, we propose that epigenetic modifications provide a biologically plausible mechanism for translating externally experienced stressful and traumatic events into long-lasting psychological consequences.

22.1.1 Epigenetic mechanisms

The past decade has seen a blossoming of research into epigenetic factors, which offer a biologically plausible mechanism through which lived experiences are transduced into changes in mental and physical health. Broadly speaking, epigenetic factors refer to those mechanisms that regulate gene function without the alteration of underlying DNA sequence.[4] By contrast with fixed DNA sequences, epigenetic factors are subject to change in response to physical, biological, and social exposures in a manner that influences the long-term regulation of gene expression.[5]

Epigenetic mechanisms include histone modifications such as: acetylation, phosphorylation, and ubiquitination, which alter the accessibility of surrounding DNA via chromatin structural changes;[4] DNA methylation (hereafter DNAm), which often results in repression of nearby genes;[4] and non-protein-coding RNAs, which regulate chromatin modification and DNAm.[6] Among these several mechanisms, DNAm is the best studied and perhaps the most biologically important; however, the key feature among all epigenetic mechanisms is that they involve processes that regulate chromatin structure and/or DNA accessibility, thereby altering the transcriptional activity of surrounding loci and, potentially, downstream gene function. Epigenetic patterns are cell type specific and play important roles in determining cell fate during early development.[4] Indeed, for decades it was believed that following embryonic development DNAm remained stable thereafter. Recent work, however, has confirmed that stochastic, age-related, and environmental influences can alter epigenetic patterning throughout life[7-9] and that these altered patterns have implications for human health, including mental illness.

22.1.2 **Life course approach to epigenetics and mental illness**

A life course approach to understanding differential risk for mental illness can best be understood by viewing mental health as part of a lifelong developmental process that incorporates
initial gene–environment interactions into subsequent and continually operating phenotype–
environment interactions. In this framework, susceptibility/resiliency to developing mental
illness is contingent upon biological and developmental responses to earlier environmental and
social exposures (Figure 22.1); epigenetic modifications in response to lived experience modify

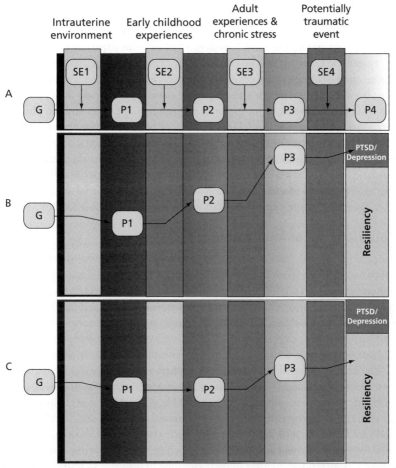

Figure 22.1 A life course model of mental illness. (A) The aetiology of mental illnesses such as
post-traumatic stress disorder (PTSD) and depression is contingent upon a series of developmental
responses, mediated by epigenetic modifications, to lifetime social experiences. Two potential
scenarios are illustrated in panels B and C. (B) Adverse childhood and adult experiences compound
to increase risk of mental illness. Arrows represent epigenetically mediated developmental responses
to social exposures. (C) Absence of childhood adversity allows for resiliency in the face of traumatic
experiences in adulthood. In the social exposure (SE) columns, light gray indicates absence of
adversity, dark gray indicates adversity. In the phenotype (P) columns, background colour gradient
represents developmental plasticity, with darker background indicating greater developmental
plasticity and thus likely greater influence over future health. G, underlying inherited genotype.

the biological determinants of mental health and dictate the pattern of epigenetic modifications made in response to future lived experience. Intergenerational inheritance of epigenetic variation, an area of keen interest in the field, requires only that we extend the concept of the life course through several generations. Although direct evidence of transgenerational epigenetic influences on mental health is currently scarce, recent work[10] suggests that biologically grounded life course approaches to mental illness should consider the possibility of such scenarios.

22.2 Epigenetics and mental health

The goal of the remainder of this chapter is to overview the life course epigenetic influences on mental health. To do so we have organized subsequent sections to echo the historical progression of work in the field. We begin by providing a summary of foundational research in rodent animal models—the first work to provide evidence that early life experiences affect mental health via lasting epigenetic changes. We then outline how this animal work has been translated into human studies, highlighting evidence for early life experience-mediated epigenetic patterns, and associations between mental health and epigenetic states. We continue the discussion of work in humans by outlining evidence for prenatal environmental effects and the phenomenon of transgenerational inheritance of mental illness that may be mediated by epigenetic mechanisms. Because post-traumatic stress disorder (PTSD) is unique among mental illnesses in requiring a lived experience as an aetiological event, it provides an ideal model for elucidating how epigenetics may mediate the connection between lived experiences and mental health; we thus focus on PTSD as an example when possible. We also draw heavily from the depression literature. We end with further discussion of specific insights that can be drawn from the study of PTSD.

22.2.1 Foundational animal studies

Direct evidence for the influence of epigenetic factors on mental illness over the life course was initially obtained through work in rodent animal models. Ground-breaking work by Meaney et al.[11] demonstrated that early life experiences have an immediate yet lasting impact on epigenetic patterning of genes involved in the stress response: rat pups born to mothers who provide a high degree of licking, grooming, and arched back nursing show reduced levels of hippocampal DNAm and increased gene expression at the NR3C1 glucocorticoid receptor locus—an important modulator of the stress response and integral component of the hypothalamic–pituitary–adrenal (HPA) axis—compared to pups born to mothers who provide less licking and grooming and non-arched back nursing.[11] These differences emerge during the first week of life, persist until adulthood, and are accompanied by increased histone H3K9 acetylation—an additional epigenetic alteration—and greater transcription factor binding in pups receiving a high level of maternal care.[11] Most importantly, these epigenetic changes are concordant with differences in HPA axis responses to stress during adulthood, whereby the offspring of the more 'attentive' mothers show a more modest increase in corticosterone in response to restraint stress compared with their peers born from less 'attentive' mothers. Collectively, these findings provided some of the first evidence of a developmentally sensitive period during which behavioural responses later in life may be epigenetically programmed.[11] Similar results have since been reported for other genes.[10,12,13]

22.2.2 Initial human studies

Foundational discoveries in animal models spurred interest in whether similar patterns of long-lasting DNAm differences, established early in life, exist in humans. Recent work on the NR3C1 locus showed increased methylation among adult suicide victims with a history of childhood abuse when compared to suicide victims without such a history and other postmortem controls.[14] This pattern of relative *NR3C1* hypermethylation has been supported by two additional human studies: one in which increased maternal depressed/anxious mood, assessed prenatally, showed an association with increased DNAm at a predicted *NGFI-A* binding site in cord blood-derived DNA, and with increased salivary cortisol stress responses at 3 months postnatally;[15] and, more recently, another study which identified increased whole blood-derived DNAm levels among healthy adults who reported exposure to childhood adversity, including childhood maltreatment, parental loss, and poor parental care.[16] Early life adversity has also been linked to DNAm changes at the serotonin transporter (*SLC6A4*) locus in DNA derived from EBV-transformed lymphoblastoid cell line samples drawn from the Iowa Adoption Study, in which child abuse was associated with significantly elevated DNAm across multiple CpG sites in the *SLC6A4* promoter region and, among females, at specific CpG sites.[17]

Complementing these focused candidate gene studies, genome-scale investigations have also detected epigenetic differences associated with exposure to early life stress. Compared with adolescents whose mothers were unexposed to high stress levels during their first year of life, adolescents whose mothers reported high stress levels during their infancy showed higher DNAm levels at 139 CpG sites in buccal cell-derived DNA.[18] Together, these data from animal and human studies suggest that early life experiences, and especially adverse early life experiences, have the potential to alter epigenetic gene regulation and downstream gene function with lasting physiological, behavioural, and psychological implications.[5,19]

22.2.3 Prenatal exposures and altered risk for mental illness

The above-described work largely focuses on postnatal exposures that are associated with DNAm-based epigenetic differences. Recent work, however, has provided evidence that prenatal exposures are also important to differential risk for, or resilience to, frequently occurring mood–anxiety disorders such as PTSD and depression, in a manner consistent with known epigenetic mechanisms. For example, using a case–control design Yehuda *et al.* determined that maternal, but not paternal, PTSD was independently associated with increased risk for PTSD in adult offspring of Holocaust survivors compared with demographically similar Jewish study participants who were born to parents free of PTSD and trauma exposure (note that the survivors' offspring were not conceived during the Holocaust).[20] Despite the overall increased risk associated with maternal PTSD, the same study also observed an association with offspring gender: females born to fathers with lifetime PTSD were more likely to develop PTSD, whereas the opposite was true among male offspring.[20] More recently, population-based sampling demonstrated that PTSD is transmitted intergenerationally such that mothers with higher levels of lifetime PTSD symptoms were observed to have children at higher risk of PTSD (this study did not assess paternal PTSD).[21] Much of this effect was mediated through elevated exposure to trauma among children of mothers with higher lifetime PTSD symptoms; however, a substantial proportion (36%) of the increased risk for PTSD was not accounted for by elevated trauma exposure, indicating that other mechanisms contribute to this risk.

The epigenetic activity that occurs early in development involves a number of events that could plausibly account for this intergenerational increased risk of PTSD. As has been previously observed,[22] early gestation is a highly sensitive period during which de-novo DNAm by DNA methyltransferases (DNMTs) occurs. DNMTs are known to be affected by inflammatory cytokines; cytokine dysregulation, in turn, has previously been associated with PTSD (reviewed by Andrews and Neises[23]). These observations suggest a hypothesis whereby the gestational milieu of women currently or previously affected by PTSD may be altered in a manner that affects the functioning of their children's epigenetic machinery in early development, producing DNAm levels that increase vulnerability to trauma in postnatal life.

22.2.4 Direct evidence of epigenetics in mental health: gene–environment interactions

Despite these suggestive observations, the most robust direct evidence regarding epigenetic influences on risk for, or resilience to, frequently occurring mood–anxiety disorders relates to within-generation epigenetic influences, with some of these influences observed at different developmental stages. As discussed in the introduction, the existence of uniformly stable DNAm levels over the life course is no longer supported by empirical evidence. Indeed, as potential regulators of DNA accessibility and activity, epigenetic factors, through influences on gene expression, offer one mechanism by which the environment can moderate the effects of genes[24]. Furthermore, epigenetic mechanisms may be involved in the mediation of some gene–environment interactions, such that individuals with particular genotype/epigenotype combinations may be especially inclined toward mental illness in the presence of specific environmental exposures. For example, numerous studies investigating variation in the serotonin transporter promoter (5HTTLPR) locus have demonstrated that carriers of the short allele are more susceptible to depression following exposure to stressful life experiences.[25] The s allele, in turn, has been associated with increased depressive symptoms in adolescents, but only among individuals who also showed relatively high methylation levels at this locus:[26] examination of DNAm levels from buccal cells in a prospective cohort of Australian adolescents found a joint effect of DNAm and s allele carriage on risk for depression, such that adolescents with the highest tertile of methylation in a subregion of the promoter-associated CpG island in the SLC6A4 locus and who also carried one or more 5HTTLPR s alleles were at approximately five-fold higher risk for persistent depressive symptoms. Transfection assays with the 5HTT promoter confirmed that methylation of as little as 10% of CpG sites within this island could silence 5HTT activity (i.e. expression), suggesting a possible mechanism by which the methylation exerts its influence among s allele carriers. By contrast, work investigating the role of epigenetic factors in vulnerability/resilience to trauma found that the long, l, allele in combination with high methylation levels in the SLC6A4 CpG island promoter region predicted more unresolved loss or trauma among adults.[27] The opposing direction of these findings compared with those reported for depression suggests the possibility that different combinations of DNAm and DNA sequence at the SLC6A4 locus may show divergent patterns depending on the outcome of interest (e.g. depression versus trauma resolution); however, additional study variables, such as developmental stage (adolescent versus adult) and DNA source (buccal versus EBV-transformed cell lines), cannot be ruled out as contributors to these opposing patterns based on the few currently available studies.

22.3 Insights from post-traumatic stress disorder

By definition, PTSD requires exposure to trauma. As such, epigenetic effects offer a plausible way in which an environmental exposure (i.e. potentially traumatic event (PTE)) may modify biological substrates (i.e. gene expression) in a manner that may increase risk of an adverse psychopathological outcome.[28]

22.3.1 **Evidence from animal models**

Animal models of PTSD have identified epigenetic differences that can discern rats with PTSD-like versus non-PTSD-like behaviours, using PTSD models that involve exposure to cats.[29] In a cat scent-based model, rats are exposed to a predator stimulus (cat scent carried on soiled litter) which serves as the PTE; seven days following the stress exposure, animals are classified as exhibiting PTSD-like and non-PTSD-like behaviour according to their performance on behavioural tests (elevated pulse-maze and acoustic startle response).[30] Assessment of DNAm changes in brain tissue following this stress paradigm identified some loci (e.g. *Dlgap2*) that showed PTSD-associated changes in both methylation and gene expression patterns in post-mortem hippocampal tissue.[31] Interestingly, *Dlgap2* gene expression was correlated with degree of behavioural stress responses in individual rats, suggesting that this locus may contribute to the molecular substrate of traumatic stress adaptation in these animals.[31] More recent work is based on a stress group of adult rats exposed to non-tactile sensory stimuli from cats (who had been primed to show gustatory activity towards the rats), along with unstable housing conditions, for 31 days. This stress paradigm was associated with significant hypermethylation in a promoter region of *BDNF* in the dorsal CA1 region of the hippocampus, a brain region important to learning and memory and implicated in PTSD aetiology in meta-analytic studies of human participants.[32] In addition, *BDNF* gene expression was significantly reduced in both the dorsal and ventral CA1 hippocampal regions. That these results were obtained from adult rats indicates that DNAm is an active process throughout the life course, modifiable by environmental exposures even in the mature central nervous system, with consequent effects on gene expression.

22.3.2 **Evidence from human studies**

Recent genome-scale work in humans has also demonstrated that DNAm profiles across multiple genes distinguish between those with versus without PTSD in samples drawn from urban, predominantly African-American population-based studies. Using whole blood-derived DNA samples from a longitudinal study of adult Detroit residents, DNAm profiles in trauma-exposed participants were shown to differ between those with versus without lifetime PTSD, with differences found predominantly in immune-system-related genes (lowered DNAm in PTSD) and in genes relating to developmental processes in general, and neurogenesis in particular (higher DNAm in PTSD).[33] Although gene expression was not directly assessed in this work, using publicly available data, the study also showed that hypermethylated genes corresponded to lower expression levels, and hypomethylated genes to higher gene expression levels, in whole blood-derived samples taken from healthy participants. In addition, to provide a direct measure of the functional significance of the DNAm results, the study assessed antibody activity to cytomegalovirus (CMV) and found that those affected by PTSD showed a significantly higher antibody response than those resilient to the disorder. Secondary analyses of the same participants, reported elsewhere,[34] found that lifetime depression status was also associated with DNAm differences in genes implicated in brain development/neurogenesis, tryptophan metabolism, and lipoprotein-related functions—i.e. pathways or processes previously implicated in the aetiology of this disorder—and that those with depression had marginally higher serum interleukin-6 (IL-6) and significantly higher C-reactive protein levels compared with controls, again demonstrating a consistency between the biological pathways identified in the methylation analyses and the inflammation-associated findings identified in the serum measures. Notably, the primary PTSD analyses showed that only a handful of genes were significantly different between those with PTSD alone compared to those with PTSD and one or more of depression and generalized anxiety disorder, suggesting that comorbidity did not unduly influence the PTSD-associated findings. Taken together, these results indicate that genome-scale analyses of DNAm, along with additional independent measures of physiological function, can discern between two frequently occurring mood–anxiety disorders whose aetiologies include stressful and traumatic experiences that accumulate across the life course.

The nature of traumatic events that result in PTSD may vary substantially among individuals; thus it is not unreasonable to expect that the epigenetic 'footprint' of such experiences may differ substantially from person to person. Nevertheless, many of the PTSD-associated DNAm differences found in the Detroit study were confirmed in an independent cohort of trauma-exposed African-Americans recruited from a clinical setting in inner-city Atlanta.[35] In this work, investigators showed that CpG sites in five genes met experiment-wide cut-offs for statistical significance, two of which (*TLR8* and *ACP5*) are known to be related to immune function. In addition, 15 genes implicated in PTSD in the earlier work[33] showed significant (uncorrected $P < 0.05$) associations with PTSD in this study, many of which are again known to be related to immune function (e.g. *CD2*, *CXCL1*, *SLAMF7* and others). Furthermore, the authors observed decreased levels of IL-4, an anti-inflammatory cytokine, in plasma from PTSD-affected participants compared with trauma-exposed controls, confirming similar findings from earlier studies.[36] Additional work based on participants from the same Atlanta-based cohort showed that post-traumatic stress symptoms are positively correlated with blood DNAm levels at the adenylate cyclase activating polypeptide 1 (pituitary) receptor type I (*ADCYAP1R1*) locus,[37] a gene involved in the stress response[38] that is also involved in transcriptional control of neurotrophic factors important to normal neural development and neurogenesis (i.e. *BDNF*).[39] These findings also echo those from the earlier study, albeit from a candidate gene perspective, and again suggest that traumatic experiences can leave a molecular footprint rendering some individuals more vulnerable to trauma. Furthermore, despite an overall focus on PTSD-associated epigenetic variation observed within generations, the Detroit-based work did note that PTSD-associated differences existed in DNAm among imprinted genes that had been previously implicated in other mental disorders, including Prader–Willi syndrome and Angelmann syndrome,[33] leaving open the possibility that prenatal (and perhaps intergenerational) exposures influence epigenetic vulnerability to such frequently occurring mood–anxiety disorders.

These studies provide some evidence of a biological embedding of post-traumatic stress within a lifetime; nevertheless, it is likely that there are also both molecular and environmental features that render some individuals more susceptible to PTSD. Potential epigenetic examples of this come from the Detroit-based study, in which investigators found that DNAm levels at *SLC6A4* and *MAN2C1*, both implicated in PTSD aetiology in earlier molecular studies,[40,41] modified the effect of cumulative trauma on risk for PTSD. In the case of *SLC6A4*, individuals with higher PTE exposure were at increased risk for PTSD at lower methylation levels but protected from this disorder at higher methylation levels; and among individuals with lower PTE exposure, this predicted pattern was reversed.[42] By contrast, at low levels of *MAN2C1* methylation, there appears to be little variation in risk for PTSD among those with lower versus higher PTE exposure; at higher *MAN2C1* methylation levels, however, the risk of PTSD is exponentially higher among those with greater numbers of PTEs. These results suggest that individuals' pre-existing DNAm levels at certain loci may moderate their experience of potentially traumatic events in a manner salient to PTSD aetiology, suggesting potential molecular signatures of increased risk for—or resilience to—this disorder.

22.3.3 **Putting it all together: a model of epigenetic modifications with PTSD**

Taken together, these genome-scale and candidate gene studies suggest a model whereby PTSD is affected by pre-trauma epigenetic differences (which may be emergent either pre- or post-natally). Following traumatic exposure, those who go on to develop PTSD experience epigenetic changes in immune system-related loci that then alter immune function, ultimately leading to PTSD (Figure 22.2). By contrast, among those who remain PTSD free, epigenetic differences in neurogenesis-related loci may occur, as suggested by cross-sectional work in humans[33,37] and experimental work in rodents,[29] consequently activating protective gene expression patterns in these loci that perhaps increase plasticity in a manner that permits and promotes resiliency to trauma. Although the model suggests that trauma induces the changes in these alternative biological pathways, we note that some of these DNAm levels probably also precede trauma. Longitudinal work, assessing pre- and post-trauma exposure levels of DNAm and other epigenetic factors, should help to clarify the relative contribution of these two scenarios.

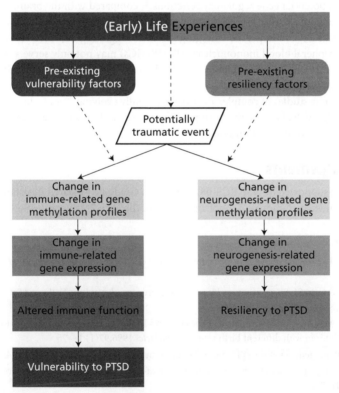

Figure 22.2 A proposed model of differential risk for/resiliency to post-traumatic stress disorder (PTSD). Exposure to a potentially traumatic event (PTE) can result in either (i) the development of altered immune function via changes in DNAm profiles and gene expression or (ii) activation of neurogenesis-related loci via DNAm changes that affect gene expression and function. Differential risk and resiliency is, in part, determined by vulnerability and resiliency factors that represent epigenetic modifications made throughout the life course in response to lived experiences. These factors pre-exist PTE exposure.

22.4 **Summary**

As may be inferred by the above review, epigenetic research holds much promise for informing a life course perspective on commonly occurring mood anxiety disorders, and mental health and illness more broadly. Nevertheless, a number of difficulties and limitations are inherent to this type of research and should be borne in mind whenever new findings are reported. Chief among these are the tissue- and cell-type specific nature of epigenetic marks, and the difficulty of obtaining repeated samples from living individuals in the target organ of illness, i.e. the brain. For example, recent work focused on assessing DNAm levels in the human prefrontal cortex found that neurons showed distinctive methylation profiles as well as higher interindividual variation compared with non-neurons, and that this pattern could not be detected using bulk cortex.[43] Although single-cell analyses of epigenetic patterns are growing in number, they are not likely to take hold in population-focused studies in the near term, even if peripheral tissues are assayed, due to the prohibitively high cost of obtaining such samples. Moreover, unlike 5-methylcytosine, which has been discussed in this review, peripheral tissues contain substantially lower concentrations of 5-hydroxymethylcytosine,[44] the so-called 'sixth base' formed from methylated cytosines which maintain potential gene regulatory functions,[45] compared with the brain. Future research seeking to elucidate epigenetic processes that operate over the life course with relevance to mental illness would thus do well to pursue emerging research suggesting that accessible peripheral tissues such as peripheral blood mononuclear cells (PBMCs) may not only serve as important biomarkers of disorders such as PTSD, but may also directly contribute to mental illness (reviewed by Andrews and Neises[23]). Despite these and other challenges, the theoretical framework for pursuing epigenetic studies of complex disorders is rapidly evolving,[46] and, along with the falling costs of assays that will allow for the testing of population-scale sample sizes, the time is ripe for addressing this important area of inquiry.

Acknowledgements

Levent Sipahi is supported by NSF BCS-0827546 and a Graduate Research Assistantship from the Wayne State University Graduate School and Office of the Vice President for Research.

References

1 MacLean K. The impact of institutionalization on child development. *Dev Psychopathol* 2003;**15**(4): 853–884.

2 Harlow HF, Suomi SJ. Social recovery by isolation-reared monkeys. *Proc Natl Acad Sci USA* 1971;**68**(7):1534–1538.

3 McCormick MC, Workman-Daniels K, Brooks-Gunn J. The behavioral and emotional well-being of school-age children with different birth weights. *Pediatrics* 1996;**97**(1):18–25.

4 Feinberg AP. Epigenetics at the epicenter of modern medicine. *JAMA* 2008;**299**(11):1345–1350.

5 Meaney MJ. Epigenetics and the biological definition of gene × environment interactions. *Child Dev* 2010;**81**(1):41–79.

6 Mattick JS, Amaral PP, Dinger ME, Mercer TR, Mehler MF. RNA regulation of epigenetic processes. *Bioessays* 2009;**31**(1):51–59.

7 Tobi EW, Slagboom PE, van Dongen J, et al. Prenatal famine and genetic variation are independently and additively associated with DNA methylation at regulatory loci within IGF2/H19. *PLoS One* 2012;**7**(5):e37933.

8 Fraga MF, Ballestar E, Paz MF, et al. Epigenetic differences arise during the lifetime of monozygotic twins. *Proc Natl Acad Sci USA* 2005;**102**(30):10604–10609.

9 Bjornsson HT, Sigurdsson MI, Fallin MD, et al. Intra-individual change over time in DNA methylation with familial clustering. *JAMA* 2008;**299**(24):2877–2883.

10 Roth TL, Lubin FD, Funk AJ, Sweatt JD. Lasting epigenetic influence of early-life adversity on the BDNF gene. *Biol Psychiatry* 2009;**65**(9):760–769.

11 Weaver IC, Cervoni N, Champagne FA, et al. Epigenetic programming by maternal behavior. *Nat Neurosci* 2004;**7**(8):847–854.

12 Champagne FA, Weaver IC, Diorio J, Dymov S, Szyf M, Meaney MJ. Maternal care associated with methylation of the estrogen receptor-alpha1b promoter and estrogen receptor-alpha expression in the medial preoptic area of female offspring. *Endocrinology* 2006;**147**(6):2909–2915.

13 Murgatroyd C, Patchev AV, Wu Y, et al. Dynamic DNA methylation programs persistent adverse effects of early-life stress. *Nat Neurosci* 2009;**12**(12):1559–1566.

14 McGowan PO, Sasaki A, D'Alessio AC, et al. Epigenetic regulation of the glucocorticoid receptor in human brain associates with childhood abuse. *Nat Neurosci* 2009;**12**(3):342–348.

15 Oberlander TF, Weinberg J, Papsdorf M, Grunau R, Misri S, Devlin AM. Prenatal exposure to maternal depression, neonatal methylation of human glucocorticoid receptor gene (NR3C1) and infant cortisol stress responses. *Epigenetics* 2008;**3**(2):97–106.

16 Tyrka AR, Price LH, Marsit C, Walters OC, Carpenter LL. Childhood adversity and epigenetic modulation of the leukocyte glucocorticoid receptor: preliminary findings in healthy adults. *PLoS One* 2012;**7**(1):e30148.

17 Beach SR, Brody GH, Todorov AA, Gunter TD, Philibert RA. Methylation at SLC6A4 is linked to family history of child abuse: an examination of the Iowa Adoptee sample. *Am J Med Genet B Neuropsychiatr Genet* 2010;**153B**(2):710–713.

18 Essex MJ, Thomas Boyce W, Hertzman C, et al. Epigenetic vestiges of early developmental adversity: childhood stress exposure and DNA methylation in adolescence. *Child Dev* 2013;**84**(1):58–75.

19 Szyf M. DNA methylation, the early-life social environment and behavioral disorders. *Journal of neurodevelopmental disorders* 2011;**3**(3):238–249.

20 Yehuda R, Bell A, Bierer LM, Schmeidler J. Maternal, not paternal, PTSD is related to increased risk for PTSD in offspring of Holocaust survivors. *J Psychiatr Res* 2008;**42**(13):1104–1111.

21 Roberts AL, Galea S, Austin SB, et al. Posttraumatic stress disorder across two generations: concordance and mechanisms in a population-based sample. *Biol Psychiatry* 2012;**72**(6):505–511.

22 Bale TL. Sex differences in prenatal epigenetic programming of stress pathways. *Stress* 2011;**14**(4): 348–356.

23 Andrews JA, Neises KD. Cells, biomarkers, and post-traumatic stress disorder: evidence for peripheral involvement in a central disease. *J Neurochem* 2012;**120**(1):26–36.

24 Rutter M, Moffit TE, Caspi A. Gene–environment interplay and psychopathology: multiple varieties but real effects. *J Child Psychol Psychiatry* 2006;**47**(3/4):226–261.

25 Caspi A, Hariri AR, Holmes A, Uher R, Moffitt TE. Genetic sensitivity to the environment: the case of the serotonin transporter gene and its implications for studying complex diseases and traits. *Am J Psychiatry* 2010;**167**(5):509–527.

26 Olsson CA, Foley DL, Parkinson-Bates M, et al. Prospects for epigenetic research within cohort studies of psychological disorder: a pilot investigation of a peripheral cell marker of epigenetic risk for depression. *Biol Psychol* 2010;**83**(2):159–165.

27 van Ijzendoorn MH, Caspers K, Bakermans-Kranenburg MJ, Beach SR, Philibert R. Methylation matters: interaction between methylation density and serotonin transporter genotype predicts unresolved loss or trauma. *Biol Psychiatry* 2010;**68**(5):405–407.

28 Yehuda R, Bierer LM. The relevance of epigenetics to PTSD: implications for the DSM-V. *J Trauma Stress* 2009;**22**(5):427–434.

29 Roth TL, Zoladz PR, Sweatt JD, Diamond DM. Epigenetic modification of hippocampal Bdnf DNA in adult rats in an animal model of post-traumatic stress disorder. *J Psychiatr Res* 2011;**45**(7):919–926.

30 Cohen H, Zohar J. An animal model of posttraumatic stress disorder: the use of cut-off behavioral criteria. *Ann NY Acad Sci* 2004;**1032**:167–178.

31 Chertkow-Deutsher Y, Cohen H, Klein E, Ben-Shachar D. DNA methylation in vulnerability to post-traumatic stress in rats: evidence for the role of the post-synaptic density protein Dlgap2. *Int J Neuropsychopharmacol* 2010;**13**(3):347–359.

32 Woon FL, Sood S, Hedges DW. Hippocampal volume deficits associated with exposure to psychological trauma and posttraumatic stress disorder in adults: a meta-analysis. *Prog Neuropsychopharmacol Biol Psychiatry* 2010;**34**(7):1181–1188.

33 Uddin M, Aiello AE, Wildman DE, et al. Epigenetic and immune function profiles associated with posttraumatic stress disorder. *Proc Natl Acad Sci USA* 2010;**107**(20):9470–9475.

34 Uddin M, Koenen KC, Aiello AE, Wildman DE, de los Santos R, Galea S. Epigenetic and inflammatory marker profiles associated with depression in a community-based epidemiologic sample. *Psychol Med* 2011;**41**(5):997–1007.

35 Smith AK, Conneely KN, Kilaru V, et al. Differential immune system DNA methylation and cytokine regulation in post-traumatic stress disorder. *Am J Med Genet B Neuropsychiatr Genet* 2011;**156**(6): 700–708.

36 von Kanel R, Hepp U, Kraemer B, et al. Evidence for low-grade systemic proinflammatory activity in patients with posttraumatic stress disorder. *J Psychiatr Res* 2007;**41**(9):744–752.

37 Ressler KJ, Mercer KB, Bradley B, et al. Post-traumatic stress disorder is associated with PACAP and the PAC1 receptor. *Nature* 2011;**470**(7335):492–497.

38 Stroth N, Holighaus Y, Ait-Ali D, Eiden LE. PACAP: a master regulator of neuroendocrine stress circuits and the cellular stress response. *Ann NY Acad Sci* 2011;**1220**:49–59.

39 Zink M, Otto C, Zorner B, et al. Reduced expression of brain-derived neurotrophic factor in mice deficient for pituitary adenylate cyclase activating polypeptide type-I-receptor. *Neurosci Lett* 2004;**360**(1–2):106–108.

40 Yehuda R, Cai G, Golier JA, et al. Gene expression patterns associated with posttraumatic stress disorder following exposure to the World Trade Center Attacks. *Biol Psychiatry* 2009;**66**(7):708–711.

41 Cornelis MC, Nugent NR, Amstadter AB, Koenen KC. Genetics of post-traumatic stress disorder: review and recommendations for genome-wide association studies. *Curr Psychiatry Rep* 2010;**12**(4):313–326.

42 Koenen KC, Uddin M, Chang SC, et al. SLC6A4 methylation modifies the effect of the number of traumatic events on risk for posttraumatic stress disorder. *Depress Anxiety* 2011;**28**(8):639–647.

43 Iwamoto K, Bundo M, Ueda J, et al. Neurons show distinctive DNA methylation profile and higher interindividual variations compared with non-neurons. *Genome Res* 2011;**21**(5):688–696.

44 Globisch D, Munzel M, Muller M, et al. Tissue distribution of 5-hydroxymethylcytosine and search for active demethylation intermediates. *PLoS One* 2010;**5**(12):e15367.

45 Jin SG, Wu X, Li AX, Pfeifer GP. Genomic mapping of 5-hydroxymethylcytosine in the human brain. *Nucleic Acids Res* 2011;**39**(12):5015–5024.

46 Relton CL, Davey Smith G. Two-step epigenetic Mendelian randomization: a strategy for establishing the causal role of epigenetic processes in pathways to disease. *Int J Epidemiol* 2012;**41**(1):161–176.

Chapter 23

Adverse childhood experiences and brain development: neurobiological mechanisms linking the social environment to psychiatric disorders

Katie A. McLaughlin, Margaret A. Sheridan, and Charles A. Nelson, III

23.1 Introduction

Increasing popularity of the life course approach in psychiatric epidemiology has led to renewed interest in the childhood determinants of mental disorders and the mechanisms through which childhood experiences increase risk of psychopathology. The main thesis of this chapter is that social and environmental experience weaves its way into the developing brain and exerts powerful effects on neural structure and function throughout childhood and into adulthood. These experiences ultimately influence the course of human development and have relevance for understanding population-level patterns of mental illness. Here we provide evidence suggesting that the influence of the early social environment on the developing brain may be a primary mechanism linking childhood social experience to later outcomes, including mental illness.

We begin by briefly reviewing recent life course epidemiology studies examining the association between the childhood social environment and psychopathology, with a focus on the lasting impact of adverse childhood experiences such as maltreatment, violence exposure, environmental deprivation, and poverty on mental health. Next, we highlight potential neurobiological mechanisms that might explain the association between these adverse childhood experiences and the later onset of psychopathology. Finally, we review existing literature examining the associations of two specific types of adverse childhood experiences: maltreatment and poverty or socio-economic status (SES), with brain structure and function. In each section, we review neuroimaging studies examining brain structure and function using electroencephalogram (EEG) and both structural and functional magnetic resonance imaging (MRI), focusing on studies that have been conducted in children and adolescents. Although numerous studies have examined brain structure and function in adults who have experienced childhood adversity,[1] the accumulation of life experiences from childhood into adulthood makes it difficult to assume that alterations in brain structure and function observed in adults are the result of early experiences. We conclude by discussing the implications of integrating developmental cognitive neuroscience methods into life course epidemiology and population health approaches to mental disorders.

23.2 **Childhood adversity and mental disorders**

Adverse childhood experiences are robust determinants of psychiatric disorders with effects that persist across the life course.[2] Exposure to maltreatment, environmental deprivation, family violence, and parental instability have lasting detrimental effects on mental health.[2,3] Retrospective studies consistently identify higher rates of these childhood adversities among individuals with a psychiatric disorder,[2,4] and prospective data confirm these associations.[5,6] High rates of mental disorders among individuals with a history of adverse childhood experiences are evident not only in childhood but also in adolescence and adulthood.[7,8] Importantly, childhood adversities are associated with new disorder onsets in adulthood,[7,8] even after accounting for the effects of early onset disorders[2] as well as greater chronicity and severity of lifetime mental disorders.[9,10]

From a population health perspective, childhood adversities are an important set of exposures for several reasons. First, these experiences are common. National surveys estimate that 25–50% of children are exposed to violence or other victimization.[7,11] Second, the association between adverse childhood experiences and psychopathology is strong. Across numerous studies, individuals with a history of childhood adversities are at least twice as likely to develop a mental disorder as those with no exposure.[5,12] Finally, childhood adversities account for a substantial proportion of mental disorders in the population. Recent evidence suggests that >30% of lifetime mental disorder onsets in the USA are directly attributable to exposure to childhood adversities,[7] underscoring the significance of these exposures as a population health problem.

23.3 **Potential neurobiological mechanisms**

There are various neurobiological mechanisms through which exposure to adverse childhood experiences might increase risk for psychopathology. One central pathway involves a network of brain and bodily systems that respond to stress (e.g. changes in the environment that require psychological or physiological adaptation). Many of the adverse childhood experiences reviewed here are considered to be psychologically stressful or traumatic, particularly because they are unpredictable and uncontrollable and have the potential to overwhelm a child's coping resources. Physiological responses to stress involve activation of both the sympathetic nervous system and the hypothalamic–pituitary–adrenal (HPA) axis. Activation of the HPA axis initiates a cascade of neuroendocrine responses that culminate in increased levels of circulating cortisol. Two structures in the brain, the hippocampus and the amygdala, are necessary to initiate and modulate the stress response and can be influenced by chronic stress exposure. The hippocampus provides a negative-feedback mechanism, which modulates the HPA axis response.[13] During a typical HPA axis response to stress, glucocorticoids are released and bind to hippocampal glucocorticoid receptors, activating a negative-feedback loop and decreasing the HPA axis response. Chronic stress disrupts hippocampal function, which may in turn disrupt this negative feedback, resulting in extended HPA axis activation following stressful events and increasing the possibility of damage as a result of excessive glucocorticoid exposure.[14] Damage to the hippocampus via exposure to stress disrupts both modulation of the HPA axis response and memory formation and is mediated through glucocorticoid exposure.[15]

The amygdala plays an important role in recognizing and learning about emotion, particularly in fear acquisition and interpretation of emotional information such as facial expressions.[16] Humans and non-human primates with bilateral amygdala lesions exhibit indiscriminate friendliness and overly trusting behaviour,[17,18] and have compromised identification of emotional facial expressions.[19] The amygdala also plays a role in fear conditioning[20] by preparing the body for negative stimuli even prior to conscious awareness. Heightened amygdala activity and larger amygdala volume have been documented among both children and adults with anxiety disorders.[21,22]

A second pathway through which childhood adversity may influence brain development and psychopathology is through deprivation, or absence of experience. Children who are neglected or raised in institutional settings—and potentially even children raised in extreme poverty—confront social and environmental circumstances that deviate from the expectable environments necessary for normal brain development. During sensitive periods of brain development, expected environmental inputs are necessary to guide neural differentiation and pruning. The environmental inputs necessary for proper development of the visual system and for language acquisition, for example, are well characterized.[23] When the expected environmental conditions necessary for proper neurodevelopment are either absent or inadequate, brain development is likely to be affected in important ways.

The primary neural substrate of executive functioning is the prefrontal cortex (PFC), a large expanse of association cortex that plays a central role in complex cognitive functions including inhibition, planning, and decision-making. When children experience damage to the PFC, they have immediate deficits in executive function and fail to develop typically as adults.[24] The PFC has a long developmental trajectory;[25] gross changes in volume and connectivity begin at birth and continue through early adulthood. This protracted development is reflected in children's increasing competence in behavioural tests of executive functions[26] and changes in PFC functioning across childhood.[27–30] Given the long developmental trajectory of the PFC and its central role in complex cognitive function, inadequate exposure to cognitive inputs in childhood may disrupt its development in ways that influence risk for psychopathology, particularly externalizing disorders.

23.4 **Neuroimaging studies of childhood adversity**

23.4.1 **Child maltreatment**

Child maltreatment involves acts of commission or omission that have the potential to harm a child or result in actual harm to a child, regardless of whether harm was intended, and typically includes four broad categories: physical abuse, sexual abuse, emotional abuse, and neglect.[31] Child maltreatment is perpetrated by parents or other caregivers in the vast majority of cases.[9] The following sections review neuroimaging studies that examine potential neurodevelopmental mechanisms through which child maltreatment increases risk for psychopathology.

23.4.1.1 **Brain structure**

Global differences in brain structure have been consistently reported in studies comparing children with and without exposure to maltreatment. Specifically, maltreated children have been found to have smaller total brain volume than non-maltreated children.[32–35] Although most studies reporting reduced total brain volume in maltreated youths are based on samples of children with maltreatment-related PTSD, at least one study reported a similar finding in a sample of maltreated children with a low prevalence of mental disorders.[10] Larger ventricles have also been observed among maltreated children relative to controls.[36]

The structure of the hippocampus and amygdala has frequently been examined in studies of child maltreatment given their central role in the regulation of stress response systems. However, studies of children have not found an association between maltreatment exposure and hippocampal volume.[37,38] Differences in the volume of the amygdala as a function of maltreatment history have also not been observed. Despite considerable interest in the effects of stress and trauma on limbic areas, the global structure of the hippocampus and amygdala appear to be preserved in children exposed to maltreatment.

Structural differences in the PFC among maltreated children have been reported, although the results have been inconsistent across studies. In one study, children exposed to physical abuse had smaller total brain volumes than children with no maltreatment exposure and smaller volume of the right orbitofrontal cortex, right ventral–medial PFC, and bilateral dorsolateral PFC.[10] A study of maltreated children with PTSD also reported globally smaller volume of the PFC in this group relative to controls, although this difference disappeared after adjusting for total brain volume.[36] Two studies found an opposite pattern of findings, however, with children with maltreatment-related PTSD exhibiting larger gray matter volume in the PFC relative to non-maltreated children.[39]

Maltreatment is also associated with structural changes in the cerebellum. Smaller volume of the vermis has been observed in physically abused children and children with maltreatment-related PTSD relative to controls.[39] Reduced overall volume of the cerebellum among children with maltreatment-related PTSD relative to controls has also been documented.[40]

One of the most consistently identified structural differences between maltreated and non-maltreated children is the corpus callosum, a white matter structure with dense fibres connecting the left and right hemispheres. Reduced corpus callosum volume—specifically in the anterior and posterior mid-body and splenium—in children who have been maltreated has been reported in several studies.[36,39] This pattern is consistent with findings from a diffusion tensor imaging study that documented reduced fractional anisotropy—a marker of structural connectivity and myelination in white matter tracts—in the corpus callosum of maltreated compared with non-maltreated children.[41]

23.4.1.2 Brain function

Disruptions in neural function related to child maltreatment have been studied using a variety of tasks designed to assess emotional processing and more global aspects of cognitive functioning. We first review studies that have utilized EEG and event-related potentials (ERPs) in response to specific visual stimuli. The EEG records electrical activity at the scalp, and the signal is decomposed into oscillations that occur in different frequency bands. The frequency bands that have been most frequently examined in developmental studies are beta (13–20 Hz), alpha (7–12 Hz), and theta (4–6 Hz). ERPs assess scalp-derived changes in brain electrical activity, measured using EEG, occurring in a time-locked fashion following presentation of a stimulus. ERP analysis typically examines the amplitude and latency of responses to specific stimuli.

EEG methods have been used to examine the influence of child maltreatment on patterns of frontal EEG asymmetry. Frontal regions of the cerebral cortex are differentially lateralized to process positive and negative stimuli and underlie behavioural and expressive responses to emotional information. The left frontal region is activated by positive emotional stimuli and promotes approach behaviour, whereas the right frontal region is activated by negative stimuli and underlies withdrawal or avoidance behaviour.[13,42] Individual differences in relative hemispheric activation of the frontal cortex—as indexed by EEG alpha power—are associated with emotional reactivity, behavioural inhibition, and psychopathology.[15] Poor quality maternal caregiving is associated with a pattern of asymmetry characterized by greater activation in the right relative to the left frontal cortex in infants.[43] This pattern has also been observed among adolescents exposed to child maltreatment.[44]

EEG methods have also been used to examine whether child maltreatment influences patterns of cortical differentiation. EEG coherence provides a measure of the degree of spatial synchrony between electrical signals measured at different parts of the scalp. Higher coherence indicates greater synchrony in the oscillations across scalp regions and is thought to reflect greater strength or coupling of cortical synaptic connections.[45] Reduced coherence reflects a pattern of greater cortical differentiation associated with more complex neuronal networks.[46] At least two studies have observed increased left hemisphere EEG coherence in maltreated children and adolescents relative to non-maltreated youths.[47] In both studies, this pattern of EEG coherence was interpreted as a sign of reduced left hemisphere cortical differentiation in maltreated children.

Cognitive processing of facial emotion provides important social information that is necessary to facilitate appropriate social interactions and can be disrupted by child maltreatment. Pollak et al. documented differences in ERPs in response to facial displays of emotion among maltreated and non-maltreated youths.[48] Children exposed to physical abuse and/or neglect exhibited larger ERP amplitudes to angry faces compared with happy faces and larger amplitudes to angry faces than controls, whereas non-maltreated children displayed similar ERP amplitude to both types of emotional stimuli.[16] These alterations in neural processing of facial emotion are consistent with behavioural findings, suggesting that physically abused children identify facial displays of anger more quickly and with less sensory information than non-maltreated children.[17]

Although the vast majority of fMRI studies of child maltreatment and neural function have been conducted in adults,[18] several recent studies have examined neural function in maltreated youths using fMRI. The first documented deficits in cognitive control in maltreated children with PTSD.[19] Non-maltreated children had greater activation in the middle frontal gyrus during response inhibition trials, whereas maltreated children exhibited greater activation in the anterior cingulate, a region activated by response conflict, and the medial frontal gyrus.[19] These findings suggest that different areas of the PFC are engaged during tasks involving sustained attention and response inhibition for children with maltreatment-related PTSD than controls. A second study documented lower right hippocampal activation among children with maltreatment-related PTSD than non-maltreated children during retrieval trials on a verbal declarative memory task,[49] suggesting that maltreatment exposure is associated with reduced hippocampal functioning in children.

23.4.2 Socio-economic status

There are strong social gradients in mental disorders according to socio-economic status (SES), such that lower SES is associated with greater psychopathology across the entire income distribution.[32] SES is an aggregate measure intended to capture social standing, which is often estimated with measures of family income, educational attainment, and occupational status. Measures of family SES are strongly linked to child emotional and behavioural problems[50–54] and risk of mental disorders.[55] These inequalities in mental health are evident early in childhood and persist or worsen across development into adulthood.[56]

Socio-economic status is a broad variable that is measured using numerous indicators[33,34] and predicts exposure to a broad array of experiences.[57,58] As such, there are numerous pathways through which childhood SES may influence brain development in ways that increase risk for psychopathology. These include deprivation in material resources needed to sustain health, such as nutrition, clothing, shelter, and health care; differential exposure to childhood traumatic events; parental psychopathology; deficits in the complexity and amount of language exposure within the home, school, and community; and differences in the degree of structure in educational and home settings.[55,59,60] We now review studies that examine SES differences in brain structure and function in children.

23.4.3.1 Brain structure

Several reviews have emphasized the importance of the stress response system as a mechanism by which SES influences neural structure and function, suggesting that low SES will be associated with decreased hippocampus volume and increased amygdala volume.[61,62] However, the associations between childhood SES and limbic structure volume are complex. In a recent study, a positive association was observed between family income-to-needs ratio and child hippocampal volume, such that greater resources were associated with larger hippocampal volume, but a negative association was found between hippocampal volume and parental education.[53] Although the divergent associations of hippocampal volume with different measures of SES are perplexing, a similar pattern has been reported in other studies. Family income was positively associated with child hippocampal volume in one of these studies.[54] In a second study, hippocampal volume was negatively associated with parental nurturance and unrelated to degree of enrichment in the home.[55] One interpretation of this pattern of results is that measures that directly or indirectly assess parenting behaviour are negatively associated with hippocampal volume, whereas markers of environmental enrichment are positively associated with hippocampal volume. Amygdala volume has been inconsistently associated with SES in children. In the recent study by Noble et al., the associations between amygdala volume and SES were reported to be similar to those found in the hippocampus.[53] However, these were not replicated in two other studies.[54,55]

The consistent finding that children from low SES families perform more poorly on tests of executive functioning than children from middle-class families has led some to argue that childhood SES may influence the development of the PFC.[56,63–65] This hypothesis was supported by a recent study in young adults. Subjective social status was positively associated with anterior cingulate cortex volume, a part of the PFC involved in conflict monitoring.[58] However, a subsequent study did not observe an association between PFC structure and SES in children.[54]

23.4.3.2 Brain function

Recent fMRI studies have documented associations between childhood SES and function of the limbic system. Children whose parents reported low subjective social status activated the hippocampus less in a long term memory encoding paradigm than children whose parents had high subjective social status.[59] These findings extend previous work demonstrating decrements in performance on long term memory tasks in children from low SES families.[65] Childhood SES has also been related to amygdala function. Low parental SES, as rated by adolescent participants, was associated with greater amygdala activation during a task that involved passive viewing of emotional faces.[60]

Parental SES has been consistently associated with PFC function in neuroimaging studies. Using EEG methods, Otero et al.[61] reported higher levels of low frequency brain electrical activity (theta) in frontal regions among children living in low SES families relative to children living in middle-class families. This pattern is similar to the pattern of brain electrical activity observed in children raised in institutional settings[66] and likely represents a delay in maturation of the PFC. Poor PFC function among children raised in low SES families was also reported in two ERP studies such that low SES was associated with reduced a reduced ability to suppress neural responses to distracting stimuli.[63,67]

Two recent studies examined the association between SES and PFC function using fMRI methods. Children from low-SES families exhibited an inefficient pattern of PFC recruitment involving greater activation of the right PFC while learning a complex stimulus–response association despite worse task performance compared to children from middle-class families.[68] Activation of the lateral PFC during this task was associated with complexity of parental language used in the home environment. In a related study of adults, parental education during childhood was associated with greater activation of both the anterior cingulate and of the lateral PFC during a complex card guessing game, even after controlling for the participant's own educational attainment.[69] Taken together these results are consistent with the idea that childhood SES may influence the development of the PFC, potentially through both enrichment and stress exposure pathways.

23.5 **Summary**

We have presented converging evidence that different types of adverse childhood experience influence brain development via three neurodevelopmental pathways. The first of these is a stress-related pathway involving disruptions in emotional processing and limbic structures, including the hippocampus and amygdala. The second pathway implicated in the association between childhood adversity and psychopathology involves the PFC and associated executive functions. Finally, diverse forms of childhood adversity are associated with decrements in white matter volume, corpus callosum volume, and both structural and functional connectivity. To better inform interventions aimed at preventing the onset of mental disorders in children exposed to adverse childhood environments, the specific psychological, neurobiological, and social mechanisms linking these experiences to the onset of mental disorders must be identified. Incorporating methods from developmental cognitive and affective neuroscience into population health approaches provides the opportunity to investigate these central neurobiological mechanisms linking the social environment to the propensity for mental disorders, thereby elucidating potential targets of intervention.

References

1 **Teicher MH, Anderson CM, Polcari A.** Childhood maltreatment is associated with reduced volume in the hippocampal subfields CA3, dentate gyrus, and subiculum. *Proc Natl Acad Sci USA* 2012;**109**:E563–572.

2 **Green JG, McLaughlin KA, Berglund P, et al.** Childhood adversities and adult psychopathology in the National Comorbidity Survey Replication (NCS-R) I: associations with first onset of DSM-IV disorders. *Arch Gen Psychiatry* 2010;**62**:113–123.

3 **Chapman DP, Whitfield CL, Felitti VJ, Dube SR, Edwards VJ, Anda RF.** Adverse childhood experiences and the risk of depressive disorders in adulthood. *J Affect Disord* 2004;**82**:217–225.

4 **Collishaw S, Pickles A, Messer J, Rutter M, Shearer C, Maughan B.** Resilience to adult psychopathology following childhood maltreatment: evidence from a community sample. *Child Abuse Negl* 2007;**31**:211–229.

5 **Dong M, Giles WH, Felitti VJ, et al.** Insights into causal pathways for ischemic heart disease: adverse childhood experiences study. *Circulation* 2004;**110**:1761–1766.

6 **Fantuzzo JW, DePaola LM, Lambert L, Martino T, Anderson G, Sutton S.** Effects of interparental violence on the psychological adjustment and competencies of young children. *J Consult Clin Psychol* 1991;**59**:258–265.

7 **Fergusson DM, Horwood LJ, Lynskey MT.** Childhood sexual abse and psychiatric disorder in young adulthood: II. Psychiatric outcomes of childhood sexual abuse. *J Am Acad Child Adolesc Psychiatry* 1996;**35**:1365–1374.

8 **Kessler RC, Davis CG, Kendler KS.** Childhood adversity and adult psychiatric disorder in the US National Comorbidity Survey. *Psychol Med* 1997;**27**:1101–1119.

9 McLaughlin KA, Green JG, Gruber M, Sampson NA, Zaslavsky A, Kessler RC. Childhood adversities and adult psychopathology in the National Comorbidity Survey Replication (NCS-R): II. Associations with persistence of DSM-IV disorders. *Arch Gen Psychiatry* 2010;**62**:124–132.

10 McLaughlin KA, Green JG, Gruber M, Sampson NA, Zaslavsky A, Kessler RC. Childhood adversities and adult psychopathology in the National Comorbidity Survey Replication (NCS-R): III. Associations with severity of DSM-IV disorders. *Psychol Med* 2010;**40**:847–859.

11 Zeanah CH, Egger HL, Smyke AT, et al. Institutional rearing and psychiatric disorders in Romanian preschool children. *Am J Psychiatry* 2009;**166**:777–785.

12 Edwards VJ, Holden GW, Felitti VJ, Anda RF. Relationship between multiple forms of childhood maltreatment and adult mental health in community respondents: results from the adverse childhood experiences study. *Am J Psychiatry* 2003;**160**:1453–1460.

13 Kim JJ, Yoon KS. Stress: metaplastic effects in the hippocampus. *Trends Neurosci* 1998;**21**(12):505–509.

14 Mullen PE, Martin JL, Anderson JC, Romans SE, Herbison GP. The long-term impact of the physical, emotional, and sexual abuse of children: a community study. *Child Abuse Negl* 1996;**20**:7–21.

15 de Quervain DJ-F, Roozendaal B, McGaugh JL. Stress and glucocorticoids impair retrieval of long-term spatial memory. *Nature* 1998;**394**:787–790.

16 Monk CS, Grillon C, Baas JM, et al. A neuroimaging method for the study of threat in adolescents. *Dev Psychobiol* 2003;**43**(4):359–366.

17 De Bellis MD, Casey BJ, Dahl RE, et al. A pilot study of amygdala volumes in pediatric generalized anxiety disorder. *Biol Psychiatry* 2000;**48**:51–57.

18 Etkin A, Wager TD. Functional neuroimaging of anxiety: a meta-analysis of emotional processing in PTSD, social anxiety disorder, and specific phobia. *Am J Psychiatry* 2007;**164**:1476–1488.

19 Thomas KM, Drevets WC, Dahl RE, et al. Amygdala response to fearful faces in anxious and depressed children. *Arch Gen Psychiatry* 2001;**58**:1057–1063.

20 Cyander MS, Frost BJ. Mechanisms of brain development: neuronal sculpting by the physical and social environment. In: Keating DP, Hertzmann C, editors. *Developmental health and the wealth of nations: social, biological, and educational dynamics.* New York: Guilford Press; 1999.

21 Scott KM, Smith DR, Ellis PM. Prospectively ascertained childhood maltreatment and its associations with DSM-IV mental disorders in young adults. *Arch Gen Psychiatry* 2010;**67**:712–719.

22 Dube SR, Felitti VJ, Dong M, Chapman DP, Giles WH, Anda RF. Childhood abuse, neglect, and household dysfunction and the risk of illicit drug use: the adverse childhood experiences study. *Pediatrics* 2003;**111**:564–572.

23 Jaffee SR, Moffit TE, Caspi A, Fombonne E, Poulton R, Martin J. Differences in early childhood risk factors for juvenile-onset and adult-onset depression. *Arch Gen Psychiatry* 2002;**58**:215–222.

24 De Bellis MD, Keshavan MS, Clark DB, et al. Developmental traumatology. Part II: Brain development. *Biol Psychiatry* 1999;**45**:1271–1284.

25 De Bellis MD, Keshavan MS, Shifflett H, et al. Brain structures in maltreatment-related posttraumatic stress disroder: a sociodemographically matched study. *Biol Psychiatry* 2002;**52**:1066–1078.

26 Hanson JL, Chung MK, Avants BB, et al. Early stress is associated with alterations in the orbitofrontal cortex: a tensor-based morphometry investigation of brain structure and behavioral risk. *J Neurosci* 2010;**30**:7466–7472.

27 De Bellis MD, Hall J, Boring AM, Frustaci K, Moritz G. A pilot londitudinal study of hippocampal volumes in pediatric maltreatment-related posttraumatic stress disorder. *Biol Psychiatry* 2001;**50**:305–309.

28 Tottenham N, Sheridan MA. A review of adversity, the amygdala and the hippocampus: consideration of developmental timing. *Front Hum Neurosci* 2010;**3**:Article 68.

29 Carrion VG, Weems CF, Watson C, Eliez S, Menon V, Reiss AL. Converging evidence for abnormalities of the prefrontal cortex and evaluation of midsagittal structures in pediatric posttraumatic stress disorder: an MRI study. *Psychiatry Res Neuroimaging* 2009;**172**:226–234.

30 Richert KA, Carrion VG, Karchemskiy A, Reiss AL. Regional differences of the prefrontal cortex in pediatric PTSD: an MRI study. *Depress Anxiety* 2006;**23**:17–25.

31 De Bellis MD, Kuchibhatla M. Cerebellar volumes in pediatric maltreatment-related posttraumatic stress disorder. *Biol Psychiatry* 2006;**60**:697–703.

32 Jackowski AP, Douglas-Paulmberi H, Jackowski M, et al. Corpus callosum in maltreated children with posttraumatic stress disorder: a diffusion tensor imaging study. *Psychiatry Res Neuroimaging* 2008;**162**:256–261.

33 Davidson RJ. Emotion and affective style: hemispheric substrates. *Psychol Sci* 1992;**3**:39–43.

34 Davidson RJ, Ekman P, Saron CD, Senulis JA, Friesen WV. Approach–withdrawal and cerebral asymmetry: emotional expression and brain physiology. *J Pers Soc Psychol* 1990;**58**:330–341.

35 Davidson RJ, Fox NA. Asymmetrical brain activity discriminates between positive and negative affective stimuli in human infants. *Science* 1982;**218**(4578):1235–1237.

36 Finkelhor D, Ormrod R, Turner H, Hamby SL. The victimization of children and youth: a comprehensive, national survey. *Child Maltreatment* 2005;**10**:5–25.

37 Fox NA. If it's not left, it's right. *Am Psychol* 1991;**46**:863–872.

38 Buss KA, Malmstadt Schumacher JR, Dolski I, Kalin NH, Goldsmith HH, Davidson R. JJ. Right frontal brain activity, cortisol, and withdrawal behavior in 6-month olds. *Behav Neurosci* 2003;**117**:11–20.

39 Molnar BE, Buka SL, Kessler RC. Child sexual abuse and subsequent psychopathology: results from the National Comorbidity Survey. *Am J Public Health* 2001;**91**:753–760.

40 Afifi TO, Enns MW, Cox BJ, Asmundson GJG, Stein MB, Sareen J. Population attributable risk fractions of psychiatric disorders and suicide ideation and attempts associated with adverse childhood experiences. *Am J Public Health* 2008;**98**:946–952.

41 McLaughlin KA, Green JG, Gruber MJ, Sampson NA, Zaslavsky A, Kessler RC. Childhood adversities and first onset of psychiatric disorders in a national sample of adolescents. *Arch Gen Psychiatry* 2012;**69**(11):1151–1160.

42 Sapolsky RM, Romero LM, Munck AU. How do glucocorticoids influence stress responses? Integrating permissive, suppressive, stimulatory, and preparative actions. *Endocr Rev* 2000;**21**:55–89.

43 Sapolsky RM. The possibility of neurotoxicity in the hippocampus in major depression: a primer on neuron death. *Biol Psychiatry* 2000;**48**:755–765.

44 Shin LM, Rauch SL, Pitman RK. Amygdala, medial prefrontal cortex, and hippocampal function in PTSD. *Ann NY Acad Sci* 2006;**1071**:67–79.

45 Beesdo K, Lau JYF, Guyer AE, et al. Common and distinct amygdala-function perturbations in depressed vs anxious adolescents. *Arch Gen Psychiatry* 2009;**66**(3):275–285.

46 Bechara A, Tranel D, Damasio H, Adolphs R, Rockland C, Damasio AR. Double dissociation of conditioning and declarative knowledge relative to the amygdala and hippocampus in humans. *Science* 1995;**269**(5227):1115–1118.

47 Emery NJ, Capitanio JP, Mason WA, Machado CJ, Mendoza SP, Amaral DG. The effects of bilateral lesions of the amygdala on dyadic social interactions in rhesus monkeys (*Macaca mulatta*). *Behav Neurosci* 2001;**115**(3):515–544.

48 Adolphs R. What does the amygdala contribute to social cognition? *Ann NY Acad Sci* 2010;**1191**:42–61.

49 Bauer PM, Hanson JL, Pierson RK, Davidson RJ, Pollak SD. Cerebellar volume and cognitive functioning in children who experienced early deprivation. *Biol Psychiatry* 2009;**66**:1100–1106.

50 Nelson CA, Sheridan MA. Lessons from neuroscience research for understanding causal links between family and neighborhood characteristics and educational outcomes. In: Duncan GJ, Murnane RJ editors. *Whither opportunity? Rising inequality, schools and children's life chances.* New York: Russell Sage Foundation (in press).

51 Gianaros PJ, Manuck SB. Neurobiological pathways linking socioeconomic position and health. *Psychosom Med* 2010;**72**(5):450–461.

52 **McEwen BS, Gianaros PJ.** Central role of the brain in stress and adaptation: links to socioeconomic status, health, and disease. *Ann NY Acad Sci* 2010;**1186**:190–222.

53 **Noble KG, Houston S, Kan E, Sowell ER.** Neural correlates of socioeconomic status in the developing human brain. *Dev Sci* 2012;**15**(4):516–527.

54 **Hanson JL, Chandra A, Wolfe BL, Pollak SD.** Association between income and the hippocampus. *PloS One* 2011;**6**(5):e18712.

55 **Rao H, Betancourt L, Giannetta JM, et al.** Early parental care is important for hippocampal maturation: evidence from brain morphology in humans. *Neuroimage* 2010;**49**(1):1144–1150.

56 **Ardila A, Rosselli M, Matute E, Guajardo S.** The influence of the parents' educational level on the development of executive functions. *Dev Neuropsychol* 2005;**28**(1):539–560.

57 **Gianaros PJ, Horenstein JA, Cohen S, et al.** Perigenual anterior cingulate morphology covaries with perceived social standing. *Soc Cogn Affect Neurosci* 2007;**2**(3):161–173.

58 **Sheridan MA, How J, Araujo M, Schamberg M, Nelson CA.** What are the links between maternal social status, hippocampal function, and HPA axis function in children? *Dev Sci* (in press).

59 **Mueller SC, Maheu FS, Dozier M, et al.** Early-life stress is associated with impairment in cognitive control in adolescence: an fMRI study. *Neuropsychologia* 2010;**48**:3037–3044.

60 **Gianaros PJ, Horenstein JA, Hariri AR, et al.** Potential neural embedding of parental social standing. *Soc Cogn Affect Neurosci* 2008;**3**(2):91–96.

61 **Otero GA, Pliego-Rivero FB, Fernández T, Ricardo J.** EEG development in children with sociocultural disadvantages: a follow-up study. *Clin Neurophysiol* 2003;**114**(10):1918–1925.

62 **Kishiyama MM, Boyce WT, Jimenez AM, Perry LM, Knight RT.** Socioeconomic disparities affect prefrontal function in children. *J Cogn Neurosci* 2009;**21**(6):1106–1115.

63 **Leeb RT, Paulozzi L, Melanson C, Simon T, Arias I.** *Child maltreatment and surveillance. Uniform definitions for public health and recommended data elements.* Atlanta: Centers for Disease Control and Prevention; 2008.

64 **Farah MJ, Shera DM, Savage JH, et al.** Childhood poverty: specific associations with neurocognitive development. *Brain Res* 2006;**1110**(1):166–174.

65 **Hackman DA, Farah MJ.** Socioeconomic status and the developing brain. *Trends Cogn Sci* 2009;**13**(2):65–73.

66 **Tottenham N, Hare T, Millner A, Gilhooly T, Zevin JD, Casey BJ.** Elevated amygdala response to faces following early deprivation. *Dev Sci* 2011;**14**:190–204.

67 **Stevens C, Lauinger B, Neville H.** Differences in the neural mechanisms of selective attention in children from different socioeconomic backgrounds: an event-related brain potential study. *Dev Sci* 2009;**12**(4):634–646.

68 **Carrion VG, Weems CF, Eliez S, et al.** Attenuation of frontal asymmetry in pediatric posttraumatic stress disorder. *Biol Psychiatry* 2001;**50**:943–951.

69 **Gianaros PJ, Manuck SB, Sheu LK, et al.** Parental education predicts corticostriatal functionality in adulthood. *Cereb Cortex* 2011;**21**(4):896–910.

Chapter 24

Social–biological interplay over the life course

Kelly Skelton, Kerry Ressler, Elisabeth Binder, and Bekh Bradley-Davino

24.1 Introduction

Multiple psychiatric illnesses have been demonstrated to have a heritable, genetic component.[1–4] However, even twins who share identical DNA are still frequently discordant for a given psychiatric diagnosis, implicating factors other than genetic risk for the development of psychiatric disorders. Numerous environmental risk factors have also been identified for various psychiatric disorders. These events may impact an individual at multiple times across their developmental course—in utero (i.e. maternal stress), perinatally (i.e. low birth weight), during childhood and adolescence (i.e. physical and/or sexual abuse), or during adulthood (i.e. exposure to traumatic events).[4] Research also implicates broader social forces as environmental factors that contribute to risk for psychiatric disorders. These risk factors include residing or being raised in an urban environment, exposure to neurotoxins (e.g. lead), migration, and experiencing discrimination (e.g. racial, gender-based).

Not surprisingly, the potential impact of this range of social and environmental factors is broad. The combined impact of multiple types of adverse early life experiences increases risk for a wide range of psychiatric disorders and other behavioural problems.[5] Similarly, data from human and translational research show that exposure to enriched/positive early environmental factors decreases risk for the development of mental health problems.[6,7]

Despite the demonstrated association between these environmental risk factors and subsequent risk and resilience, no single environmental factor or specific combination of environmental factors determines psychiatric outcomes. Likewise, there are multiple 'biological pathways' to any given psychiatric diagnosis. In this way, genetic and environmental factors seem to co-influence one another in a manner that suggests both equifinality (multiple pathways to one disorder) and multifinality (multiple outcomes resulting from a given genetic or environmental factor) in psychiatric risk and resilience. Despite the awareness of this complexity, the research on the genetics of psychiatric disorders has not been fully integrated with research on social risk factors for psychiatric disorders. Moreover, even less research has focused on understanding the neurobiological mechanisms that account for the combined influence of environmental and genetic factors on risk for psychiatric disorders. This chapter presents a life course perspective on understanding the interplay of genes and environments in producing psychiatric disorders. Post-traumatic stress disorder (PTSD) is a psychiatric disorder that requires exposure to a specific environmental event for diagnosis (i.e. a Criterion A trauma), and individuals vary in their phenotypic response to that event based on biological characteristics and trauma characteristics.

Therefore, we focus on PTSD in our review of the interplay of biology and environment over the life course in part because it is the area of our own work.

24.2 **Gene-by-environment interactions**

Some of the first reports of a specific genotype moderating the response to environmental risk factors were published by Caspi et al.[8,9] This research suggested that variations in the serotonin transporter (*5HTT*) gene, a functional polymorphism in the promoter region of the gene, interact with exposure to environmental stressors to predict increased symptoms of depression including suicidality. Following these initial studies there has been an expanding literature on gene-by-environment (G × E) predicting increased risk for psychiatric disorders. Despite the promise of this research, failure of studies to replicate has raised concerns and recent review of psychiatric studies of G × E interaction points to methodological problems in this area of research.[10] Nonetheless, the variability in the development of psychiatric symptoms following exposure to adverse life events implies that consequences of environmental exposure are moderated by genetic factors.

The majority of G × E studies have focused on genetic variations that confer risk in the context of adverse environmental exposures (e.g. childhood abuse). Another perspective suggests that the degree to which an individual is affected by an environment is an inherited phenotype.[10] Under this model, genetic polymorphisms are seen as markers of sensitivity to environmental context rather than serving solely as risk markers. Therefore, just as individuals who carry genetic variations associated with environmental sensitivity and plasticity are more vulnerable when exposed to detrimental social/environmental forces, these same individuals are more resilient when exposed to enriching and supportive social/environmental forces (Figure 24.1). For example, Van Ijzendoorn et al. conducted a meta-analytic review of G × E studies involving dopamine-related genes in children.[11] They found that children with the less efficient dopamine-related genetic variations showed increased risk for poor behavioural outcomes when they were raised in negative environments, but also demonstrated increased likelihood for good behavioural outcomes

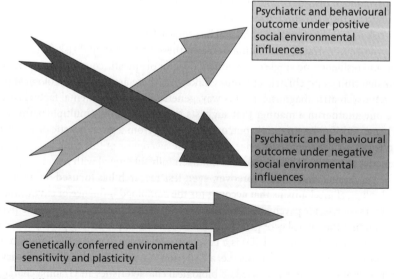

Figure 24.1 A differential sensitivity model of risk and resilience.

when they were raised in positive environments. Evidence for a differential sensitivity model has been also found in studies of the serotonin transporter gene[12,13] and in studies of oxytocin receptor genes.[13,14] However, differential sensitivity is only one theoretical model which, much like the overall body of psychiatric G × E research, is still very much debated.[15] Regardless of the ultimate verdict on this particular model of G × E interactions, the research underlying it points out the need to carefully consider and control for a range of environmental exposures in psychiatric G × E research (Figure 24.1).

Because PTSD is a psychiatric disorder that requires exposure to a specific environmental event for diagnosis, it is particularly amenable to studies of G × E interaction. Research from G × E studies of PTSD attempts to take into account not only the index trauma, but also other social–environmental factors. Several studies of adults exposed to the 2004 Florida hurricanes found that genetic risk interacted with level of social support to predict likelihood of developing post-hurricane exposure PTSD.[16,17] An additional study in this population found that a county-level environment (e.g. low county-level crime and unemployment) interacted with genetic factors to predict risk for developing PTSD.[18]

Research also demonstrates an interaction between polymorphisms in *FK506 Binding Protein 5* (*FKBP5*) and childhood maltreatment in predicting risk for PTSD. *FKBP5* is a gene that impacts the neuroendocrine stress response as co-ordinated by the hypothalamic–pituitary–adrenal axis (HPA). Feedback inhibition of the HPA axis is mediated in part by the binding of cortisol (the end product of HPA axis activation) to glucocorticoid receptors (GRs) to terminate the stress response once the exposure to the stressor has ended. A dysregulation of this response at any level may contribute to an enhanced vulnerability, with an increased susceptibility to develop stress- and trauma-related psychiatric disorders, such as PTSD (Figure 24.2). In a study of highly

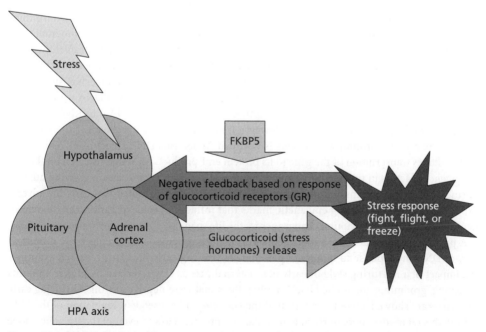

Figure 24.2 Role of glucocorticoid receptors and FK506 Binding Protein 5 (FKBP5) in the stress–response negative feedback loop. HPA, hypothalamic–pituitary–adrenal.

traumatized, inner city, African-American subjects,[9] four polymorphisms in the *FKBP5* gene were shown to interact with severity of childhood abuse to predict severity of adult PTSD symptoms. Further, these polymorphisms were demonstrated to be functional, in that those individuals with both PTSD and the risk alleles demonstrated enhanced suppression of cortisol in response to the synthetic glucocorticoid, dexamethasone.[19] Several additional studies in different cohorts have now replicated the initial finding and have extended them to other psychiatric phenotypes, including depression, risk for suicide attempts, and aggression.[20,21] This suggests that the same G × E can increase the risk for a number of psychiatric symptoms that are now classified in distinct diagnostic categories with different treatment approaches.

24.3 Developmental timing and epigenetic modification of DNA

Although studies of G × E interaction are an improvement over studying the main effects of genes alone, they do not account for the role of developmental timing of stressor exposure to producing phenotypic changes associated with exposure to environmental forces. However, investigation of the epigenetic modification of DNA can provide insight into this issue.

In the eighteenth century, Jean-Baptiste Lamarck posited that as individuals interacted with their environments they acquired adaptive characteristics and that these acquired adaptations could be genetically transmitted to the next generation. This theory of 'soft inheritance' was subsequently replaced by inherited genetic explanations. However, recent research has led to a new appreciation of the role of life experience in influencing gene expression. Research in this area, referred to as epigenetics, suggests that 'negative' environmental influences (e.g. famine, environmental toxins, and stress/trauma) and 'positive' environmental influences (e.g. good early life maternal care) alter the chemical scaffolding of DNA to change not the underlying genetic code, but rather the rate at which that code can be transcribed into mRNA and translated into proteins. These epigenetic modifications influence the interaction of 'nature' and 'nurture' in determining vulnerability to mental illness. These changes can be specific to critical developmental periods, can be stable, enduring, and site-specific, and may be intergenerationally transmitted.[22,23] Epigenetic changes begin to occur in the developing fetus and continue to accrue across the lifespan.[24] The biological mechanism of epigenetic modification involves several mechanisms. One is the addition of a chemical 'tag' (methylation) to one of the building blocks of DNA within a gene, which typically produces decreased transcription of that segment of DNA into RNA to reduce expression of the gene into a protein.[25] However, it may also involve the chemical alternation of the histone proteins around which DNA is wrapped. When this DNA structure is 'opened up', this facilitates transcription of the gene to its protein end-product. Although research on the role of epigenetic factors in psychiatric/behavioural disorders is in its early stages, a growing number of studies (in both humans and non-human animals) have demonstrated that early life adverse experiences may leave lasting epigenetic marks that influence gene expression and associated neurobiological and behavioural changes across the life span.

A particularly elegant set of experiments in rodents has demonstrated epigenetic modification of DNA in response to quality of parental care during early life. This research examines the impact of a nurturing style of early life maternal care as characterized by higher amounts of licking, grooming, and arched back nursing. Pups that were deprived of this nurturing early maternal care showed altered expression of the *GR* gene and subsequent regulation of the HPA axis. In this rat model, more nurturing maternal care produced lower levels of the stress hormone corticosterone in the rat pups, but only if this variation in maternal care occurred during a specific, early developmental window. These rat pups also demonstrated enhanced suppression of corticosterone in response to dexamethasone, as well as greater expression of the *GR* gene and a greater number of hippocampal GRs as a result of hypomethylation in promoter region of the hippocampal *GR* gene.[26,27] Moreover, these epigenetic changes were stable over time and were associated with enhanced nurturing maternal behaviour displayed by the female pups when they reached adulthood and gave birth to their own offspring. This pattern of behaviour then induced similar epigenetic changes in their offspring, allowing for the associated phenotype to be transmitted from one generation to the next.[28,29]

Some human research has shown similar patterns of maternal mood state impacting the expression and function of the glucocorticoid receptor in the offspring. Prenatal exposure to maternal depression/anxiety specifically during the third trimester, but not during second trimester or at birth, has been shown to be associated with increased DNA methylation of the *GR* gene (*NR3C1*) at birth, and this was functionally correlated with increased salivary cortisol concentrations in response to novel visual stimuli at age 3 months.[30] Postnatally, adverse early rearing environment has also been associated with increased methylation of the promoter region of this same gene, along with decreased levels of GR mRNA expression in the hippocampus of suicide victims with a history of childhood abuse.[31]

The neuroendocrine alterations described in this animal model parallel those of PTSD, with low basal cortisol and enhanced suppression of cortisol in response to a synthetic glucocorticoid. One caveat of these studies is that it has not been possible to follow the state of methylation over time in a given individual or animal. Thus, although the interpretation is that there are early developmental methylation changes that are long-lasting and enduring, it cannot yet be ruled out that methylation may represent a state-dependent effect. In this alternative view, other causal factors in the adult animals and suicide victims (e.g. ongoing adult stress or depression) may lead to similar methylation effects as seen during development or in the previous generation, even if they were not maintained consistently over time in these individuals.

Epigenetic modification of the *FKBP5* gene may also play a role in the regulation of GR activity and susceptibility to stress-related psychopathology. A recent study in adult mice demonstrated transient de-methylation of glucocorticoid response elements (GREs) within the *FKBP5* gene locus in both peripheral blood and brain tissue following chronic stress hormone (corticosterone) exposure.[32] The *FKBP5* alleles that have been associated with higher risk for PTSD symptoms following exposure to early trauma are also the ones associated with stronger induction of *FKBP5* by GR activation which leads to an impaired negative feedback of the stress response by increasing GR resistance.[19] Exposure to child abuse leads to a demethylation of functional GREs in the *FKBP5* gene, further depressing its activity, but only in carriers of the risk allele.[21] These epigenetic changes interfere with the GR/*FKBP5* ultra-short feedback loop and thus the regulation of the stress hormone system. Interestingly, using human embryonic neuronal precursor cells, the demethylation of the *FKBP5* locus upon activation of the *GR* only remains stable when the *GR* is activated in proliferating neurons, but not when activated in neurons that have already differentiated. This suggests that the epigenetic changes mediating the G × E interaction need to be installed during a certain developmental window. This parallels G × E studies in PTSD, where only exposure to child abuse, but not adult trauma, interacted with the *FKBP5* polymorphisms to predict risk. More recently, FKBP5 mRNA expression was found to be reduced in survivors of the World Trade Center attacks on 11 September 2001 who had a diagnosis of PTSD[33] as well as in a second independent cohort, but here only in *FKBP5* risk allele carriers.[34] Such epigenetic changes may also underlie other G × E. A recent study found an interaction between level of trauma exposure and serotonin transporter gene (*SLC6A4*) methylation levels in predicting risk for PTSD.[35]

Our research group has recently examined the impact of the type and timing of trauma exposure on genome-wide gene expression and DNA methylation in peripheral blood cells in adults with PTSD (D. Mehta, personal communication). When compared with a sample of trauma-exposed adults who did not develop PTSD ($n = 108$), the gene expression profile of adults diagnosed with PTSD who did not experience childhood maltreatment were almost completely non-overlapping with the gene expression profile of adults with PTSD and a history of childhood maltreatment as well as adult trauma. Moreover, these gene expression changes were accompanied by alterations in DNA methylation in the same transcripts in a much larger proportion in the individual with a history of childhood as compared with those who experience trauma only during adulthood.

Whereas epigenetic changes can be enduring, recent research has demonstrated that there may be ways to reverse these changes after they occur. Drugs (so-called HDAC inhibitors) which block an enzyme that removes acetyl groups from DNA-binding histone proteins help to keep the DNA in a more 'open' structure which is more readily transcribed. This can counteract the effect of over-methylation which tends to reduce gene expression. Such manipulations have been found to promote nurturing behaviour in the rat model studied by Meaney et al.[36,37] As such, these drugs hold the potential to reverse the detrimental impact of early, negative environmental events on the epigenome.[38]

24.4 Effect of the environment on brain structure and function

In order to manifest behaviourally, the interplay between genetics and social/environmental influences must be expressed as changes in brain structure and function. Early experiences influence gene expression and ultimately brain architecture and neuronal function. Environmental influences on neural plasticity may be negative, such as childhood abuse, or positive, such as exercise, psychotherapy, or social support.

Multiple types of stress including abuse and neglect, malnutrition, neighbourhood environment, exposure to neurotoxins, poverty, and living in an urban environment have all been shown to be associated with important changes in the development of brain structure and function.[39] In animal models, stress has been shown to physically alter neuronal structures in a number of ways including changes in dendritic spine density, length and degree of branching. These types of stress-related changes have been shown to occur in multiple areas of the brain that have been demonstrated to play a key role in behaviour, anxiety, and mood.[40]

Neuroimaging studies and neurobiological research have strongly implicated these three brain regions in the neurocircuitry of PTSD. The amygdala is composed of several nuclei located within the temporal lobe of the brain and plays a key role in emotional learning, the development and consolidation of fear conditioning and expression of the fear response.[41] Increased activation of the amygdala in the presence of fear/threat-related stimuli is a consistent finding in individuals diagnosed with PTSD.[42] By contrast with the amygdala 'driving' the fear response, the medial prefrontal cortex (mPFC), is essential for extinction of fear conditioning and, in general, for balancing lower-level limbic processing (the 'emotional brain') with higher-order cognitive processing (the 'rational brain'). Decreased volume of the mPFC regions, a failure of the mPFC to activate in response to trauma narratives, and an inverse relationship between activation of the amygdala and the mPFC have all been demonstrated in PTSD.[43–45] The hippocampus is another neuronal region that can act as the 'brakes' on the fear response. It is a brain region central to PTSD because of involvement in explicit memory processes and encoding context during fear conditioning, and has been demonstrated to have decreased volume and neuronal integrity in individuals diagnosed with PTSD.[46,47]

Exposure to adverse experiences early in development appears have particular impact on elements of this fear neurocircuitry, and may represent a neuronal mechanism by which earlier exposure to stressors increases later vulnerability to the development of PTSD. In a study of children who were reared in impoverished orphanages in Eastern Europe and Asia during infancy, those who were adopted later in life (aged >15 months) were found to have significantly larger amygdala volume compared with those adopted earlier.[48] Conversely, stress has also been shown to reduce neuronal size in the mPFC and to reduce volume in the orbitofrontal cortex of abused children.[49] In addition to volumetric changes, a relative functional decoupling of mPFC inhibition from the amygdala[50] has been demonstrated in individuals with the *s* allele polymorphism of the *5HTTLPR* serotonin transporter gene. This is the same polymorphism that has been associated with a G × E risk for adult depression and PTSD in those with a history of childhood trauma.[9] Interactions between this polymorphism and a history of trauma have been found to be predictive of PTSD.[18] The hippocampus appears to be particularly vulnerable to the deleterious effects of stress, with evidence of atrophy and impaired neurogenesis in both animals and humans, and the magnitude of this impact is related to both the developmental timing and chronicity of exposure to stress.[51,52]

Emerging evidence also indicates that positive environmental influences can produce beneficial changes in these same brain circuits. Rats placed into an enriched environment have demonstrated increased cortical thickness. Similarly, both environmental enrichment and physical activity have been shown to increase neurogenesis in the dentate gyrus of the hippocampus.[53] In humans, studies suggest that psychotherapy including cognitive therapy and mindfulness-based stress reduction enhances function of the PFC while inhibiting function of the amygdala.[54,55] It is also encouraging to note that even exposure to early, mild stress may also have beneficial effects. Squirrel monkeys exposed to mild stress during postnatal weeks 17–27 exhibited reduced HPA axis responsivity to stress, in conjunction with increased volume and white matter myelination of the ventromedial prefrontal cortex (vmPFC), as well as enhanced vmPFC-dependent response inhibition as adults.[56–59] These findings have been described as representing a form of adaptive stress inoculation. The previously described rat pups who received greater nurturing maternal behaviour during their early rearing also demonstrated increased synaptic plasticity of their hippocampal dentate gyrus neurons in vitro, in association with the epigenetically mediated increases in hippocampal GR mRNA expression.[60]

24.5 **Impact of social risk factors**

Whereas most of the data presented here have been on the impact of exposure to specific types of trauma or stress, broader social risk factors—particularly those associated with low socio-economic status–also influence brain development. Research has demonstrated an association between lower levels of perceived socio-economic status and a reduction in PFC gray matter volume.[61] Similarly, lower socio-economic status has been found to correlate with smaller hippocampal volumes.[62] By contrast, higher levels of poverty during development is associated with increased amygdala reactivity to the negative emotional stimuli of sad and angry faces.[63] Taken together, these findings suggest that adverse social environments are associated with changes in the fear neurocircuitry of the brain that would be expected to increase risk for fear and anxiety disorders, such as PTSD.

A number of factors have been proposed to explain the association between decreased economic resources and increased psychiatric risk including factors likely to impact brain development. These include home environment, nutritional deficits, toxin exposure, and chronic stress that both directly impacts developing children and also negatively impacts parenting capacities, thereby further impacting children's social and biological development.[64] Most likely it is not any one of these individual factors that accounts for the relationship of socio-economic status and increased risk for impaired brain development. Rather, it is likely the combination of factors which add up over time. Frequent activation of the body's stress response as a result of trauma and PTSD can cause a cumulative strain on the body, a concept referred to as allostatic load.[65]

24.6 Summary and future directions

Biology does not occur in isolation, but rather is shaped by the social environment that the individual experiences across their developmental course. Similarly, biological factors impact on an individual's perception of, and reaction to, that social environment. Recent research has shown the impact of both 'negative' and 'positive' social environmental effects during development on psychiatric risk and resilience. These data highlight the importance of understanding multiple levels and types of environmental experiences. Environmental exposures need to be understood in the context of many factors including the timing and severity of environmental exposure, other concurrent environmental exposures, socio-economic status, developmental history, as well as the gender and genetic inheritance of individuals exposed to any given social or environmental force. For example, although 'stress' is generally considered to be a 'negative' environmental factor, its impact is instead more likely to be a matter of degree.

One model of the impact of stress[66] posits three levels of stress exposures experienced by children during the course of development—positive stress exposure, tolerable stress exposure, and toxic stress exposure. The degree to which a stressor is positive depends on both degree and duration of the stress (generally mild-to-moderate and short-lived) and the availability of supportive caregivers who assist in responding effectively to the stressor which both allows for the physiological stress response system to return to baseline and also encourages the development of a sense of competence that will facilitate adaptation to future stressors. At the other end of the continuum, toxic stress involves repeated exposure to multiple types of severe stressors without the presence of supportive adult caregivers to assist in negotiating the stress.

Future work to best understand the interplay of social–environmental and biological factors will need to integrate what we have learned from research on G × E interactions, epigenetics, and brain development and function, as well as take into account the importance of gender and the developmental timing of these exposures. An example of a translational experimental approach that incorporates this is found in the studies of pituitary adenylate cyclase-activating polypeptide (PACAP), which has been demonstrated in humans to be associated with PTSD risk in a gender-specific manner.[67] In this study, blood levels of PACAP were found to correlate with PTSD symptom severity and enhanced acoustic startle response in women, but not in men. Further investigation revealed that this finding is likely related to sexually dimorphic regulation of a specific single nucleotide polymorphism located within an estrogen response element in the PAC1 receptor. Complementary data were obtained in mice demonstrating that both fear conditioning and estrogen induce expression of the mRNA for this receptor. These data suggest that the PACAP-PAC1 pathway may be regulated by estrogen in a gender-specific manner to moderate the biological responses to stress and fear conditioning that underlie risk for the development of PTSD.

In summary, there is clearly a bidirectional interplay between biological factors and environmental exposures in mediating psychiatric outcomes. Furthermore, the developmental timing of these environmental exposures upon the underlying neurobiological substrate significantly impacts the phenotypic result of the exposure. Whereas adverse early life experiences can produce negative and potentially enduring detrimental impacts on an individual's stress response and psychiatric functioning, positive social interventions can have similarly prolonged benefit and mitigate against these outcomes. Thus, the relationship between biology and environment is dynamic rather than static and does not produce outcomes that are 'written in stone', but instead are plastic in nature and subject to future interventions.

References

1 **Kendler KS.** Genetics of schizophrenia. *Am Psychiatr Assoc Annu Rev* 1986;**5**:25–41.

2 **Sullivan PF, Neale MC, Kendler KS.** Genetic epidemiology of major depression: review and meta-analysis. *Am J Psychiatry* 2000;**157**(10):1552–1562.

3 **Hettema JM, Neale MC, Kendler KS.** A review and meta-analysis of the genetic epidemiology of anxiety disorders. *Am J Psychiatry* 2001;**158**(10):1568–1578.

4 **Caspi A, Moffitt TE.** Gene–environment interactions in psychiatry: joining forces with neuroscience. *Nat Rev Neurosci* 2006;**7**(7):583–590.

5 **Anda RF, Felitti VJ, Bremner JD, et al.** The enduring effects of abuse and related adverse experiences in childhood. *Eur Arch Psychiatry Clin Neurosci* 2006;**256**(3):174–186.

6 **Fox C, Merali Z, Harrison C.** Therapeutic and protective effect of environmental enrichment against psychogenic and neurogenic stress. *Behav Brain Res* 2006;**175**(1):1–8.

7 **Laviola G, Hannan AJ, Macrì S, Solinas M, Jaber M.** Effects of enriched environment on animal models of neurodegenerative diseases and psychiatric disorders. *Neurobiol Dis* 2008;**31**(2):159–168.

8 **Caspi A, McClay J, Moffitt TE, et al.** Role of genotype in the cycle of violence in maltreated children. *Science* 2002;**297**(5582):851–854.

9 **Caspi A, Sugden K, Moffitt TE, et al.** Influence of life stress on depression: moderation by a polymorphism in the 5-HTT gene. [See comment.] *Science* 2003;**301**(5631):386–389.

10 **Belsky J, Jonassaint C, Pluess M, Stanton M, Brummett B, Williams R.** Vulnerability genes or plasticity genes? *Mol Psychiatry* 2009;**14**(8):746–754.

11 **van Ijzendoorn M, Belsky J, Bakermans-Kranenburg M.** Serotonin transporter genotype 5HTTLPR as a marker of differential susceptibility? A meta-analysis of child and adolescent gene-by-environment studies. *Transl Psychiatry* 2012;**2**(8):e147.

12 **Homberg JR, Lesch KP.** Looking on the bright side of serotonin transporter gene variation. *Biol Psychiatry* 2010;**69**:513–519.

13 **Cicchetti D, Rogosch FA.** Gene × Environment interaction and resilience: effects of child maltreatment and serotonin, corticotropin releasing hormone, dopamine, and oxytocin genes. *Dev Psychopathol* 2012;**24**(02):411–427.

14 **Bradley B, Westen D, Mercer KB, et al.** Association between childhood maltreatment and adult emotional dysregulation in a low-income, urban, African American sample: moderation by oxytocin receptor gene. *Dev Psychopathol* 2011;**23**(02):439–452.

15 **Pluess M, Belsky J.** Conceptual issues in psychiatric gene–environment interaction research. *Am J Psychiatry* 2012;**169**(2):222–223.

16 **Kilpatrick DG, Koenen KC, Ruggiero KJ, et al.** The serotonin transporter genotype and social support and moderation of posttraumatic stress disorder and depression in hurricane-exposed adults. *Am J Psychiatry* 2007;**164**(11):1693–1699.

17 **Amstadter A, Koenen K, Ruggiero K, et al.** Variant in RGS2 moderates posttraumatic stress symptoms following potentially traumatic event exposure. *J Anxiety Disord* 2009;**23**(3):369–373.

18 **Koenen K, Aiello A, Bakshis E, et al.** Modification of the association between serotonin transporter genotype and risk of posttraumatic stress disorder in adults by county-level social environment. *Am J Epidemiol* 2009;**169**(6):704.

19 Binder E, Bradley R, Liu W, et al. Association of FKBP5 polymorphisms and childhood abuse with risk of posttraumatic stress disorder symptoms in adults. *JAMA* 2008;**299**(11):1291.

20 Xie P, Kranzler H, Poling J, et al. Interaction of FKBP5 with childhood adversity on risk for posttraumatic stress disorder. *Neuropsychopharmacology* 2010;**35**(8):1684–1692.

21 Klengel T, Mehta D, Anacker C, et al. Allele-specific FKBP5 DNA demethylation mediates gene–childhood trauma interactions. *Nat Neurosci* 2013;**16**(1):33–41.

22 Meaney M, Szyf M. Maternal care as a model for experience-dependent chromatin plasticity? *Trends Neurosci* 2005;**28**(9):456–463.

23 Yehuda R, Bierer L. The relevance of epigenetics to PTSD: implications for the DSM-V. *J Traum Stress* 2009;**22**(5):427–434.

24 Fraga MF, Ballestar E, Paz MF, et al. Epigenetic differences arise during the lifetime of monozygotic twins. *Proc Natl Acad Sci USA* 2005;**102**(30):10604.

25 Novik K, Nimmrich I, Genc B, et al. Epigenomics: genome-wide study of methylation phenomena. *Curr Iss Mol Biol* 2002;**4**:111–128.

26 Francis D, Diorio J, Liu D, Meaney M. Nongenomic transmission across generations of maternal behavior and stress responses in the rat. *Science* 1999;**286**(5442):1155.

27 Weaver I, Szyf M, Meaney M. From maternal care to gene expression: DNA methylation and the maternal programming of stress responses. *Endocr Res* 2002;**28**(4):699.

28 Seckl J, Meaney M. Glucocorticoid "programming" and PTSD risk. *Ann NY Acad Sci* 2006;**1071**(1): 351–378.

29 Weaver I. Epigenetic programming by maternal behavior and pharmacological intervention. Nature versus nurture: let's call the whole thing off. *Epigenetics* 2007;**2**(1):22.

30 Oberlander TF, Weinberg J, Papsdorf M, Grunau R, Misri S, Devlin AM. Prenatal exposure to maternal depression, neonatal methylation of human glucocorticoid receptor gene (NR3C1) and infant cortisol stress responses. *Epigenetics* 2008;**3**(2):97–106.

31 McGowan P, Sasaki A, D'Alessio A, et al. Epigenetic regulation of the glucocorticoid receptor in human brain associates with childhood abuse. *Nat Neurosci* 2009;**12**(3):342–348.

32 Lee RS, Tamashiro KLK, Yang X, et al. Chronic corticosterone exposure increases expression and decreases deoxyribonucleic acid methylation of Fkbp5 in mice. *Endocrinology* 2010;**151**(9): 4332–4343.

33 Yehuda R, Cai G, Golier JA, et al. Gene expression patterns associated with posttraumatic stress disorder following exposure to the World Trade Center attacks. *Biol Psychiatry* 2009;**66**(7): 708–711.

34 Mehta D, Gonik M, Klengel T, et al. Using polymorphisms in FKBP5 to define biologically distinct subtypes of posttraumatic stress disorder: evidence from endocrine and gene expression studies. *Arch Gen Psychiatry* 2011;**68**(9):901–910.

35 Koenen KC, Uddin M, Chang SC, et al. SLC6A4 methylation modifies the effect of the number of traumatic events on risk for posttraumatic stress disorder. *Depress Anxiety* 2011;**28**(8):639–647.

36 Szyf M. Epigenetics, DNA methylation, and chromatin modifying drugs. *Annu Rev Pharmacol Toxicol* 2009;**49**:243–263.

37 Champagne FA, Curley JP. Epigenetic mechanisms mediating the long-term effects of maternal care on development. *Neurosci Biobehav Rev* 2009;**33**(4):593–600.

38 Nestler EJ. Hidden switches in the mind. *Scient Amer* 2011;**305**(6):76–83.

39 Middlebrooks JS, Audage NC. *The effects of childhood stress on health across the lifespan*. Atlanta: Centers for Disease Control and Prevention; 2008.

40 McEwen BS. Physiology and neurobiology of stress and adaptation: central role of the brain. *Physiol Rev* 2007;**87**(3):873–904.

41 Davis M. The role of the amygdala in fear and anxiety. *Annu Rev Neurosci* 1992;**15**(1):353–375.

42 Rauch SL, Whalen PJ, Shin LM, et al. Exaggerated amygdala response to masked facial stimuli in posttraumatic stress disorder: a functional MRI study. *Biol Psychiatry* 2000;**47**(9):769–776.

43 Thomaes K, Dorrepaal E, Draijer N, et al. Reduced anterior cingulate and orbitofrontal volumes in child abuse-related complex PTSD. *J Clin Psychiatry* 2010;**71**(12):1636.

44 Shin LM, Rauch SL, Pitman RK. Amygdala, medial prefrontal cortex, and hippocampal function in PTSD. *Ann NY Acad Sci* 2006;**1071**(1):67–79.

45 Shin LM, Orr SP, Carson MA, et al. Regional cerebral blood flow in the amygdala and medial prefrontal cortex during traumatic imagery in male and female Vietnam veterans with PTSD. *Arch Gen Psychiatry* 2004;**61**(2):168.

46 Bremner JD. Traumatic stress: effects on the brain. *Dialog Clin Neurosci* 2006;**8**(4):445.

47 Woon FL, Sood S, Hedges DW. Hippocampal volume deficits associated with exposure to psychological trauma and posttraumatic stress disorder in adults: a meta-analysis. *Prog Neuropsychopharmacol Biol Psychiatry* 2010;**34**(7):1181.

48 Tottenham N, Hare TA, Quinn BT, et al. Prolonged institutional rearing is associated with atypically large amygdala volume and difficulties in emotion regulation. *Dev Sci* 2009;**13**(1):46–61.

49 Hanson JL, Chung MK, Avants BB, et al. Early stress is associated with alterations in the orbitofrontal cortex: a tensor-based morphometry investigation of brain structure and behavioral risk. *J Neurosci* 2010;**30**(22):7466–7472.

50 Pezawas L, Meyer-Lindenberg A, Drabant E, et al. 5-HTTLPR polymorphism impacts human cingulate–amygdala interactions: a genetic susceptibility mechanism for depression. *Nature* 2005;**8**(6):828–834.

51 Stein MB, Koverola C, Hanna C, Torchia M, McClarty B. Hippocampal volume in women victimized by childhood sexual abuse. *Psychol Med* 1997;**27**(4):951–959.

52 Bremner JD, Narayan M. The effects of stress on memory and the hippocampus throughout the life cycle: implications for childhood development and aging. *Dev Psychopathol* 1998;**10**(4):871–885.

53 Brown J, Cooper-Kuhn CM, Kempermann G, et al. Enriched environment and physical activity stimulate hippocampal but not olfactory bulb neurogenesis. *Eur J Neurosci* 2003;**17**(10):2042–2046.

54 DeRubeis RJ, Siegle GJ, Hollon SD. Cognitive therapy versus medication for depression: treatment outcomes and neural mechanisms. *Nat Rev Neurosci* 2008;**9**(10):788–796.

55 Hölzel BK, Carmody J, Evans KC, et al. Stress reduction correlates with structural changes in the amygdala. *Social Cogn Affect Neurosci* 2010;**5**(1):11–17.

56 Parker KJ, Buckmaster CL, Schatzberg AF, Lyons DM. Prospective investigation of stress inoculation in young monkeys. *Arch Gen Psychiatry* 2004;**61**(9):933.

57 Parker KJ, Buckmaster CL, Justus KR, Schatzberg AF, Lyons DM. Mild early life stress enhances prefrontal-dependent response inhibition in monkeys. *Biol Psychiatry* 2005;**57**(8):848–855.

58 Lyons DM, Parker KJ. Stress inoculation-induced indications of resilience in monkeys. *J Traum Stress* 2007;**20**(4):423–433.

59 Katz M, Liu C, Schaer M, et al. Prefrontal plasticity and stress inoculation-induced resilience. *Dev Neurosci* 2009;**31**(4):293–299.

60 van Hasselt FN, Cornelisse S, Yuan Zhang T, et al. Adult hippocampal glucocorticoid receptor expression and dentate synaptic plasticity correlate with maternal care received by individuals early in life. *Hippocampus* 2012;**22**(2):255–266.

61 Gianaros PJ, Horenstein JA, Cohen S, et al. Perigenual anterior cingulate morphology covaries with perceived social standing. *Social Cogn Affect Neurosci* 2007;**2**(3):161–173.

62 Hanson JL, Chandra A, Wolfe BL, Pollak SD. Association between income and the hippocampus. *PloS One* 2011;**6**(5):e18712.

63 Gianaros PJ, Horenstein JA, Hariri AR, et al. Potential neural embedding of parental social standing. *Social Cogn Affect Neurosci* 2008;**3**(2):91–96.

64 **Hackman DA, Farah MJ, Meaney MJ.** Socioeconomic status and the brain: mechanistic insights from human and animal research. *Nat Rev Neurosci* 2010;**11**(9):651–659.

65 **McEwen BS, Seeman T.** Protective and damaging effects of mediators of stress: elaborating and testing the concepts of allostasis and allostatic load. *Ann NY Acad Sci* 2006;**896**(1):30–47.

66 **Shonkoff JP.** Building a new biodevelopmental framework to guide the future of early childhood policy. *Child Dev* 2010;**81**(1):357–367.

67 **Ressler KJ, Mercer KB, Bradley B, et al.** Post-traumatic stress disorder is associated with PACAP and the PAC1 receptor. *Nature* 2011;**470**(7335):492–497.

New directions in the life course epidemiology of mental illness

Chapter 25

Intergenerational transmission

Virginia Warner and Myrna M. Weissman

25.1 Introduction

Multigenerational, also referred to as transgenerational, family studies examining transmission of mental illness among biological relatives were popular in the 1980s and 1990s but became less so as attention turned to molecular genetic studies. Information on familial transmission, comorbidity, subtypes (e.g. early onset recurrent depression), and early risk factors of later disease (e.g. pre-pubertal fear predicting later adolescent onset depression) have been derived from multigenerational studies.[1,2] From the beginning, family studies have provided evidence demonstrating high familial loading and specificity of transmission of diagnosis for multiple disorders. These findings provided the basis for the use of multigenerational studies to examine endophenotypes.[3,4] The interest in multigenerational, longitudinal studies for depression, in particular, was stimulated in part by the strong findings that that the disorder was highly familial and began in adolescence. Therefore, the question was raised about the course of the disorder in high risk versus low risk families. Multigenerational studies have yielded insights into how familial characteristics, such as acute and chronic stress generated by lower socio-economic status, racial discrimination, and abusive parental behaviour, which play a role in the transmission of mental illness and are also transmitted across generations.[5]

High risk studies are a variant of family studies that focus on biological offspring at increased risk for a disorder usually by virtue of the presence of the same disorder in one or more parent. Such studies allow assessment to begin in the high risk offspring before the onset of symptoms and therefore identify risk factors that are premorbid to, rather than concomitant with, the disorder or a particular manifestation of it.[6,7] High risk samples are also populated with non-ill but at-risk individuals; therefore the high risk design is well-suited for discovering endophenotypes (i.e. biological trait markers associated with the diseases but that can be measured independently of the disease state). The measurement and understanding of endophenotypes has led to a much greater understanding of the multigenerational transmission of mental illness.[8]

25.2 What is intergenerational transmission and how is it associated with life course epidemiology?

Life course epidemiology attempts to elucidate the mechanisms by which biological, environmental, and social characteristics alter the risk for mental illness by exposure during all phases of life and how transmission of these characteristics increases risk across generations. Intergenerational studies attempt to describe associations across generations, elucidate mechanisms underlying associations, and to quantify the extent to which different mechanisms explain associations across generations.[9] Intergenerational studies obtain information from multiple family members from at least two generations and examine associations between these characteristics[9] Intergenerational, family studies offer a much broader understanding of the critical impact of family environment and its transmission on mental illness in families. Family studies also provide feedback from multiple family members on the same characteristic such as parental behaviour leading to a more valid interpretation of the family environment. In addition, it allows clinical assessments of multiple family members which provide a more accurate determination of whether the disorder is transmitted across generations, clustering within families, the proportion of family members affected, and the key characteristics involved in the transmission. Many different characteristics can be transmitted across generations and can affect mental health outcomes. Genetic characteristics, parenting behaviour, educational status, cigarette smoking, socio-economic status, sexual abuse, emotional abuse, physical abuse, and other traumatic events are merely examples of a few such characteristics, most of which can increase exposure to acute and chronic stress which plays an important role with regard to endophenotypes and risk for mental illness. Not taking these factors into account can easily lead to inaccurate conclusions when attempting to determine the risk for mental illness, how to prevent it, how to treat it, and how to define it.

Three- or more generation studies, particularly if they are longitudinal, allow examination of whether mechanisms that may be involved in the transmission of mental illness from generation 1 (G1) to generation 2 (G2) are replicated when examining transmission from generation 2 to generation 3 (G3), which in turn strengthens the findings. Multigenerational studies allow extension of the life course. The life course of a parent and/or grandparent can easily contribute to, and possibly be replicated by, the life course of the child and grandchild. Examining genes and endophenotypes makes it possible to better understand the steps in the life course of mental illness prior to its onset.

Figure 25.1 provides an example of the intergenerational transmission of mental illness in a family with three generations and is focused on the pathways to mental illness in G3. Box 25.1 includes risk factors, symptoms and diagnoses that could be transmitted from G1 to G2 and/or G3. Box 25.2 includes the same information for G2. Box 25.3 includes exposure of G3 to risk factors by developmental phase. Box 25.4 demonstrates changes in biological measures, the onset of symptoms and of diagnoses by developmental phase. Box 25.5 points out the potential importance of community factors. The shaded arrows demonstrate that some of the transmission from G1 to G3 may be direct and not all is indirect via G2. It is important for the study to be longitudinal so that prodromal symptoms and the impact of exposures by developmental phase can be evaluated. For example, Figure 25.1 illustrates how G3 was exposed to risk factors for mental illness that varied by developmental phase that in turn led to the onset of prodromal symptoms and subsequently the onset of diagnoses that met criteria. This figure also demonstrates how important it is to know the mental health history of prior generations. The high rates of mental illness, poor parenting skills, and genotypes known to increase the risk for mental illness in G1 is transmitted to G2 and G3 directly and indirectly. This emphasizes that there are multiple pathways from parent to child mental illness. The figure also illustrates the importance of community environment and biological contributions. For instance, sexual abuse from age 7 to 13 years may be associated with G3 decreased hippocampal volume. It has been shown that the impact of abuse on the brain varies by developmental phase, and decreased hippocampal volume has been shown to be associated with familial depression.[10,11] Lastly, the figure demonstrates that the G1 mental illness and behavioural issues impact the risk for G3 mental illness directly, moderate the effect of G2 on G3, and the effect of G1 on G3 can be mediated by G2 characteristics. The fact that both G1 and G2 have alcohol use disorder could have an additive effect on the risk of substance abuse in G3. The effect of G1's poor parenting on mental illness in G3 could be mediated by G2's poor parenting

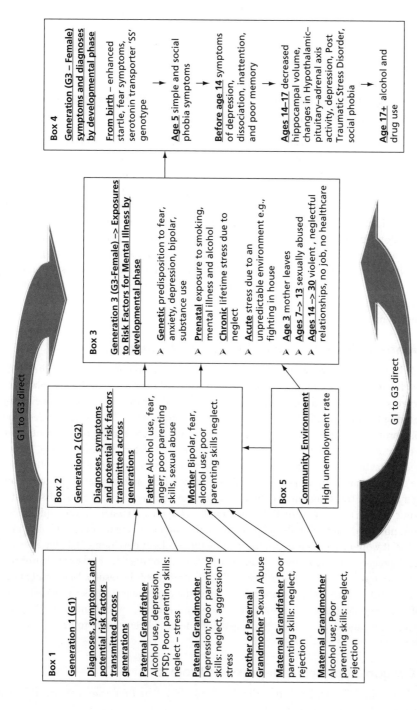

Figure 25.1 Example of intergenerational transmission of mental illness: three generations.

skills. The genotypes of G1 and G2 can interact with chronic and acute stress, increasing the risk for mental illness in G3. In addition, environmental stress due to factors such as changes in the unemployment rates in the population can be important moderators of the association between G2 and G3 mental illness.

In Section 25.3 we review and summarize actual longitudinal, multigenerational studies that have tested some of the hypotheses that are generated from Figure 25.1.

25.3 Multigenerational, longitudinal studies of mental illness and risk factors for mental illness

Table 25.1 includes descriptions of multigenerational studies of mental illness and risk factors for mental illness. The table includes sample size, age, gender, ethnicity, socio-economic status, whether the study includes biological measures, the number of generations, and length of follow-up. The predominant focus is on major depressive disorder, but disorders shown to be comorbid with depression such as substance use, prodromal symptoms, and a variety of risk factors for multiple mental illnesses are also examined. Relatively few multigenerational studies have included endophenotypes. The ones that do not include endophenotypes nevertheless provide vital information regarding possible causal factors in familial transmission of mental illness. The table describes studies with and without endophenotypes or biological measures. For each study we review the findings regarding intergenerational transmission, their association with life course epidemiology, and the limitations of each study. First, we review multigenerational studies without biological markers.

25.3.1 Mater-university study of pregnancy, Australia

The study tested hypotheses of the intergenerational transmission of stress and depression, and examined the role of early childhood adversity and maternal depression in the interplay between youth depression and stress over 20 years.[5] Stress, acute and chronic, was shown to be important with regard to the intergenerational transmission of mental illness. This study, as described in Table 25.1, provides evidence that youth of depressed mothers are at risk not only for depression but also for continuing experiences of acute and chronic stress from childhood to age 20 years. It also suggests that the intergenerational transmission of depression from mothers to offspring may be in the earliest years of the child's life (birth to 5 years). Not only are there long-term patterns of intergenerational transmission of depression, but also intergenerational transmission of acute and chronic stress.[5] Limitations include: the sample is largely Caucasian, lower-middle income, and the number of depressed male offspring is small. Therefore, the results could vary in other populations. It would have been useful to examine the results at developmental phases critical to brain development and to examine prenatal stress. The role of the father was not examined. The examination of more than two generations could also strengthen the results. Neurobiological and genetic factors likely play an important role in understanding the mechanisms, as well as occurrence, of stress and depression. For example, endophenotypes such as enhanced startle response, cortical thinning, and decreased hippocampal volume have been shown to be associated with stress and depression.[12–14]

25.3.2 Oregon Adolescent Depression Project

Two studies from this sample are described in Table 25.1. The first examines the influence of grandparental (G1) and parental (G2) substance use disorder on grandchild (G3) emotional disorder (EmD).[15] The second study examines the influence of G1 and G2 major depressive

Table 25.1 Multi-generational, longitudinal studies of mental illness and risk factors for mental illness

Study	No. of participants	Age	Gender, ethnicity, and socio-economic status	Biological measures	No. of generations	Length of follow-up
Mater-University Study of Pregnancy, Australia[43]	815 families G2 = 705; 62 exposed to maternal depression birth to 5 years of age	G2: birth to 5 years 15 years of age 20 years of age	G2: 52% females; 92% Caucasian lower middle class	No	2	20 years
Oregon Adolescent Depression Project (OADP).[15,16]	284 families G2 probands: 55.2% one or more G1 with substance use; 54.9% with emotional disorder. G2: 40.1% and 65.8% lifetime substance use and emotional disorders. G3: n = 284	Grandfather (G1): mean 50.69 (SD 5.47) years. Grandmother (G1): 48.71 (4.37) years. G2: 27.38 (2.72) years. G3: 4.74 (2.43) years	G2: 65.5% females. G3: 50.4% females. 90% Caucasian middle class	No	3	14 years

Table 25.1 (continued) Multi-generational, longitudinal studies of mental illness and risk factors for mental illness

Study	No. of participants	Age	Gender, ethnicity, and socio-economic status	Biological measures	No. of generations	Length of follow-up
Iowa Family Transitions Project: Angry and Aggressive Behaviour Across Three Generations[17]	G2: probands n = 75 G3: n = 74	G2: mean 22 years G3: mean 2.4 years	G2: 65% female. G3: 37% female. 100% Caucasian lower middle or middle class	No	3	First G1 and G2 assessments 1989 to 1991, then annually through 1999; G3 began in 1997
Inner City London[19]	G1 = probands; 276 mother–offspring pairs; 172 low risk, 104 high risk with vulnerable (conflict with partner or child, lack of support or low self-esteem) mothers	Mean (SD) offspring average: 20 (3.7) years; mothers 38 (5.8) years	G2: 48% females; 85% Caucasian; 55% working class	No	2	Prospectively over a year, lifetime history obtained
Cambridge Study in Delinquent Development (CSDD)[18]	G1: n = 408 males, n = 411 females. G2 probands: n = 411, 178 with children. G3: n = 322	G2: assessed at ages 16, 18, 21, 25, and 32 years. G3: assessed at ages 3–15, mean 7 years	G2: 100% male. G3: 47.5% female. G2: 92% Caucasian working class	No	3	24 years

Table 25.1 (continued) Multi-generational, longitudinal studies of mental illness and risk factors for mental illness

Study	No. of participants	Age	Gender, ethnicity, and socio-economic status	Biological measures	No. of generations	Length of follow-up
Sexually abused females from Child Protective Service agencies and non-abused females in the greater Washington DC metropolitan area[23,24]	G2 = proband females; 84 G2 sexually abused; 89 G2 not sexually abused; 67 G3 with sexually abused mothers, 56 without sexually abused mothers	G2: median age 11 years at the first assessment and median age 25 years at the sixth assessment. G3: mean (SD) abused mother 4.60 (3.35) years comparison: 3.56 (2.57) years female caregiver (G1) 96% were biological mothers the mean age was 35.4 (SD 5.5) years	G2: 100% females. G3: offspring of abused mothers = 56% females. G3: offspring of comparison mothers = 49% females. G2: 49% Caucasian, 46% African-American, 4% Hispanic, and 1% Asian. G3: 53.7% minority mostly African-American with 3% Hispanic and 1% Asian working class	G2: ECG, vagal tone and withdrawal and cortisol from saliva samples during relaxation and a 10 min cognitive stressor. Incorrect responses were followed by a loud, aversive noise	3	23 years
EEG, sleep and hypothalamic–pituitary–adrenal (HPA) activity and depression[25]	48 adolescents (G2) with no personal history of depression at high risk for depression due to parental depression (G1) and 48 low risk adolescents with no personal or family history of depression	G2: ~15 years of age in both groups	G2: 60% of controls female, 56% of high risk females; 48% Caucasian, remainder African-American, Asian and Hispanic middle and upper middle classes	G2: EEG, sleep and HPA salivary cortisol prior to sleep and nocturnal urinary free cortisol measures	2	6-month intervals for first year, annual for 5 years

Table 25.1 (continued) Multi-generational, longitudinal studies of mental illness and risk factors for mental illness

Study	No. of participants	Age	Gender, ethnicity, and socio-economic status	Biological measures	No. of generations	Length of follow-up
Stanford High-Risk Project[27,28]	200 never-disordered girls (G2), half of whom are at familial risk for the development of major depressive disorder	G2 between the ages of 10 and 14 years	G2: 100% female	G2: saliva samples during the laboratory stress paradigm, genotyping, structural and functional MRI	2	Six years
Pittsburgh Multigenerational Study of Depression[30–32]	3 parental groups (G1): those with child onset depression, those with childhood onset bipolar, and normals—with no major psychiatric disorder	G2 subsample 1: mean age 7.8 years, SD 80 years.[13] G2 subsample 2: mean age, years: 3.7, SD 2.1 at initial assessment, 4/5 assessment, last at age ~9 years.[14] G2 subsample 3: age, mean (SD), years, low risk mean (SD): 7.93 (2.06); high risk mean (SD): 7.36 (1.53)[15]	G2 subsample 1: 39% females; 39% Caucasian; parents primarily high school graduates.[13] G2 subsample 2: 47% females; 62%; Caucasian G2 subsample 3: 48% of mothers some college education.[14] sex (% male) low risk: 55 high risk: 51. Race (% Caucasian) low risk: 54; high risk: 55. Parental education level (% high school diploma or above) low risk: 91, high risk: 93[15]	G2 subsample 1: behavioural reaction time, event-related potential[13] G2 subsample 2: seven annual, structured laboratory tasks that were designed to elicit positive affect and negative affect.[4] G2 subsample 3: EEG frontal; EEG was recorded while participant watched emotion-eliciting films[15]	2	14 years

Table 25.1 (continued) Multi-generational, longitudinal studies of mental illness and risk factors for mental illness

Study	No. of participants	Age	Gender, ethnicity, and socio-economic status	Biological measures	No. of generations	Length of follow-up
Stony Brook Temperament Study[33,44]	556 families, children G2 without mood disorders. G2 with at least one parent (G1) with mood disorder (high risk), n = 219, 41%[17]	G2: mean age was 43.5 months (SD = 2.8). Age, mean (SD), months, low risk: 43.82 (2.71); high risk: 42.88 (3.00)	G2: 50% females; 88% Caucasian; 98% middle-class families. G2 subsample: sex, male (%), low risk: 56; high risk: 41; ≥1 parent college graduate (%), low risk: 28; high risk: 2	G2 subsample: Stress-inducing laboratory tasks, and four salivary cortisol samples were obtained	2	6 years
Children at High and Low Risk for Depression[14,39–42]	G1: n = 188. G2: n = 295; 208 high risk (one or more parent depressed) 87 low risk (neither parent depressed). G3: n = 181; 110 high risk; 71 low risk	G2 mean (SE) age: 35.3 (1.5) years. G3 mean (SE) age: 14.6 (1.1) years[18]	G2: 53% female. G3: 53% female; 100% Caucasian; 74% lower/middle class	DNA samples: G1, G2, G3. G2 and G3 subsample: Fear and Anxiety Potentiated Startle[18] G2 and G3 subsample: structural MRI.[19] G2 and G3 subsamples: quantitative EEG[21,22]	3	30 years

G1, Generation 1; G2, Generation 2; G3, Generation 3; MRI, magnetic resonance imaging; EEG electroencephalogram.

disorder (MDD) on behaviour problems in young children.[16] In the three-generation sample, results indicated that MDD in G1 is associated with increased risk for depression in G3, even in the absence of G2 MDD, G1 and G2 substance use, and independent of G1 and G2 emotional disorder.[15] These findings point out the importance of taking into account multiple generations as well as comorbid disorders such as substance use in the life course of mental illness. This study had several limitations: (i) they were unable to obtain diagnostic information on all G1 and G2 participants; (ii) the Child Behavior Check List (CBCL) was used for the measurement of EmD in G3; (iii) the role of parental informants; (iv) the sample may not be representative of the general population; (v) information on the timing, onset, and course of disorders was not considered; (vi) the age range of G3 was limited; and (vii) G3 offspring had not passed through peak risk period for EmD onset. The study provides heritability information on only 50% of the G2 parents and G1 grandparents. There was insufficient power to examine whether risk differed depending on the gender of grandchildren.

25.3.3 Iowa Family Transitions

This study examined intergenerational transmission and interaction of both angry, aggressive parenting and angry, aggressive behaviour of children and adolescents.[17] Whereas this does not deal directly with the transmission of mental illness, it examines the transmission of an important potential risk factor (aggressive parenting) for mental illness. G1 aggressive parenting predicted G2 aggressive parenting, and G2 aggressive parenting increased the risk of G3 aggressive behaviour. Aggressive behaviour was therefore transmitted across three generations. The generalizability of the results was limited because the sample of G2 parents and G3 children was relatively small and of singular ethnicity. The transmission of parental behaviour plays a substantial role in the intergenerational transmission of mental illness; however, the study could be greatly strengthened by the addition of mental illness outcomes.

25.3.4 Inner City London

This study addresses the extent to which antisocial behaviour in parents predicts antisocial behaviour in children in two successive generations; the degree to which a man's childhood antisocial behaviour predicts antisocial behaviour in his own children; the extent to which parenting problems are related to child antisocial behaviour similarly in two successive generations; and the extent to which intergenerational continuities in antisocial behaviour are mediated by parenting variables.[18] An investigation of intergenerational factors associated with psychiatric disorder in late adolescence/early adulthood attempted to elucidate the influences from maternal disorder, maternal poor psychosocial functioning and poor parenting, on offspring.[19] Maternal characteristics including psychosocial vulnerability and depression were examined in relation to risk transmission. The results demonstrated that abuse and neglect of the child and maternal vulnerability increased the risk of offspring disorder whereas maternal depression did not. To fully understand intergenerational transmission and life course of disorders, factors such as these must be measured, not just mental illness diagnoses. Limitations include: information was only available on two generations; and the collection of information on potential endophenotyes would help to understand the findings.

25.3.5 Cambridge Study in Delinquent Development (CSDD)

The CSDD includes data on 411 Inner London males (Generation 2, or G2), their female partners, their parents (G1) and their children (G3).[18] This study, like the others with three generations, provides a longer timeline and a better understanding of the life course of externalizing disorders. It demonstrates the role of the transmission of behaviour (such as aggressive parenting and poor supervision) as well as the importance of assortative mating in the transmission of mental illness across generations. Some limitations include: additional unmeasured G2 maternal characteristics may have contributed to the transmission of conduct problems in G3; and the incorporation of stress measurements and the measurement of endophenotypes could also help explain the results.

25.4 Multigenerational studies with endophenotypes and other biological markers

25.4.1 Endophenotypes

Biological markers can be either state or trait markers; endophenotypes are trait markers.[20] An endophenotype is a measured component unseen by the unaided eye along the causal pathway from gene to mental illness disease. An endophenotype can be neurophysiological, biochemical, endrocrinological, neuroanatomical, or neuropsychological.[21] Some endophenotypes may be associated with genetic variants or with neural circuitry affected by risk gene variants.[22] Endophenotypes not only help target aetiology and mechanisms, but can also help identify persons who are at increased risk, so that they can be targeted for appropriate intervention. They can also be used to strengthen classifications of clinical phenotypes, or to differentiate possible biological subtypes that may in turn have different clinical or treatment profiles. A majority of studies thus far, however, have targeted state markers by comparing depressed with non-depressed, or sometimes non-ill, subjects. What these comparisons yield, however, are correlates of illness measured at an end stage. The more rigorous definition requires it to lie in the causal pathway to disease (that is, it should not arise as a result of the disease); it should be heritable or familial; and state independent (that is, it should be observed in subjects who are at risk but not currently symptomatic).[21] Because the high risk (cohort) design (unlike case–control studies) conditions subjects based on their risk for, rather than presence of, the outcome of interest, it is particularly well suited to meet these requirements.

The next studies reviewed include biological markers.

25.4.2 Three-generation, longitudinal study of the impact of sexual abuse: Child Protective Service agencies in the greater Washington DC metropolitan area

This 23-year, three-generation, longitudinal study examined the impact of intrafamilial sexual abuse on female development.[23] Participants included females with substantiated sexual abuse predominately by the father and a demographically similar comparison group. The study also examined a potential endophenotype (hypothalamic–pituitary–adrenal axis (HPA) activity). A prior history of childhood sexual abuse predicted a simultaneous vagal withdrawal, the change in vagal tone from the relaxation condition to the cognitive stressor condition ($V_w = V_{relax} - V_{stressor}$), and blunted cortisol response to a cognitive stressor 7 years after the documented sexual abuse in late adolescence. This response predicted both higher levels of depression and antisocial behaviours in young adulthood.[24] The study also indicated that childhood maltreatment was transmitted across the generations which, as in G2, will likely lead to high rates of mental illness in G3. The question remains as to whether HPA activity in G3 may be altered in the same way as in G2 due to maltreatment, and in addition may act as a predictor of increased mental illness in

G3. The generalizability of the findings could be limited, partially due to the fact that the study does not examine the impact of sexual abuse on male children.

25.4.3 Electroencephalogram (EEG), sleep, and HPA changes in healthy adolescents at high risk for depression

The aim of this study was to identify depression-related EEG sleep and HPA changes in healthy adolescents at high risk for depression, and to examine the relationship between EEG sleep (or HPA) changes and the onset of depression. In the Rao and Hammen study of adolescent girls at high risk for depression due to having a parent with depression and low risk females with no personal or family history of depression, EEG, sleep, and HPA were studied for 5 years at regular intervals.[25] Adolescents at high risk had shorter latency to rapid eye movement (REM) sleep, increased phasic REM sleep, more REM sleep, and elevated nocturnal urinary-free cortisol (NUFC) excretion at baseline. In addition, shorter REM latency, higher REM density, and elevated NUFC and elevated HPA activity occurred before the onset of depression and were associated with the subsequent onset of depression. These changes suggest that they may serve as vulnerability markers for depression that could contribute to familial transmission of depression. Limitations include a relatively small sample size, only females in the study, relatively short follow-up, and symptom and functional measures that did not always coincide with the onset of the depressive episode.

25.4.4 Stanford High Risk Project

Over the past 6 years, a sample of never-disordered girls, half of whom are at familial risk for the development of MDD, were recruited, carefully diagnosed, and—to elucidate mechanisms that might underlie the intergenerational transmission of risk for depression—cognitive biases, biological stress reactivity, emotion (dys)regulation, neural function and structure, and reward processing have been assessed.[26] Although the high risk girls were asymptomatic at entry to the study, it was found that they nevertheless already resembled individuals diagnosed with MDD in several important ways. Girls who were homozygous for the *s* allele produced higher and more prolonged levels of cortisol in response to a stressor than did girls with an *l* allele. These findings indicate that the *5HTTLPR* polymorphism is associated with biological stress of stressful life events.[26] While the association of the *s* allele could be related to intergenerational transmission, it was not examined due to the lack of a statistically significant difference in the rates of the allele in the high and low risk groups. Similar to the Rao study, reduced sleep quality was also found in the healthy girls of mothers with a history of recurrent MDD compared with girls of 21 mothers with no history of MDD.[27] Daughters of depressed mothers required greater intensity than did daughters of control mothers to accurately identify sad facial expressions; they also made significantly more errors identifying angry expressions.[28] In the same sample, during sad mood induction, high risk girls exhibited greater activation than did low risk girls, including the amygdala and ventrolateral prefrontal cortex. By contrast, during automatic mood regulation, low risk daughters exhibited greater activation than did their high risk daughters in brain areas that have frequently been associated with top-down regulation of emotion, including the dorsolateral prefrontal cortex and dorsal anterior cingulate cortex. These results suggest that anomalies in neural functioning precede the onset of a depressive episode and may contribute to intergenerational transmission.[29] The greatest limitations in this study are that these tests were not done on the entire sample, were only done on females, and did not have follow-up data to determine if they predicted onset of depression. Furthermore, in the *5HTTLPR* study, despite the fact that there was no statistically significant difference in the rate of *s* allele across the high and low risk groups, there was a difference in the proportion in each group. Although the difference was not significant, it might have made sense to examine the two groups separately to determine whether, over time, the rates of depression in the two groups might vary by presence of the *s* allele.

25.4.5 Pittsburgh Multigenerational Study of Depression

In a series of studies using subsamples from a larger study of children of parents with childhood onset depression (COD) compared to children without a major psychiatric disorder, numerous vulnerability factors for depression have been examined. With the introduction of an affective stressor, COD children appear to perform similarly to children without a familial history of COD; however they deploy greater processing resources (increased frontal event-related potential amplitudes) and take greater care (increased reaction times) to do so.[30] In laboratory tests eliciting positive affects (PA) and negative affects (NA), attenuated PA (rather than excessive NA) was shown to be a possible early vulnerability factor for eventual unipolar depressive disorder in COD children and may represent one pathway through which depression is transmitted.[31] This study also examined whether frontal alpha EEG asymmetry moderates the association between stressful life events and depressive symptoms in children at familial risk for depression.[32] In COD children, greater relative left lateral frontal activation moderated the effects of stressful events on internalizing symptoms in at-risk children.[32] The limitations include: internalizing symptoms and life events were reported by the parent; the number of specific life events was also not recorded; and all of the findings in this study identify factors that could be involved in transgenerational transmission.

25.4.6 Stony Brook Temperament Study

The HPA axis is thought to play an important role in stress and the aetiology of depression. One hundred and sixty pre-school-age children in a study conducted by Dougherty et al. were exposed to stress-inducing tasks, and salivary cortisol samples were obtained.[33] Parents completed clinical interviews and a parent–child interaction task. The offspring who had high and increasing cortisol levels were those who were exposed to maternal depression during the first few years of life and who were exposed to parental hostility.[33] The greatest limitation of this particular study is that it was a cross-sectional design; however, it is a long term study and follow-up data could very likely be obtained. Other limitations include: the parent reported on child symptoms; the families were Caucasian and had two parents, so it was not a diverse sample; and there was no cortisol sample obtained under a situation without stress. It is more than likely that high cortisol, in an environment with hostile parenting, and familial predisposition to depression will significantly increase the likelihood of intergenerational transmission of depression and anxiety in these families.

25.4.7 Children at High and Low Risk for Depression

This is a 30-year, six-wave, and now four-generation, longitudinal study.[34] This family study of depression was initiated in 1982 to study patterns of transmission of MDD across generations of families. The project began with recruitment of two sets of probands. The first, selected from outpatient specialty clinics in the New Haven, Connecticut, area had moderate-to-severe major depression with impairment. Subsequently, at year 2, the first group was redefined as one or more parent with depression. The second group, selected concurrently and from the same community, was required to have no lifetime history of psychiatric illness as determined through multiple interviews. At year 2, this group was redefined as both parents without depression. The two groups were matched by age and gender.[35] Both proband groups (G1) were followed over time, along with their biological children (G2), grandchildren (G3) and more recently great-grandchildren (G4). The families where one or more parent (G1) had depression formed the 'high-risk' group, by virtue of their familial loading for depression, and those families where neither parent had depression (G1) formed the 'low risk' group. The overall study design is illustrated in Figure 25.2; further details can be found elsewhere.[34,36–38] These families have now been followed through five completed assessment waves (baseline, 2, 10, 20, and 25 years), with a sixth wave currently underway (Table 25.2). The first and second generations have been followed for the longest time (>30 years) and have now passed the age of highest risk for most psychopathology.

The clinical findings from this study document a clear transmission of MDD and anxiety across generations. Specifically, offspring of depressed parents were at increased risk for depression, anxiety, and substance use disorders.[34,36] The anxiety disorders began before puberty, with mood disorders emerging around puberty, especially in girls.[34] As the offspring aged, there was also a greater incidence of medical problems, particularly cardiovascular, in the high risk group.[34] As the third generation aged, similar patterns were found: they had high rates of early onset simple and social phobia, parental depression severity increased the likelihood of a mood disorder in the offspring, and offspring from families with two generations—i.e. both a parent and a grandparent—previously affected were at greatest risk for psychopathology.[37] Panic and phobic disorders also mediated the relationship between parental and offspring depression for both G2 and G3, whereas other disorders related to anxiety did not indicate that disorders associated with fear could play a role in transgenerational transmission in these families.[1]

Given the consistent patterns across waves and generations, we were interested in further identifying endophenotypes that may help explain why the offspring of depressed parents are at high risk. Furthermore, it is not only important to examine endophenotypes but their transmission across generations. At year 20 we collected startle data on G2 and G3. Enhanced anxiety-potentiated startle in G2 and G3 was shown to be associated with parental depression independent of G2 and G3 diagnoses of mental illness.[39] We are currently examining whether anxiety-potentiated startle measures brain activity that meets criteria for an endophenotype for a subtype of depression with comorbid childhood panic and/or phobia that is transmitted across generations.[1]

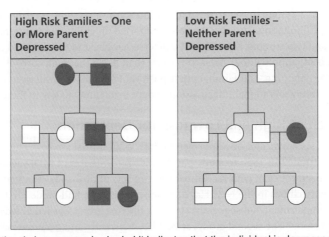

If the circle or square is shaded it indicates that the individual is depressed.

Figure 25.2 Study design.

Table 25.2 Assessments by year of data collection

	Year					
	Baseline	**2**	**10**	**20**	**25**	**≥30[a]**
Generation 1 (probands)	Clinical battery	Clinical battery	Clinical battery		Clinical battery DNA MRI	Clinical battery DNA EEG MRI
Generation 2 (children)	Clinical battery	Clinical battery		Clinical battery EEG Startle	Clinical battery DNA MRI	Clinical battery DNA EEG MRI
Generation 3 (grandchildren)	Clinical battery	Clinical battery	Clinical battery	Clinical battery EEG Startle	Clinical battery DNA MRI	Clinical battery DNA EEG MRI

MRI, magnetic resonance imaging; EEG electroencephalogram.

[a] A small number of Generation 4 (great-grandchildren) have participated so far in years ≥30.

Clinical battery: includes the SADS, the KSADS, self-reports, and symptom scales.

MRI: the assessment includes functional and structural MRI, neuropsychiatry measures, and IQ.

Adapted with permission from Talati A, Weissman MM, Hamilton SP, Using the high risk design to identify biomarkers for depression, *Philosophical Transactions in Biology*, 5 April 2013; Volume 368, Number 1615, Copyright © 2013 The Author(s). Published by the Royal Society. All rights reserved.

We have also collected data on other potential endophenotypes. At year 20 and currently we are collecting EEG data. Offspring (G2) with both parents having MDD showed greater alpha asymmetry at medial sites, with relatively less activity (more alpha) over right central and parietal regions, compared with offspring having one or no parent with MDD.[40] Similarly, G3 with both depressed parent and grandparent showed greater alpha asymmetry, with relatively less right than left hemisphere activity, when compared with those with neither depressed parent nor grandparent.[41] Both findings were independent of a diagnosis of mental illness.

At year 25, and currently, we are collecting structural and functional magnetic resonance imaging (MRI) data and DNA samples. We compared cortical thickness across high and low risk groups, detecting large expanses of cortical thinning across the lateral surface of the right cerebral hemisphere in persons at high risk.[14] Thinning correlated with measures of current symptom severity, inattention, and visual memory for social and emotional stimuli. EEG evidence of reduced cortical activity was associated with increased cortical thinning.[42] All of the endophenotypes in this study are currently being examined in an attempt to determine whether they are associated with anxiety-, stress-, and depression-related genes; and whether they predict new onsets of depression or anxiety as well as meet other criteria for endophenotypes.

The primary limitation of the study is that the depressed parents came from outpatient clinics, which limits the generalization of the study results to families with parents with moderate-to-severe depression, who have received treatment. Furthermore, the families are all Caucasian, predominantly of Irish or Italian origin, and working class; therefore, the results are likely to vary in more diverse populations.

25.5 **Summary and future directions**

The results of all the studies reviewed here consistently and clearly demonstrate key factors involved in the transmission of mental illness and risk factors for mental illness across generations. Consistent with Figure 25.1, they explicate the complexity of intergenerational transmission. Focusing only on the rates of a disorder gives a distorted view of transmission. Stress (chronic and acute), parental behaviour (e.g. neglect, aggression, hostility), and the timing of exposure to parental mental illness (in the first 5 years of life) in these studies appear to play important roles in intergenerational transmission.[5,17,43] The results from the studies with biological markers are also consistent with these factors being critical. Changes in HPA activity, sleep, startle reactivity, cortical thinning, and other factors shown in children at high risk for mental illness (in particular depression) are also shown to be associated with stress.[13,14,26,27,33,39]

It is important to include as many generations as possible to fully understand transmission. A three- as opposed to a two-generation study provides a much greater understanding of intergenerational transmission of mental illness, particularly since it has been shown that for some illnesses (i.e. depression) having a grandparent with depression—even if the parent does not have depression—puts the grandchild at higher risk for depression.[16] It is inaccurate to assume that only parents contribute to transmission of mental illness. The assessment of multiple generations gives a broader understanding of genetic, environmental and biological factors that play a role in transmission. G1 can have a direct impact on G3; for example, if G1 was diagnosed with bipolar disorder and G2 was not, this does not mean that related symptoms will not be expressed in G3. G1 can also provide valuable information about G2 that is not reported by G2, such as prenatal exposures to smoking, alcohol, or antidepressants, all of which might contribute to transmission of mental illness to G3.

One important future direction to pursue is the transmission of stress reactivity which has been shown to be consistent cross-species.[8] Meaney has shown that variations in maternal care alter the expression of genes that regulate behavioural and endocrine responses to stress, as well as hippocampal synaptic development. Maternal care also influences the maternal behaviour of female offspring, which appears to be related to oxytocin receptor gene expression, and forms the basis for the intergenerational transmission of individual differences in stress reactivity. These findings provide evidence for the importance of parental care as a mediator of the effects of environmental adversity on neural development.[8] Another important future direction is a greater focus on biological markers, in particular endophenotypes, and their role in the prevention of intergenerational transmission of mental illness. For studies collecting data on endophenotypes, it would be helpful if larger samples were collected, including more data on fathers and more generations. It would not be possible to unravel these mechanisms without taking a life course approach to multigenerational studies of mental illness.

References

1 **Warner V, Wickramaratne P, Weissman MM.** The role of fear and anxiety in the familial risk for major depression: a three-generation study. *Psychol Med* 2008;**38**(11):1543–1556.

2 **Levinson DF, Zubenko GS, Crowe RR, et al.** Genetics of recurrent early-onset depression (GenRED): design and preliminary clinical characteristics of a repository sample for genetic linkage studies. *Am J Med Genet B Neuropsychiatr Genet* 2003;**119B**(1):118–130.

3 **Weissman MM, Merikangas KR, John K, Wickramaratne P, Prusoff BA, Kidd KK.** Family-genetic studies of psychiatric disorders. Developing technologies. *Arch Gen Psychiatry* 1986;**43**(11):1104–1116.

4 **Weissman MM, Wickramaratne P, Merikangas KR, et al.** Onset of major depression in early adulthood. Increased familial loading and specificity. *Arch Gen Psychiatry* 1984;**41**(12):1136–1143.

5 **Hammen C, Hazel NA, Brennan PA, Najman J.** Intergenerational transmission and continuity of stress and depression: depressed women and their offspring in 20 years of follow-up. *Psychol Med* 2012;**42**(5):931–942.

6 **Hammen C, Burge D, Burney E, Adrian C.** Longitudinal study of diagnoses in children of women with unipolar and bipolar affective disorder. *Arch Gen Psychiatry* 1990;**47**(12):1112–1117.

7 **Lieb R, Isensee B, Hofler M, Pfister H, Wittchen HU.** Parental major depression and the risk of depression and other mental disorders in offspring: a prospective-longitudinal community study. *Arch Gen Psychiatry* 2002;**59**(4):365–374.

8 **Meaney MJ.** Maternal care, gene expression, and the transmission of individual differences in stress reactivity across generations. *Annu Rev Neurosci* 2001;**24**:1161–1192.

9 **Lawlor DA, Leary, S, Smith, GD.** Theoretical underpinnings for the use of intergenerational studies in life course epidemiology. In: Lawlor DA, Mishra, Gita D, editors. *Family matters*. New York: Oxford University Press; 2009. pp. 13–56.

10 **Andersen SL, Tomada A, Vincow ES, Valente E, Polcari A, Teicher MH.** Preliminary evidence for sensitive periods in the effect of childhood sexual abuse on regional brain development. *J Neuropsychiatry Clin Neurosci* 2008;**20**(3):292–301.

11 **Rosenberg DR, MacMaster FP, Mirza Y, Easter PC.** Imaging and neurocircuitry of pediatric major depression. *Clin Neuropsychiatry* 2006;**3**:219–229.

12 **Grillon C.** Startle reactivity and anxiety disorders: aversive conditioning, context, and neurobiology. *Biol Psychiatry* 2002;**52**(10):958–975.

13 **McEwen BS.** Protective and damaging effects of stress mediators: central role of the brain. *Dialogues Clin Neurosci* 2006;**8**(4):367–381.

14 **Peterson BS, Warner V, Bansal R, et al.** Cortical thinning in persons at increased familial risk for major depression. *Proc Natl Acad Sci USA* 2009;**106**(15):6273–6278.

15 **Leventhal AM, Pettit JW, Lewinsohn PM.** Familial influence of substance use disorder on emotional disorder across three generations. *Psychiatry Res* 2011;**185**(3):402–407.

16 **Olino TM, Pettit JW, Klein DN, Allen NB, Seeley JR, Lewinsohn PM.** Influence of parental and grandparental major depressive disorder on behavior problems in early childhood: a three-generation study. *J Am Acad Child Adolesc Psychiatry* 2008;**47**(1):53–60.

17 **Conger RD, Neppl T, Kim KJ, Scaramella L.** Angry and aggressive behavior across three generations: a prospective, longitudinal study of parents and children. *J Abnorm Child Psychol* 2003;**31**(2):143–160.

18 **Smith CA, Farrington DP.** Continuities in antisocial behavior and parenting across three generations. *J Child Psychol Psychiatry* 2004;**45**(2):230–247.

19 **Bifulco A, Moran PM, Ball C, et al.** Childhood adversity, parental vulnerability and disorder: examining inter-generational transmission of risk. *J Child Psychol Psychiatry* 2002;**43**(8):1075–1086.

20 **Ritsner MS, Gottesman, Irving I.** Where do we stand in the quest for neuropsychiatric biomarkers and endophenotypes and what next? In: Ritsner MS, editor. *The handbook of neuropsychiatric biomarkers, endophenotypes, and genes*. London: Springer; 2009. pp. 3–22.

21 **Gottesman, II, Gould TD.** The endophenotype concept in psychiatry: etymology and strategic intentions. *Am J Psychiatry* 2003;**160**(4):636–645.

22 **Meyer-Lindenberg A, Weinberger DR.** Intermediate phenotypes and genetic mechanisms of psychiatric disorders. *Nat Rev Neurosci* 2006;**7**(10):818–827.

23 **Trickett PKN, Jennie G, Putnam, Frank W.** The impact of sexual abuse on female development: Lessons from a multigenerational, longitudinal research study. *Dev Psychopathol* 2011;**23**(2):453–476.

24 Shenk CE, Noll JG, Putnam FW, Trickett PK. A prospective examination of the role of childhood sexual abuse and physiological asymmetry in the development of psychopathology. *Child Abuse Negl* 2010;**34**(10):752–761.

25 Rao U, Hammen CL, Poland RE. Risk markers for depression in adolescents: sleep and HPA measures. *Neuropsychopharmacology* 2009;**34**(8):1936–1945.

26 Gotlib IH, Joormann J, Minor KL, Hallmayer J. HPA axis reactivity: a mechanism underlying the associations among 5-HTTLPR, stress, and depression. *Biol Psychiatry* 2008;**63**(9):847–851.

27 Chen MC, Burley HW, Gotlib IH. Reduced sleep quality in healthy girls at risk for depression. *J Sleep Res* 2012;**21**(1):68–72.

28 Joormann J, Gilbert K, Gotlib IH. Emotion identification in girls at high risk for depression. *J Child Psychol Psychiatry* 2010;**51**(5):575–582.

29 Joormann J, Cooney RE, Henry ML, Gotlib IH. Neural correlates of automatic mood regulation in girls at high risk for depression. *J Abnorm Psychol* 2012;**121**(1):61–72.

30 Perez-Edgar K, Fox NA, Cohn JF, Kovacs M. Behavioral and electrophysiological markers of selective attention in children of parents with a history of depression. *Biol Psychiatry* 2006;**60**(10):1131–1138.

31 Olino TM, Lopez-Duran NL, Kovacs M, George CJ, Gentzler AL, Shaw DS. Developmental trajectories of positive and negative affect in children at high and low familial risk for depressive disorder. *J Child Psychol Psychiatry* 2011;**52**(7):792–799.

32 Lopez-Duran NL, Nusslock R, George C, Kovacs M. Frontal EEG asymmetry moderates the effects of stressful life events on internalizing symptoms in children at familial risk for depression. *Psychophysiology* 2012;**49**(4):510–521.

33 Dougherty LR, Klein DN, Rose S, Laptook RS. Hypothalamic–pituitary–adrenal axis reactivity in the preschool-age offspring of depressed parents: moderation by early parenting. *Psychol Sci* 2011;**22**(5):650–658.

34 Weissman MM, Wickramaratne P, Nomura Y, Warner V, Pilowsky D, Verdeli H. Offspring of depressed parents: 20 years later. *Am J Psychiatry* 2006;**163**(6):1001–1008.

35 Weissman MM, Gershon ES, Kidd KK, et al. Psychiatric disorders in the relatives of probands with affective disorders. The Yale University–National Institute of Mental Health Collaborative Study. *Arch Gen Psychiatry* 1984;**41**(1):13–21.

36 Weissman MM, Warner V, Wickramaratne P, Moreau D, Olfson M. Offspring of depressed parents 10 years later. *Arch Gen Psychiatry* 1997;**54**(10):932–940.

37 Weissman MM, Wickramaratne P, Nomura Y, et al. Families at high and low risk for depression: a 3-generation study. *Arch Gen Psychiatry* 2005;**62**(1):29–36.

38 Warner V, Weissman MM, Fendrich M, Wickramaratne P, Moreau D. The course of major depression in the offspring of depressed parents. Incidence, recurrence, and recovery. *Arch Gen Psychiatry* 1992;**49**(10):795–801.

39 Grillon C, Warner V, Hille J, et al. Families at high and low risk for depression: a three-generation startle study. *Biol Psychiatry* 2005;**57**(9):953–960.

40 Bruder GE, Tenke CE, Warner V, et al. Electroencephalographic measures of regional hemispheric activity in offspring at risk for depressive disorders. Biol Psychiatry 2005;**57**(4):328–335.

41 Bruder GE, Tenke CE, Warner V, Weissman MM. Grandchildren at high and low risk for depression differ in EEG measures of regional brain asymmetry. *Biol Psychiatry* 2007;**62**(11):1317–1323.

42 Bruder GE, Bansal R, Tenke CE, et al. Relationship of resting EEG with anatomical MRI measures in individuals at high and low risk for depression. *Hum Brain Mapp* 2012;**33**(6):1325–1333.

43 Hammen C, Brennan PA, Le Brocque R. Youth depression and early childrearing: stress generation and intergenerational transmission of depression. *J Consult Clin Psychol* 2011;**79**(3):353–363.

Chapter 26

Mental disorders and the emergence of physical disorders

Laura D. Kubzansky and Ashley Winning

26.1 Introduction

[T]he origin or cause of most men and women's sickness, disease and death, is first some great
discontent which brings a habit of sadness of mind

John Archer 1673[1]

Interest in the connection between the mind and the body, between mental health and physical
health, has existed since ancient times, although beliefs about the nature of the connection has
shifted over time. For example, Hippocrates (460–370 BCE) considered melancholic temperament
to be produced by excess black bile that led first to depression and then physical illness.[2] In 1628,
Sir William Harvey—a pioneer in cardiovascular physiology—declared that mental disturbances
influenced the heart.[3] Psychoanalytic theory of the early and mid-twentiethth century proposed
that physical symptoms and disease were manifestations of underlying psychological conflicts.[4]
When these ideas were tested empirically with the limited measures and methods available, findings were inconsistent and the notion that mental states might influence physical health fell out of
favour. However, interest in this relationship revived as more data and methods became available
to conduct better empirical tests and more consistent findings emerged. With the recognition that
high levels of healthcare utilization accompany high levels of distress and the unmet public health
challenge this creates, there is now added urgency for understanding the relation between mental
disorders and physical health.[5]

Given the substantial body of evidence demonstrating a consistent association between emotion, emotion-related disorders, and health, scholarly attention is increasingly focused on the
potential importance of mental health in *determining* physical health. A relationship between
mental and physical health can be considered from numerous angles, and evidence that physical
illness may lead to distress and subsequent poor mental health (e.g. depression following cancer
diagnosis) is well established.[6,7] Whether mental disorders actually influence the development
of physical disease is more controversial. However, a more comprehensive understanding of the
interrelationship between mental and physical health would substantially improve our ability to
devise targeted prevention and intervention strategies to improve population health.

Thus, in this chapter we evaluate whether psychological disorders contribute to the development of physical disorders. If psychological disorders are true causal factors, this has a number of
implications for population health, prevention research, and medicine. For example, many psychological disorders onset and become apparent earlier in the life course than chronic diseases of
adulthood. This would suggest that early surveillance and prevention strategies might effectively

reduce or delay the burden of not only psychological but also physical disorders. However, limited resources have been allocated to such efforts, as biomedicine often considers mental health as separate from, or an artefact of, physical health. Moreover, due to scepticism around whether individuals with high levels of distress are truly more vulnerable to physical disease, many physicians dismiss such patients as 'worried well',[8] thereby missing additional opportunities for intervention. Scepticism stems from several sources. Primary concerns revolve around potential reverse causality (e.g. physical illness leads to psychological distress); the third variable problem (e.g. a gene or combination of genes lead to both psychological and physical disturbances); and that physical symptoms may simply be by-products of affect.

Mental disorders have been linked to numerous diseases, including cancer,[9] respiratory,[10] and gastrointestinal[11] disorders. However, the most extensive and rigorous research has been conducted in relation to cardiovascular disease (CVD), a leading cause of death worldwide.[12] Accordingly, for the remainder of the chapter we consider the role of mental disorders in relation to development of two primary forms of CVD: stroke and coronary heart disease (CHD). Research on CVD has been particularly active in part because onset, triggering, and exacerbation can each be clearly identified, and also because other risk factors are well known, so the role of potential confounders can be carefully considered.

26.2 Mental disorder and the emergence of CVD

The international INTERHEART study reported a population attributable risk for acute myocardial infarction of 32.5% for psychosocial distress after accounting for eight other frequently occurring risk factors.[13] This places psychological distress behind only lipids and smoking in importance among the nine major modifiable CHD risk factors. Various forms of psychological distress are widespread in the population, with estimates of lifetime prevalence of anxiety or mood disorders ranging from 20% to 30% in the USA.[14] Thus, these and related psychological disorders have tremendous population health importance not only because they signal poor mental health but also because they influence physical health. If chronic psychosocial distress could be reliably alleviated or prevented, a significant proportion of new cases of CVD might also be prevented.

The growing field of life course epidemiology has brought increasing attention to the early childhood roots of adult health and disease.[15] In a recent national policy statement, the American Heart Association highlighted evidence that early manifestations of cardiometabolic disease are detectable even in childhood.[16] A stronger emphasis on primordial prevention with the goal of preventing the development of CVD risk factors in the first place has heightened awareness of the importance of childhood risk factors. Generally the focus has been on behavioural and lifestyle factors, not on mental disorders or psychological distress. However, a primordial prevention perspective is highly consistent with consideration of the role of mental disorders in CVD, as many mental disorders onset relatively earlier in life and also increase the likelihood of risk related behaviours and physiological dysregulation that contribute to CVD.[17]

Much of the evidence linking mental disorders with CVD comes from adult populations, with more limited work considering whether early manifestations of mental disorders may lead to subsequent cardiovascular dysregulation. Thus, we begin with an overview of the adult literature, prioritizing prospective epidemiological studies that use the strongest methods available for assessing associations. These include measuring psychological disorder in otherwise healthy individuals, and assessing disease risk or endpoints over multiple years of follow-up. We then consider the emerging literature that investigates the impact of psychological functioning earlier in life on subsequent cardiovascular risk markers and pre-disease conditions. Finally, we highlight key issues remaining to be resolved including the degree to which timing of onset and chronicity of psychological distress influence CVD risk, and how early in life physiological dysregulation due to psychological dysfunction becomes evident.

26.3 **Mental disorders and CVD risk in adult populations**

Much of the research on mental disorders and CVD has focused on depression. By 2002, a meta-analysis including 11 published studies demonstrated a strong positive association between depression and incident CHD, with a relative risk (RR) of 2.69 (95% confidence interval (CI): 1.63–4.43) for individuals with clinically relevant levels of depression and a RR of 1.49 (95% CI: 1.16–1.92) for individuals with depressed mood.[18] These risk estimates are comparable to risk conferred by active and passive smoking (RRs of 2.5 and 1.25 respectively).[19] Since this meta-analysis, more than 30 new prospective studies and numerous new meta-analyses or reviews of the relationship between depression and stroke or CHD have been conducted, all with highly similar findings.[20] Most studies have identified a dose–response relationship whereby risk is increased as depressive symptoms increase, and effects are evident not only among those with clinically relevant levels of depression (as initially hypothesized), but also among those with sub-clinical levels of depressive symptoms.

Though less research has examined this association, anxiety has also been consistently linked with increased risk of CVD, and some studies have suggested that it is as potent or perhaps more potent a risk factor for CVD than is depression.[21] The first meta-analysis to consider prospective studies of anxiety with incident CHD recently identified 21 studies comprising almost 250,000 persons followed over a mean of 11.2 years.[22] Independent of demographic, biological, and behavioural factors, individuals with anxiety consistently had significantly higher risk of incident CHD (pooled hazard ratio (HR): 1.26; 95% CI: 1.15–1.38) and cardiac death (HR: 1.48; 95% CI: 1.14–1.92). Findings from studies conducted since the meta-analysis are highly consistent with these estimates. For example, in a prospective study conducted among more than 49,000 Swedish men (aged 18–20 years at baseline), compared to those with no anxiety at baseline, men with physician-diagnosed anxiety had more than double the risk of developing CHD during 37 years of follow-up (adjusted HR: 2.17; 95% CI: 1.28–3.67).[21] A key strength of this study is the young age of participants at baseline among whom subclinical atherosclerosis is less likely to be present, which renders reverse causation less probable.

PTSD is linked closely with both anxiety and depression and has long been hypothesized to be associated with development of CVD; however, the prospective association of PTSD and CHD has been rigorously examined in only three population-based studies. Findings in these three studies are highly consistent with those from studies on anxiety or depression and CHD.[23–25] More limited work has considered other psychological disorders in relation to CVD risk. Several cross-sectional studies report a strong association of CVD with bipolar disorder,[26] and schizo-phrenia;[27] compared with the general population, individuals with these disorders have shorter life expectancies, mostly due to excess cardiovascular mortality.[28] However, such effects may be because patients with serious mental illness are less commonly monitored or treated for cardio-vascular risk factors such as high blood pressure or cholesterol.[29] Though rare, findings from pro-spective studies in this area are consistent with the cross-sectional evidence. For example, a recent birth cohort study (n = 12,939) with more than 30 years of adult follow-up, found that individuals with schizophrenia had increased risk of hospitalization for CHD (HR: 1.63; 95% CI: 1.03–2.57), CHD mortality (HR: 2.92; 95% CI: 1.70–5), and a trend among women to have increased stroke-related mortality (HR: 3.84; 95% CI: 0.92–15.96).[30]

Most studies consider each mental disorder in isolation as a risk factor, although many of these disorders are highly comorbid. Whether each disorder is uniquely associated with CVD or if associations are due to features the disorder shares with other forms of emotional dysregulation has not been established. Studies of PTSD have generally found an association with CVD even after adjusting for levels of depression.[24,31] A few studies have considered effects of mania as separate from major depression; one study found that a history of manic or hypomanic episodes was prospectively associated with increased incidence of myocardial infarction or congestive heart failure (OR: 2.97; 95% CI: 1.40–6.34), independent of major depressive episodes.[32] However, due to methodological challenges and data limitations, studies in this area are few and additional work is needed to more fully assess these relationships.

26.4 **A life course perspective on mental disorders and CVD risk**

Investigators have begun to consider whether risk of CVD-related conditions can be identified earlier in the life course by evaluating early psychological functioning.[33] A life course approach provides a number of advantages. First, such evidence can help to reduce concerns about reverse causality by more convincingly establishing the temporal ordering. In addition, this approach can make it easier to account for potential time-varying confounding that may bias estimates of the effect. Such bias is possible when the behaviours and risk factors that are affected by psychological disorders may also increase risk of these disorders. Finally, life course approaches are essential to intervention design, as they help to identify where and when exposures have the highest impact.[34]

Most of the ongoing prospective cohorts with psychological measures obtained early in life are still too young to present with clinical CVD endpoints. Thus, existing studies have used various methods to evaluate when effects may become apparent. Some work has considered whether psychological disorders in younger adult samples are associated with dysregulated cardiovascular biological function prior to onset of manifest CVD. To assess how early risk may become evident, recent work considers measures of psychological functioning in childhood in relation to dysregulated cardiovascular biological function in adulthood. Frequently used biomarkers of cardiovascular risk include measures of inflammation (e.g. C-reactive protein (CRP), interleukin-6 (IL-6), fibrinogen), metabolic function (e.g. lipids such as high density lipoprotein cholesterol, triglycerides), and cardiovascular function (e.g. blood pressures).

Studies of depression and inflammatory markers provide the strongest evidence linking mental disorders with cardiovascular risk biomarkers. A recent meta-analysis reported an overall effect size of 0.15 for CRP (95% CI: 0.10–0.21) and 0.25 for IL-6 (95% CI: 0.18–0.31) across 51 cross-sectional clinical and community studies.[35] However, cross-sectional studies cannot determine the direction of effects. One of the few available prospective studies reported a unidirectional effect of depression on CRP in a population-based study of youths with repeated measures of depression and CRP during nine waves.[36] Other prospective studies have documented a bidirectional relationship[37] or a unidirectional effect from CRP to depression.[38] Varying findings may be due in part to differences in the age of participants, methods of assessing depression, or number and timing of measurements across studies.

Relationships between mental health and other markers of cardiovascular risk have also been documented among adults. For example, several studies have found that depression is prospectively associated with biological components of the metabolic syndrome.[39] While some evidence has suggested that anxiety symptoms (or disorders) are associated with elevated inflammation,[40] and cholesterol levels,[41] findings are somewhat inconsistent. For example, several studies have reported an *inverse* association between anxiety and inflammation.[42]

Other longitudinal studies have assessed the relationship between aspects of childhood psychological functioning and cardiovascular risk biomarkers in adulthood. In one study, poor emotional functioning assessed at age 7 years was associated with higher CRP at age 42 years even after adjustment for relevant covariates, including child health status.[17] Additionally, prospective studies have found associations between child mental health problems and cardiovascular-related conditions assessed in adulthood. For example, childhood hyperactivity among 708 girls aged 3–9 years predicted greater systolic blood pressure and carotid artery intima media thickness 21 years later.[43] Numerous studies have also examined whether childhood or adolescent distress is associated with greater risk of obesity in adulthood, with findings generally indicating that associations are robust and in the expected direction.[44]

These suggest a potential childhood origin for adult cardiovascular risk associated with psychological functioning/mental disorder. Additional work has begun to assess how early in life physiological alterations and cardiovascular risk related to dysregulated psychological functioning may become evident. In cross-sectional studies, plasma IL-6 was marginally elevated in adolescents with a diagnosis of major depressive disorder[45] and higher levels of salivary IL-6 in children aged 7–12 years was associated with more depression, anxiety, impulsivity, withdrawal and distress symptoms.[46] In a prospective study of children aged 7–13 years, depression and IL-6 were measured on three occasions 6 months apart, but no main effect was found.[47] The association may be less robust in children or develop slowly over time, possibly requiring chronic poor psychological functioning or cumulative episodes.

26.5 **Mechanisms**

There are several plausible mechanisms by which poor psychological functioning could increase risk of CVD, comprising two primary pathways: biological and behavioural. For instance, mental disorders may have direct pathophysiological effects on disease risk via biological perturbations. Mental disorders may also influence disease risk indirectly by motivating harmful behaviours such as smoking, physical inactivity, or non-adherence to medical recommendations. Additionally, the link between mental disorders and CVD could be partially explained by common genetic background, changes in brain development, and epigenetic processes. In this section, however, we will focus on the best-understood links that could explain how mental disorders increase risk of CVD.

Mental disorders are characterized by high levels of distress and dysregulated emotions. Chronically dysregulated emotions and recurring high distress activate the hypothalamic–pituitary–adrenal (HPA) axis and sympathetic nervous system (SNS). In the short term, HPA activation enhances vascular reactivity, maintains blood volume, transiently activates immune system responses (and then suppresses immune response to bring immune function back to baseline), temporarily inhibits non-essential functions (e.g. growth, reproduction), and increases fuel sources in the blood including amino acids and glucose which provide energy and aid tissue repair.[48] SNS activation decreases skeletal muscle fatigue, enhances cardiac function, and also provides a quick source of glucose through increased hepatic and muscle glycogenolysis.[48] These combined actions enable the body to respond to acute stress by 'fight or flight'. However, a prolonged state of 'action preparation' can damage biological systems[49] by leading to excess 'wear and tear', and further compromising stress system elasticity (capacity to respond and rebound in response to challenge). As alterations in biological stress-regulatory systems brought on by prolonged or recurrent psychological distress might be irreversible,[50] it may be particularly important to attend to psychological functioning early in the life course.

Behaviours and lifestyle factors such as smoking, unhealthy diet, and sedentary lifestyle are widely accepted risk factors for CVD. Because these factors are consistently more prevalent among those with mental disorders compared with the general population,[51] they are frequently posited to be on the pathway between mental disorders and CVD. However, risk estimates of effects of mental disorders on CVD are typically derived from studies that control for such behaviours, and therefore are likely to be underestimates. It is generally assumed that mental disorders *lead* to poor health behaviours,but, research suggests that the relationship is likely bidirectional. There have been surprisingly few prospective studies aiming to establish more clearly the temporal ordering of these associations. However, examination of the literature using a life course approach is informative. For example, a systematic review of longitudinal studies on adolescent smoking and depression revealed a bidirectional association between depression and smoking in adolescents, with a stronger effect of depression predicting later smoking.[52] In prospective studies with younger samples, childhood externalizing problems are often associated with subsequent smoking and problem drinking in adulthood.[15]

26.6 Summary and future directions

Evidence is highly suggestive that mental disorders increase risk of developing CVD. However, much of the positive evidence is derived from observational studies, which are subject to a number of methodological criticisms, chiefly revolving around their ability to make clear causal inferences. Thus, a critical next step is to establish whether treatment (or prevention) of mental disorders may reduce CVD incidence. This would not only provide strong evidence that mental disorders indeed contribute to the development of CVD but would also have important clinical implications.

Most clinical trials have focused on depressive disorders, and findings have often been disappointing.[34] For example, in the Enhancing Recovery in Coronary Heart Disease (ENRICHD) trial, researchers randomized 2481 acute myocardial infarction patients to cognitive behavioural therapy (CBT) or usual care.[53] Though depression was significantly reduced in the CBT group compared with the usual care group, there were no differences in subsequent cardiovascular events or mortality. These kinds of trials present a number of challenges. Most are conducted within CVD patient populations rather than initially healthy individuals.[54] This is a conservative test of the hypothesis, as it is unclear whether mitigating distress at this late stage could effectively limit or reverse further damage. We know of no studies that have examined whether successful treatment of mental disorder within a CVD-free population effectively reduces risk of developing CVD.

The possible role of psychotropic medications in the association between mental disorders and CVD is also controversial. Some studies have found individuals on anti-depressants to be at *higher* risk of developing CHD.[55] Such findings could indicate either that psychotropic medication itself increases CVD risk directly, that use of psychotropic medication is an indicator of more severe mental disorder which drives CVD risk, or that once mental disorder is established treatment cannot mitigate risk (e.g. biological damage is irreversible). However, distinguishing between these possibilities is difficult as findings are largely obtained from observational studies in which individuals are not randomly assigned to antidepressant treatment and treatment effectiveness is not evaluated. One meta-analysis of four rigorous randomized controlled trials in depressed patients with CHD has suggested that selective serotonin reuptake inhibitor (SSRI) use is not associated with increased CVD risk,[56] whereas other work has suggested that SSRI use may be associated with *lower* risk.[57] Investigators have speculated that antidepressants may induce an anti-inflammatory response regardless of whether depressive symptoms effectively resolve.[58] Such studies, however, cannot assess whether successful resolution of depressive symptoms (non-pharmacologically) would also lead to reduced inflammation.

A longstanding hypothesis on the association between depression or anxiety and CVD is that it is an artefact of shared genetic factors. Affective and anxiety disorders as well as CVD are multi-factorial diseases and are likely influenced by numerous genes and their interactions. However, it has been difficult to locate reliable genetic influences of phenotypes related to anxiety or depres-sive disorders in recent genome-wide association studies.[59] Moreover, no studies to date have provided clear evidence that the association between mental disorders and CVD is primarily due to shared genetic influences. Thus, the limited evidence casts doubt on the likelihood that shared genetic pathways will provide a strong explanation of the association.

Investigators have increasingly highlighted the importance of applying a life course perspective when assessing the relationship between mental and physical disorders and devising strategies for prevention and intervention.[34] For example, findings from clinical trials may be mixed because we do not yet know the most appropriate aetiological window for treatment. We know little about whether there is a sensitive period during which onset of mental disorder is particularly toxic for subsequent physical health, whether effects are largely a function of chronicity of the disorder, or what happens if the mental disorder resolves. This is because even among the studies that consider timing of onset of mental disorder, most have relied on a single snapshot measure of childhood mental health and could not assess whether effects of sustained dysfunction differ from more limited exposure.

A life course approach, by integrating across a range of evidence gathered during both child-hood and adulthood, may also sharpen the focus on key elements in the relationship between mental disorders and CVD. For example, this perspective suggests the importance of emotion regulation. Dysregulation, a core feature of many mental disorders, may emerge early, as a major task of childhood is developing the ability to regulate emotions.[60] Several recent studies that have considered capacity to regulate emotions more explicitly have documented that individuals with better regulatory capacity have a significantly reduced risk (20–60% less) of developing CHD.[61,62] A life course approach also permits consideration of the role of the broader social environment. Extensive research documents the relationship between early social adversity and adult dis-ease,[63] as well as the relationship between early adversity and adult mental disorders.[64] Whether social adversity and mental disorders have independent effects on adult cardiovascular health or whether effects of early social environments are expressed in part through mental health remains to be determined.

In summary, it is well established that mental and physical disorders are highly comorbid. Evidence strongly indicates that mental disorders often precede and contribute to the develop-ment of physical disorders, and research seeking to establish a causal role of mental disorders in the emergence of physical disorders is coming of age. This work suggests several further steps for the next generation of research, including: the incorporation of a life course perspective to address key issues regarding how early in the life course cardiotoxic effects of mental disorders become evident; whether there are sensitive periods for these effects; and the role of duration, chronic-ity and, more generally, trajectory of mental disorders in relation to whether and when physical disorders emerge. Early identification of CVD (and other chronic disease) risk may be possible by careful monitoring of individuals at high risk for mental disorders. Treatment of mental disorders may directly reduce risk of CVD. Even if completely successful treatment of mental disorders is not possible, persons with these disorders may benefit from greater surveillance of CVD risk factors and early interventions (e.g. statins) to prevent the development of CVD. Thus, a focus on mental disorders as potential early indicators of physical morbidity and premature mortality could provide a number of exciting new directions for prevention and intervention. Benefits of understanding this relationship may stretch well beyond reducing the burden of CVD to numerous other chronic disease outcomes. In addition, greater appreciation of the interplay between mental and physical disorders might encourage additional allocation of funds to treat mental disorders in the service of reducing health care costs related to both mental and physical health.

References

1 Archer J. *Every man his own doctor*. London; 1673.

2 Allport GW. *Pattern and growth in personality*. New York: Holt, Rinehart & Winston; 1961.

3 Harvey W. *Exercitatio anatomica de motu cordis et sanguinis* [An anatomical exercise concerning the movement of heart and blood]. London: Baillière, Tindall & Cox; 1928.

4 Alexander FG, French TM, Pollock GH. *Psychosomatic specificity: experimental study and results*. Chicago: University of Chicago Press; 1968.

5 Walker J, Sharpe M, Wessely S. Commentary: symptoms not associated with disease: an unmet public health challenge. *Int J Epidemiol* 2006;**35**(2):477–478.

6 Scott KM, Bruffaerts R, Tsang A, et al. Depression–anxiety relationships with chronic physical conditions: results from the World Mental Health Surveys. *J Affect Disord* 2007;**103**(1–3):113–120.

7 van't Spijker A, Trijsburg RW, Duivenvoorden HJ. Psychological sequelae of cancer diagnosis: a meta-analytical review of 58 studies after 1980. *Psychosom Med* 1997;**59**(3):280–293.

8 Gurmankin Levy A, Maselko J, Bauer M, Richman L, Kubzansky L. Why do people with an anxiety disorder utilize more nonmental health care than those without? *Health Psychol* 2007;**26**(5):545–553.

9 Knekt P, Raitasalo R, Heliovaara M, et al. Elevated lung cancer risk among persons with depressed mood. *Am J Epidemiol* 1996;**144**(12):1096–1103.

10 Goodwin RD, Sourander A, Duarte CS, et al. Do mental health problems in childhood predict chronic physical conditions among males in early adulthood? Evidence from a community-based prospective study. *Psychol Med* 2009;**39**(2):301–311.

11 Drossman DA, Camilleri M, Mayer EA, Whitehead WE. AGA technical review on irritable bowel syndrome. *Gastroenterology* 2002;**123**(6):2108–2131.

12 World Health Organization. *Cardiovascular diseases: fact sheet 317 2012*. <http://www.who.int/mediacentre/factsheets/fs317/en/index.html>

13 Yusuf S, Hawken S, Ounpuu S, et al. Effect of potentially modifiable risk factors associated with myocardial infarction in 52 countries (the INTERHEART study): case–control study. *Lancet* 2004;**364**(9438):937–952.

14 Kessler RC, Berglund P, Demler O, Jin R, Merikangas KR, Walters EE. Lifetime prevalence and age-of-onset distributions of DSM-IV disorders in the National Comorbidity Survey Replication. *Arch Gen Psychiatry* 2005;**62**(6):593–602.

15 von Stumm S, Deary IJ, Kivimaki M, Jokela M, Clark H, Batty GD. Childhood behavior problems and health at midlife: 35-year follow-up of a Scottish birth cohort. *J Child Psychol Psychiatry* 2011;**52**(9): 992–1001.

16 Lloyd-Jones DM, Hong Y, Labarthe D, et al. Defining and setting national goals for cardiovascular health promotion and disease reduction: the American Heart Association's strategic Impact Goal through 2020 and beyond. *Circulation* 2010;**121**(4):586–613.

17 Appleton AA, Buka SL, McCormick MC, et al. Emotional functioning at age 7 years is associated with C-reactive protein in middle adulthood. *Psychosom Med* 2011;**73**(4):295–303.

18 Rugulies R. Depression as a predictor for coronary heart disease. *Am J Prev Med* 2002;**23**(1):51–61.

19 Wulsin LR, Singal BM. Do depressive symptoms increase the risk for the onset of coronary disease? A systematic quantitative review. *Psychosom Med* 2003;**65**(2):201–210.

20 Van der Kooy K, van Hout H, Marwijk H, Marten H, Stehouwer C, Beekman A. Depression and the risk for cardiovascular diseases: systematic review and meta analysis. *Int J Geriatr Psychiatry* 2007;**22**(7):613–626.

21 Janszky I, Ahnve S, Lundberg I, Hemmingsson T. Early-onset depression, anxiety, and risk of subsequent coronary heart disease: 37-year follow-up of 49,321 young Swedish men. *J Am Coll Cardiol* 2010;**56**(1):31–37.

22 Roest AM, Martens EJ, de Jonge P, Denollet J. Anxiety and risk of incident coronary heart disease: a meta-analysis. *J Am Coll Cardiol* 2010;**56**(1):38–46.

23 Boscarino JA. A prospective study of PTSD and early-age heart disease mortality among Vietnam veterans: implications for surveillance and prevention. *Psychosom Med* 2008;**70**(6):668–676.

24 Kubzansky LD, Koenen KC, Jones C, Eaton WW. A prospective study of posttraumatic stress disorder symptoms and coronary heart disease in women. *Health Psychol* 2009;**28**(1):125–130.

25 Dirkzwager AJ, van der Velden PG, Grievink L, Yzermans CJ. Disaster-related posttraumatic stress disorder and physical health. *Psychosom Med* 2007;**69**(5):435–440.

26 Beyer J, Kuchibhatla M, Gersing K, Krishnan KR. Medical comorbidity in a bipolar outpatient clinical population. *Neuropsychopharmacology* 2005;**30**(2):401–404.

27 Bresee LC, Majumdar SR, Patten SB, Johnson JA. Prevalence of cardiovascular risk factors and disease in people with schizophrenia: a population-based study. *Schizophr Res* 2010;**117**(1):75–82.

28 Hennekens CH, Hennekens AR, Hollar D, Casey DE. Schizophrenia and increased risks of cardiovascular disease. *Am Heart J* 2005;**150**(6):1115–1121.

29 Hippisley-Cox J, Parker C, Coupland C, Vinogradova Y. Inequalities in the primary care of patients with coronary heart disease and serious mental health problems: a cross-sectional study. *Heart* 2007;**93**(10):1256–1262.

30 Callaghan RC, Khizar A. The incidence of cardiovascular morbidity among patients with bipolar disorder: a population-based longitudinal study in Ontario, Canada. *J Affect Disord* 2010;**122**(1–2):118–123.

31 Kubzansky LD, Koenen KC, Spiro A, 3rd, Vokonas PS, Sparrow D. Prospective study of posttraumatic stress disorder symptoms and coronary heart disease in the Normative Aging Study. *Arch Gen Psychiatry* 2007;**64**(1):109–116.

32 Ramsey CM, Leoutsakos JM, Mayer LS, Eaton WW, Lee HB. History of manic and hypomanic episodes and risk of incident cardiovascular disease: 11.5 year follow-up from the Baltimore Epidemiologic Catchment Area Study. *J Affect Disord* 2010;**125**(1–3):35–41.

33 Miller GE, Chen E, Parker KJ. Psychological stress in childhood and susceptibility to the chronic diseases of aging: moving toward a model of behavioral and biological mechanisms. *Psychol Bull* 2011;**137**(6):959–997.

34 Berkman LF. Social epidemiology: social determinants of health in the United States: are we losing ground? *Annu Rev Public Health* 2009;**30**:27–41.

35 Howren MB, Lamkin DM, Suls J. Associations of depression with C-reactive protein, IL-1, and IL-6: a meta-analysis. *Psychosom Med* 2009;**71**(2):171–186.

36 Copeland WE, Shanahan L, Worthman C, Angold A, Costello EJ. Cumulative depression episodes predict later C-reactive protein levels: a prospective analysis. *Biol Psychiatry* 2012;**71**(1):15–21.

37 Matthews KA, Schott LL, Bromberger JT, Cyranowski JM, Everson-Rose SA, Sowers M. Are there bi-directional associations between depressive symptoms and C-reactive protein in mid-life women? *Brain Behav Immun* 2010;**24**(1):96–101.

38 Gimeno D, Kivimaki M, Brunner EJ, et al. Associations of C-reactive protein and interleukin-6 with cognitive symptoms of depression: 12-year follow-up of the Whitehall II study. *Psychol Med* 2009;**39**(3):413–423.

39 Vanhala M, Jokelainen J, Keinanen-Kiukaanniemi S, Kumpusalo E, Koponen H. Depressive symptoms predispose females to metabolic syndrome: a 7-year follow-up study. *Acta Psychiatr Scand* 2009;**119**(2):137–142.

40 Pitsavos C, Panagiotakos DB, Papageorgiou C, Tsetsekou E, Soldatos C, Stefanadis C. Anxiety in relation to inflammation and coagulation markers, among healthy adults: the ATTICA study. *Atherosclerosis* 2006;**185**(2):320–326.

41 Peter H, Hand I, Hohagen F, et al. Serum cholesterol level comparison: control subjects, anxiety disorder patients, and obsessive–compulsive disorder patients. *Can J Psychiatry* 2002;**47**(6):557–561.

42 Toker S, Shirom A, Shapira I, Berliner S, Melamed S. The association between burnout, depression, anxiety, and inflammation biomarkers: C-reactive protein and fibrinogen in men and women. *J Occup Health Psychol* 2005;**10**(4):344–362.

43 Keltikangas-Jarvinen L, Pulkki-Raback L, Puttonen S, Viikari J, Raitakari OT. Childhood hyperactivity as a predictor of carotid artery intima media thickness over a period of 21 years: the cardiovascular risk in young Finns study. *Psychosom Med* 2006;**68**(4):509–516.

44 Blaine B. Does depression cause obesity? A meta-analysis of longitudinal studies of depression and weight control. *J Health Psychol* 2008;**13**(8):1190–1197.

45 Gabbay V, Klein RG, Alonso CM, et al. Immune system dysregulation in adolescent major depressive disorder. *J Affect Disord* 2009;**115**(1–2):177–182.

46 Keller PS, El-Sheikh M, Vaughn B, Granger DA. Relations between mucosal immunity and children's mental health: the role of child sex. *Physiol Behav* 2010;**101**(5):705–712.

47 Caserta MT, Wyman PA, Wang H, Moynihan J, O'Connor TG. Associations among depression, perceived self-efficacy, and immune function and health in preadolescent children. *Dev Psychopathol* 2011;**23**(4):1139–1147.

48 Widmaier EP, Raff H, Strang KT, Vander AJ. *Vander's human physiology: the mechanisms of body function.* Boston, MA: McGraw-Hill; 2008.

49 Brosschot JF, Gerin W, Thayer JF. The perseverative cognition hypothesis: a review of worry, prolonged stress-related physiological activation, and health. *J Psychosom Res* 2006;**60**(2):113–124.

50 McEwen BS. Protective and damaging effects of stress mediators. *N Engl J Med* 1998;**338**(3):171–179.

51 Compton MT, Daumit GL, Druss BG. Cigarette smoking and overweight/obesity among individuals with serious mental illnesses: a preventive perspective. *Harv Rev Psychiatry* 2006;**14**(4):212–222.

52 Chaiton MO, Cohen JE, O'Loughlin J, Rehm J. A systematic review of longitudinal studies on the association between depression and smoking in adolescents. *BMC Public Health* 2009;**9**:356.

53 Berkman LF, Blumenthal J, Burg M, et al. Effects of treating depression and low perceived social support on clinical events after myocardial infarction: the Enhancing Recovery in Coronary Heart Disease Patients (ENRICHD) Randomized Trial. *JAMA* 2003;**289**(23):3106–3116.

54 Lesperance F, Frasure-Smith N, Koszycki D, et al. Effects of citalopram and interpersonal psychotherapy on depression in patients with coronary artery disease: the Canadian Cardiac Randomized Evaluation of Antidepressant and Psychotherapy Efficacy (CREATE) trial. *JAMA* 2007;**297**(4):367–379.

55 Whang W, Kubzansky LD, Kawachi I, et al. Depression and risk of sudden cardiac death and coronary heart disease in women: results from the Nurses' Health Study. *J Am Coll Cardiol* 2009;**53**(11):950–958.

56 Pizzi C, Rutjes AW, Costa GM, Fontana F, Mezzetti A, Manzoli L. Meta-analysis of selective serotonin reuptake inhibitors in patients with depression and coronary heart disease. *Am J Cardiol* 2011;**107**(7):972–979.

57 Taylor CB, Youngblood ME, Catellier D, et al. Effects of antidepressant medication on morbidity and mortality in depressed patients after myocardial infarction. *Arch Gen Psychiatry* 2005;**62**(7):792–798.

58 O'Brien SM, Scott LV, Dinan TG. Antidepressant therapy and C-reactive protein levels. *Br J Psychiatry* 2006;**188**:449–452.

59 Glahn DC, Curran JE, Winkler AM, et al. High dimensional endophenotype ranking in the search for major depression risk genes. *Biol Psychiatry* 2012;**71**(1):6–14.

60 National Research Council and Institute of Medicine. Committee on Integrating the Science of Early Childhood Development. *From neurons to neighborhoods: the science of early child development.* Shonkoff J, Phillips D, editors. Washington DC: National Academy Press; 2000.

61 **Kubzansky LD, Thurston RC.** Emotional vitality and incident coronary heart disease: benefits of healthy psychological functioning. *Arch Gen Psychiatry* 2007;**64**(12):1393–1401.

62 **Kubzansky LD, Park N, Peterson C, Vokonas P, Sparrow D.** Healthy psychological functioning and incident coronary heart disease: the importance of self-regulation. *Arch Gen Psychiatry* 2011;**68**(4): 400–408.

63 **Shonkoff JP, Garner AS.** The lifelong effects of early childhood adversity and toxic stress. *Pediatrics* 2012;**129**(1):e232–246.

64 **Clark C, Caldwell T, Power C, Stansfeld SA.** Does the influence of childhood adversity on psychopathology persist across the lifecourse? A 45-year prospective epidemiologic study. *Ann Epidemiol* 2010;**20**(5):385–394.

Part 6

Conclusions

Chapter 27

Public health, policy, and practice: implications of life course approaches to mental illness

Demetris Pillas, Kiyuri Naicker, Ian Colman,
and Clyde Hertzman

27.1 Introduction

Over the last few decades, a large theoretical and empirical evidence base has accumulated which supports the adoption of a life course approach to mental illness. This evidence has covered the different micro- and macro-levels of influence on mental illness and their varying temporal effects over the life course, as well as the pathways through which such influences operate. Knowledge of the multiple, and complexly inter-related, life course influences on mental illness is imperative as it informs us of the possibilities, and the constraints, of following a life course approach to understanding, preventing, and treating mental illness. This chapter synthesizes the evidence base and overviews the implications of adopting a life course approach to mental health policy and practice.

27.2 The multiple types of life course influences on mental illness

Scientific studies have identified multiple types of life course influences on mental illness. These can be clustered into three different types of influences: (i) influences arising from sensitive and critical periods of early life development; (ii) cumulative influences; and (iii) pathway influences.

Life course influences on mental illness arising from sensitive and critical periods of early life development comprise influences which are the product of suboptimal development of key physical, cognitive, or socio-emotional competencies during this period of the life course. Since optimal development of these specific competencies is important for the life course mental health of individuals, failure or delay in the achievement of these competencies is likely to influence an individual's long-term mental health status. In this context, 'sensitive' periods in early childhood represent the time-frame in an individual's life during which the long-term mental health effects of exposures are particularly strong, whereas 'critical' periods in early childhood refer to the time-frame in an individual's life during which the effects of experiences are not only strong but vital for the achievement of normal mental health later in the life course; if the appropriate exposures are not provided during this specific time-frame, it will ultimately be less successful, or even impossible, to achieve a healthy psychological development later in the life course.

Cumulative influences refer to multiple exposures over the life course whose effects on mental health outcomes accumulate or combine. Such effects can be cumulative because: (i) there exist multiple exposures to a single factor (e.g. a persistent negative health behaviour), or (ii) there exists a series of exposures to different factors (e.g. a persistent negative health behaviour and poverty throughout childhood and adolescence).

Pathway influences represent dependent sequences of exposures in which exposure at one stage of the life course influences the probability of exposures later in the life course, as well as associated expressions. For example, maternal postpartum depression may lead to delays in a pre-school child's socio-emotional development which may reduce that child's readiness for school, which may in turn affect school performance, which would affect later employment opportunities and the probability of developing depression and/or anxiety in adult life.

Although in the abstract sense it may be possible to differentiate between the effects of sensitive and critical periods of early life development, cumulative effects and pathway effects over the life course, in practical terms they may not be so easily distinguishable because they are strongly interconnected. Yet they provide an easily understood framework that can inform the development of an evidence-based mental health policy and practice to study, understand, prevent and treat mental illness.

27.3 Influences arising from sensitive and critical periods of early life development

Knowledge of the key periods during the life course that have the most profound influence on an individual's physical, cognitive or socio-emotional development is fundamental, as they can inform us of strategically appropriate times during which measures could be taken to prevent or limit adverse mental health outcomes. Sensitive periods in early life development highlight the time-period during which interventions must take place in order to have a stronger impact on an individual's mental health later in the life course.[1] Critical periods in early life development highlight the time-period during which the adverse effects of negative exposures may not be able to be fully remediated by providing more positive exposures at a subsequent time-point in later life. Hence, if a positive outcome is to be expected, any intervention must be performed before the termination of that time-frame.[2]

27.3.1 Importance of prevention/early intervention

Although a full understanding of how sensitive and critical periods of early life development operate in terms of mental health/illness development has yet to be achieved, evidence has now accumulated supporting the claim that many mental health conditions have their roots in early childhood. Such longitudinal associations have primarily been traced back either to a delayed neurodevelopment or to an adverse child-rearing environment.

During the last 30 years, multiple studies have established that some of the key mental illnesses, such as schizophrenia and other psychoses, depression, and anxiety are neurodevelopmental disorders whose roots can be tracked back to as early as the period of infancy.[3–9] Although such studies have not yet established a causal connection between the two time-points, they have highlighted independent associations between key indicators of delayed neurodevelopment in infancy, such as delayed achievement of independent locomotion or speech, and adolescent and adult mental health.

An adverse child-rearing environment has also been shown to be connected to subsequent risk for developing mental illness. For example, studies from North America, Western Europe, and

New Zealand have shown that poor parenting and disturbances in the relationship between the parents and the child, such as parental death, divorce or separation, inter-parental violence, and child abuse and neglect, may confer increased risk for developing mental illnesses such as panic disorder, post-traumatic stress disorder, schizophrenia, and depression and mental health problems such as suicide, violence, crime, and drug and alcohol dependence.[3,5,10-16]

Hence, providing preventive measures or intervening at an early stage of life in order to reduce the risk of developing mental illness (or alleviate the symptoms once such an illness develops), is an idea which has been steadily gaining ground within the scientific community, practitioners, and policy makers. Although the potential benefits of early intervention in reducing mental health problems have not yet been fully evaluated, an important evidence base is now being established indicating the clinical effectiveness of such interventions. This clinical effectiveness suggests improved outcomes in a number of factors which are either indicators of mental illness or which are assumed to be on the causal (life course) pathway of mental illness development, such as incidence of maltreatment and abuse, behavioural problems and developmental delay in childhood, and crime/delinquency in adolescence and adulthood.[17] For example, the High/Scope Perry Preschool Project, an early education programme targeting 3- and 4-year-old African-American children who were living in poverty and had low IQ scores, improved cognitive and educational outcomes throughout childhood and adolescence, and socio-economic and criminal outcomes, such as number of arrests for violent crimes and incarcerations in jail or prison, in adulthood.[17] This early childhood intervention was based on an active learning model with emphasis on promoting the children's intellectual, social, and emotional development through a 2.5 h daily (Monday to Friday) pre-school attendance, a weekly 1.5 h home visitation by a teacher, and monthly small-group meetings between parents.

27.3.2 The economic case for early intervention

Since public health policy decisions are always made under resource constraints, the value of public health investments must be judged, at least in part, in terms of economic efficiency. In deciding how funds should be allocated, one needs to know not only which intervention or type of treatment is the most effective, but also which of these choices brings the greatest benefits for a given set of resources. Hence, aside from the clinical effectiveness of early childhood interventions, of key importance to practitioners and policy-makers is the fact that such interventions have demonstrated cost-effectiveness and high rates of return to investment.

Recent evidence suggests that early childhood interventions are clinically effective (in terms of improved mental health outcomes) and, if adequately planned and implemented, may be cost-effective with substantial returns to investment. Early childhood interventions which were systematically evaluated in the long term, while the participating children became adults, indicated that economic benefits were maintained as the children transitioned to adulthood through performing better in direct indicators of mental health, such as criminal behaviour, as well as in factors associated with higher risk of mental illness, such us unemployment, lower earnings, and lower educational attainment.[17] Despite the non-inclusion of important mental health outcomes (aside from criminal behaviour) in such evaluations, early childhood interventions were found to accrue returns to investment which ranged from (US)$1.76 to $17.07 per $1 invested, suggesting that they are worthwhile investments.[17-23] These high rates of return, which range from 7% to 20% after adjustment for inflation, were largely due to juvenile justice savings, and are considered high enough to indicate that early childhood interventions should be portrayed not only as health development initiatives but also as economic development initiatives.[20,24,25] Although these initial findings are very encouraging, more research is necessary in this area as, aside from criminal behaviour, no published studies have included effects on mental health outcomes over such a long period in their evaluations.[26] The non-inclusion of such important, and costly, mental health outcomes in the various economic evaluations suggests that these (high) benefit-cost estimates are very likely to be underestimates.

The economic argument for early intervention gains further support if one considers the cost to society of failing to prevent a mental illness early in life or of failing to intervene during the early stages of disease onset, as the resulting cost may become disproportionate compared with the cost of investing in remediation early on. Not preventing or intervening early on can result in very high costs. For example, mental illness in children and adolescents in the UK, such as emotional and behavioural disturbances and antisocial behaviour, can accrue costs ranging from €13,000 to €65,000 annually per child.[27] These costs are disproportionately higher than the cost of early prevention or intervention, as has been highlighted in a UK-based study which estimated £70,000 per head direct societal costs of children with severe conduct disorder, but only a £600 per child cost of parent training programmes which could alleviate the disease burden.[28] Although such comparisons do not suggest cost-effectiveness, they highlight the very low costs of prevention and early intervention compared with later expenditures when the mental health problem is not addressed.

27.4 Cumulative influences

Cumulative influences are the product of cumulative exposure to risk or protective factors over the life course and can develop through different processes (Table 27.1).[29] Such influences confer cumulative risk (or cumulative protection) for developing mental illness and, hence, a large proportion of mental illness incidence is attributable to accumulation of risk. Accumulation of risk and disadvantage can have either an additive or a multiplicative effect on the incidence of mental illness. When an additive effect is produced, the incidence and/or severity of illness increase in a graded fashion with the number, frequency or intensity of adversities experienced. Multiplicative effects entail a more pronounced impact due to risk accumulation, as the combined presence of a number of risks is associated with markedly worse outcomes. For example, early life exposure to two risk factors related to child psychiatric disorders (such as maternal psychopathology, paternal criminality, severe marital discord) is associated with a four-fold increase in mental illness, whereas exposure to four risk factors is associated with a 10-fold increase.[34]

27.4.1 Targeting cumulative risk and disadvantage

Knowledge of the processes through which risk/disadvantage accumulates and interacts throughout the life course leading to mental illness provides us with the tools to predict, prevent, and treat mental illness. Despite the many challenges still surrounding the identification and quantification of risk and disadvantage, the creation of cumulative risk indices can be advantageous in terms of enhancing the mental health assessment of an individual or a group and in predicting their increased or reduced probability of developing mental illness.[35] Tools for detection of individuals or groups under cumulative risk still need refinement, although—since accumulation of risk is known to be embedded within families, ethnic groups, neighborhoods, and social classes[36,37]— prevention and treatment initiatives should aim to identify such 'clustering' of risk prior to developing and delivering a 'holistic' treatment against all identified risks.

Such advances in multivariate prediction tools for mental illness will ultimately translate to increased efficacy and efficiency in prevention and treatment of mental illness in a given population, at the same time reducing the mental health inequity gap between the deprived and the affluent, of which accumulation of risk and disadvantage is a key driver.[38] The provision of more

Table 27.1 Processes of accumulation of risk or protective effects

Type of cumulative effect	How the effect occurs	Examples
Dose–response Multiple-factor additive effects Interactive effects	Effect increases with exposure duration Effect increases with exposure intensity. Multiple risk/protective factors occurring at same/different life stages. An outcome depends on the coexistence of specific multiple factors (several intervening links are required before long-term sequelae become manifest). A factor specific to the outcome coexists with another life course factor which reduces or exaggerates the first factor's influence on the outcome	Persistent poverty having a stronger effect on mental health than poverty experienced only in early life.[30] The effect of severe bullying in childhood (as opposed to less severe) on psychotic symptoms.[31] The additive effect of poverty and collective violence on child mental health.[32] The adverse psychosocial effects of being reared in an institution depend on having an unsupportive marriage in adulthood.[33] Exposure to four or more risk factors in early life related to child psychiatric disorders (such as maternal psychopathology, paternal criminality, severe marital discord) is associated with a 10-fold increase of developing a clinical disorder.[34]

Source: data from Hertzman C, Power C, A life course approach to health and human development, in Heymann J, et al. editors, *Healthier societies: from analysis to action*. Oxford University Press, Inc., New York, pp. 83–106. Copyright © 2006.

precise evaluations regarding risk and vulnerability profiles of the different population groups comprising a specific society will improve the ability to tailor interventions to better address the precise needs of all groups within the overall population. This will consequently facilitate delivering the appropriate universal platforms (available to all individuals) in conjunction with targeted approaches (available to the identified at-risk populations). The concept of providing a combination of universal and targeted solutions, referred to as proportionate universality, has recently been suggested as being an effective approach in achieving greater health equity.[39]

27.5 Pathway influences: transitions, trajectories and chains of risk

Life course approaches to mental illness can also benefit from knowledge of the key pathway influences over the life course. Pathway influences may operate through trajectories, transitions, and chains of risk. Trajectories comprise the longitudinal patterns and sequences in an individual's life. Specific trajectories are associated with differential cumulative lifetime exposure to risk or protective factors, which may then lead to specific health events in adulthood. Transitions, however, are single events that occur within trajectories and are often age-graded, such as changes in social roles or societal status. Disease risk throughout the life course may be raised or lowered due to a sequence of temporally linked exposures (i.e. a series of events in which one negative experience leads to a series of subsequent negative experiences), which is known as the 'chain of risk' model. In the case of mental illness, chains of risk can confer increased or decreased risk through 'links' that may be social, biological, or psychological in nature. Chains of risk can operate in two distinct ways: (i) a precipitating exposure can increase the risk of subsequent exposures in the chain, as well as having an independent effect on risk of mental illness outside of those exposures, or (ii) the chain of risk may be conditional on a final 'trigger' exposure to precipitate disease onset. Without this trigger, the harmful effects of prior exposures are likely to remain minimal.[40]

27.5.1 Targeting key trajectories to mental illness

Given the complex aetiology of mental illnesses, which involves the interplay of genetic, dispositional, and environmental factors, multiple trajectories often exist for a single outcome. The longitudinal patterns and sequences that individuals may follow in their development of mental illness may differ substantially. However, this complexity in potential trajectories is characterized by a number of constants, such as individual factors necessarily operating in the context of social environments and socio-economic circumstances, with childhood conditions often being instrumental in the shaping of adult trajectories.

The existence of differential key trajectories leading to the same mental illness is well illustrated via the example of conduct disorder, in which early forms of disruptive or aggressive behaviour persist and develop into chronic and severe deviant and criminal acts. A peak of criminal activity is often observed during adolescence, followed by a subsequent steep decline throughout early and later adulthood.[41] This peak masks youth with two very different types of conduct disorder: (i) those who display chronic and persistent behavioural difficulties from early childhood (childhood onset); and (ii) those whose behaviour remains relatively normal during childhood but becomes overly rebellious during adolescence (adolescent onset).[42] Risk factors for the former disorder appear to centre around individual and family characteristics (e.g. gender, hyperactivity, family dysfunction), whereas the latter appears to be better predicted by societal and environmental factors (e.g. ethnic minority status or delinquent peers).[41–43] A wide body of research suggests that childhood onset conduct disorder involves more enduring vulnerabilities that lead to much more chronic and pervasive problems throughout the life course than the adolescent subtype.[44]

The knowledge that multiple trajectories leading to mental illness exist, of which a small number may be more prevalent than others, provides crucial information when planning interventions for mental illness. Specifically, elucidating the main trajectories which individuals may follow when developing a specific mental illness is fundamental, as it informs practitioners of the key risk factors and periods of the life course (associated with that specific trajectory) where interventional efforts must be emphasized in order to achieve the best results. Additionally, the knowledge that certain individuals may follow trajectories to mental illness that may be divergent from the main trajectories suggests that practitioners should occasionally follow individualized elements of intervention.

27.5.2 Targeting key periods of transition

Transitional events create the need to adapt to a new set of life circumstances and can be so sudden and influential that they transform life trajectories. Many transitional events (e.g. job loss, having a child, death of a spouse) are of elevated importance to an individual's life course mental health development, explaining why pathways to mental illness are often precipitated by major life or role transitions. Knowledge of the key transitional points over the life course that influence the development of mental illness is, therefore, imperative as it provides strategic junctions for primary prevention.

There are many examples where intervening/providing preventive measures at key transitional points in the life course alleviates the heightened risk and burden of developing mental illness. One key transitional pathway where such measures have been found to be beneficial is the pathway from job loss to impaired emotional and physical functioning. In this pathway, financial strain mediates the relationship between job loss and depression, and personal control mediates the negative effects of financial strain and depression on subsequent health outcomes.[45] Hence, interventions aimed at increasing personal control in the unemployed have the potential to minimize risk of future poor health. This has been demonstrated through the provision of tailored job-search (JOBS) workshops which resulted in participants achieving significantly higher levels of employment and monthly income, fewer depressive episodes, and better emotional functioning than the control group.[46] One of the key transitions for many children, the divorce or separation of their parents, also provides a key target period for prevention/intervention programmes. Parental divorce in early life is associated with behaviour and achievement problems in middle childhood and early adolescence, and the onset of psychiatric disorders later in life.[47,48] Programmes which focused on improving the mother–child relationship, building coping skills, improving father's access to the child, and on reducing inter-parental conflict have been associated with lower rates of psychiatric symptoms, substance abuse, and sexual partners six years later as adolescents.[49]

27.5.3 **Breaking the chain of risk**

The interlocking nature of trajectories and transitions across the life course generates many opportunities to modify the development of mental illness over the life course. A large evidence base supports the need for policies and interventions that address the multifactorial and lifelong nature of mental illness and that build on the established protective factors and the development of resilience to risk. Policies and interventions that feature these characteristics have demonstrated substantial benefits in mental health outcomes at the individual, family, community, and societal level.

27.5.3.1 Targeting the complex multifactorial nature of mental illness

For the vast majority of mental illnesses, important aetiological contributors include a host of genetic, dispositional, and environmental factors. For example, recognized risks for conduct disorder range from low serotonin levels, a low resting heart rate, and prenatal exposure to teratogens, to deficits in executive functioning, impulsivity, ineffective discipline, and association with deviant peers.[42] According to the National Institute for Mental Health, for many mental disorders, the presence of multiple risk factors is necessary, and the greater the number of risk factors an individual is exposed to, the greater the chances of developing a serious mental disorder. Also, specific risk factors are more widespread and serious than others (i.e. they have a high likelihood of leading to a number of distinct disorders).[50] This highlights the need for interventions that provide both comprehensive (i.e. able to address multiple risk factors) and individualized elements. An interdisciplinary approach to intervention is also recommended since, in addition to biological, psychological, and relational factors, it is also important to consider institutional, historical, and geographical dimensions when interpreting developmental dynamics across the life course.[51]

The complex multifactorial nature of mental illness also highlights the importance of multilevel and multimodal approaches to intervention. For example, early development interventions that combine comprehensive family support (e.g. parental skills training, material assistance, and home visits) with early education (e.g. provision of educational day-care or pre-school attendance) reveal the former component to be associated with reduced family risks, and the latter to be associated with reduced child risks.[52] Administered together, these components yield improved outcomes in regard to chronic delinquency while achieving long-term prevention through short-term protective effects on multiple risk factors.[52] Similarly, multi-faceted approaches to suicidality prevention consisting of interventions on four levels (i.e. primary care physicians, public relations campaigns, community facilitators, and affected persons/high risk groups) have demonstrated substantial reductions in suicides and suicidal behaviour in intervention regions.[53] In addition to a 24% reduction achieved during the two intervention years (a 53% reduction in the five most lethal acts), such programmes achieved a 32% decline in overall suicidality in the subsequent non-intervention year, indicating the potential for sustained and persistent effects of comprehensive, multi-pronged programmes.

27.5.3.2 Providing support over the life course

As previously discussed, precipitating risks for poor mental health may yield outcomes that manifest themselves much later in the life course. Child abuse, for example, can negatively impact one's scholastic performance, the regularity and quality of future employment, participation in leisure activities, the ability to form and maintain supportive social relationships, and the formation of healthy self-concepts throughout adulthood.[54] Similarly, although bullying victimization is a risk factor that contributes significantly to childhood psychopathology, its effects last well into late adolescence.[55] Serious stressors may exert effects later in life through the mechanism of stress proliferation, in which a single primary stressor gives rise to additional secondary stressors.[54] In support of this theory, studies show that children subjected to physical abuse or neglect experience a significantly higher number of deleterious life events (e.g. unemployment, homelessness, hospitalization) twenty years later than non-abused children.[56] The associations between early trauma and adult mental illness in this group of individuals were almost entirely accounted for by the presence of stressful life events in adulthood, indicating that proliferated secondary stressors in some cases contribute more to mental health outcomes than the primary event itself.[54]

These findings point to the need for interventionists and policy-makers to focus their efforts not entirely on addressing proximal outcomes of risk, but rather on targeting the longer-term confluence of physical, environmental, and societal difficulties faced by specific subpopulations. In support of this intervention strategy, reviews of early childhood development interventions indicate that, for these programmes to yield economic benefits, they must provide continuous support and be sustained in the long term, while maintaining an adequate level of support for at least the most disadvantaged children and families over the long term.[26] Cost-effective means of providing ongoing interventions to high risk groups may be becoming increasingly feasible through technological means, as many Internet mental health interventions (both therapist-led as well as self-directed online therapies) have reported promising results in alleviating disorder-related symptomatology[57] and have been used to provide effective follow-up care to inpatient group therapy.[58] Short message service (SMS) texts have also yielded promising results in improving the achievement of individuals suffering from schizophrenia on a number of relevant goals by compensating for the effects of cognitive impairments,[59] and provide an efficacious means of maintaining treatment gains in eating disorder patients following discharge.[60]

27.5.3.3 Building on protective factors and resilience to risk

Resilience can be defined as the process of dynamic positive adaptation in the face of adversity[61] and is linked to protective factors that are both intrinsic and extrinsic to an individual. Protective factors may mediate or moderate the effects of exposure to risk[62] and, as in the case of risk factors, can have a cumulative effect. The greater the number of protective factors to which individuals are exposed, the more resilient to a range of mental illnesses they are likely to be.[63] The concept of resilience is generally applied to three kinds of phenomena: (i) positive health outcomes despite high risk status; (ii) sustained competence under adversity; and (iii) successful recovery from trauma.[64] From a life course perspective, the question of whether resilience during development has long-term health and economic benefits remains understudied.[40] However, in light of the growing realization that the simple absence of psychological distress is not in itself indicative of good mental health or adequate social functioning,[65] it is a question that merits thorough investigation by researchers and policy-makers alike.

Protective factors may be highly context dependent and culturally specific. For example, while supportive parental relationships confer resilience to children in the face of poverty, they do not provide a buffer against high risk school systems. However, parental educational aspirations can confer educational resilience to children in low income families.[66] Similarly, whereas the presence of adequate social support is essential to psychological well-being, the protective effects of social ties do not operate uniformly across all groups in society. Social connections among women with low resources may paradoxically increase levels of mental illness symptoms, especially if these connections entail cultural obligations to provide social support to others.[67] Optimism and perceived control provide significant protection against depression in the face of stress exposure in economically disadvantaged women,[68] both of which may be successfully targeted through culturally relevant interventions. In certain cases, it is not objective socio-economic status (SES) that has a direct association with mental illness, but rather perceived social status (a subjective measure which might be more amenable to interventions than the more absolute aspects of SES).[69] While mechanisms of resilience as a whole are generally viewed as positive, they may under certain circumstances prove to be maladaptive further at a later stage of the life course. For example, foetal adaptation for survival in suboptimal early-life environments (e.g. malnutrition) can generate vulnerability to later-life psychological impairments (e.g. depression) through lasting physiological changes.[70,71]

Evidence suggests that effective prevention strategies for mental illnesses require attention to both risk and protective factors (i.e. building up protection while reducing risk), and their reach should span from individual vulnerabilities to broad social norms. For example, a multicomponent prevention strategy for adolescent drug misuse needs to support factors such as parenting skills, scholastic achievement, peer influences, and classroom or institutional attitudes towards drug use.[62] Currently, relatively few policies focus on cultivating protective factors and building resilience in individuals and children, as well as communities at large. This is partially due to the fact that mental health resources are often scarce, and largely diverted downstream to address urgent issues of intervention and treatment. In addition, departmentalized or 'silo' funding schemes (e.g. for health services, social services, or mental health services) by their nature do not support comprehensive, integrated strategies.[72] Because of the multiple factors contributing to resilience and the challenges still faced in its operationalization and assessment, it is difficult for policy-makers to focus their efforts on effective solutions.[72]

27.6 **Summary**

Life course approaches to mental illness carry important implications for mental health policy and practice. Knowledge of the multiple and complexly inter-related effects arising from sensitive and critical periods of early life development, cumulative effects, and pathway effects which influence the development of mental illness throughout the life course is imperative, as it not only provides a comprehensive understanding of how mental illness develops, but it also informs scientists, practitioners, and policy-makers of the possibilities and the constraints when aiming to prevent or alleviate the burden of mental illness.

Through providing an overview of the main ways through which life course approaches may influence mental health policy and practice, this chapter highlights a number of key approaches and strategies to improving the effectiveness, and cost-effectiveness, of policies aiming to address mental illness. Based on knowledge of sensitive and critical periods, the importance of investing in early life prevention/intervention is identified as a key strategy in reducing the probability of mental illness developing later in the life course. Identifying the processes through which risk and disadvantage accumulate and interact throughout the life course, as well as the groups where accumulation of risk is most likely to be embedded, enables mental health interventions to develop more efficient and effective approaches to tackling mental illness. Finally, targeting the relevant life course trajectories and transitions and aiming to break the chains of risk leading to mental illness improve the probability of mental health interventions being effective.

A substantial, theoretical, and practical evidence base has already accumulated in support of all the above life course approaches to mental health policy and practice. However, due to the complexity of the interrelationships of these approaches, the multifactorial nature and the context and culture specificity of mental illness, it is necessary for even more evidence-based research to be performed on this topic. Although a number of interventions following these approaches have already been performed, evaluated, and identified as being clinically effective and/or cost-effective, it is evident that this number covers only a small proportion of the potentially available interventions. The rapidly increasing interest and focus in life course approaches to mental illness, and illness in general, from both scientists and practitioners, ensures that the mechanisms of developing mental illness throughout the life course will be further elucidated in the near future, and that interventional and preventive measures will be further refined to provide the most optimal clinically effective and cost-effective solutions.

Further Reading

Elder GH, Shanahan MJ. The life course and human development. In: Lerner R, Damon W, editors. *The handbook of child psychology*, 6th ed. New York: Wiley; 2007. pp. 665–715.

Hertzman C, Power C. A life course approach to health and human development. In: Heymann J, Hertzman C, Barer ML, Evans RG, editors. *Healthier societies: from analysis to action*. New York: Oxford University Press; 2006. pp. 83–106.

Shaffer A, Yates TM. Identifying and understanding risk factors and protective factors in clinical practice. In: Compton M, editor. *Clinical manual of prevention principles in mental health*. Arlington, VA: American Psychiatric Publishing; 2010. pp. 29–48.

Acknowledgements

We would like to express our grateful thanks to Professor Glen Elder who provided feedback on the chapter outline.

References

1 Fox SE, Levitt P, Nelson CA. How the timing and quality of early experiences influence the development of brain architecture. *Child Dev* 2010;**81**(1):28–40.

2 Knudsen EI. Sensitive periods in the development of the brain and behavior. *J Cogn Neurosci* 2004;**16**(8):1412–1425.

3 Jones P, Rodgers B, Murray R, Marmot M. Child development risk factors for adult schizophrenia in the British 1946 Birth cohort. *Lancet* 1994;**344**(8934):1398–1402.

4 Isohanni M, Jones PB, Moilanen K, et al. Early developmental milestones in adult schizophrenia and other psychoses. A 31-year follow-up of the North Finland 1966 Birth Cohort. *Schizophr Res*, 2001;**52**(1–2):1–19.

5 Cannon M, Caspi A, Moffitt TE, et al. Evidence for early-childhood, pan-developmental impairment specific to schizophreniform disorder: results from a longitudinal birth cohort. *Arch Gen Psychiatry* 2002;**59**(5):449–456.

6 Isohanni M, Murray GK, Jokelainen J, Croudace T, Jones PB. The persistence of developmental markers in childhood and adolescence and risk of schizophrenic psychoses in adult life. A 34-year follow-up of the North Finland 1966 Birth Cohort. *Schizophr Res* 2004;**71**(2–3):213–225.

7 Colman I, Ploubidis GB, Wadsworth ME, Jones PB, Croudace TJ. A longitudinal typology of symptoms of depression and anxiety over the life course. *Biol Psychiatry* 2007;**62**(11):1265–1271.

8 Sørensen HJ, Mortensen EL, Schiffman J, Reinisch JM, Maeda J, Mednick SA. Early developmental milestones and risk of schizophrenia: a 45-year follow-up of the Copenhagen Perinatal Cohort. *Schizophr Res* 2010;**118**(1–3):41–47.

9 Clarke MC, Tanskanen A, Huttunen M, et al. Increased risk of schizophrenia from additive interaction between infant motor developmental delay and obstetric complications: evidence from a population-based longitudinal study. *Am J Psychiatry* 2011;**168**(12):1295–1302.

10 Kendler KS, Bulik CM, Silberg J, Hettema JM, Myers J, Prescott CA. Childhood sexual abuse and adult psychiatric and substance use disorders in women: an epidemiological and cotwin control analysis. *Arch Gen Psychiatry* 2000;**57**(10):953–959.

11 Gilman SE, Kawachi I, Fitzmaurice GM, Buka SL. Family disruption in childhood and risk of adult depression. *Am J Psychiatry* 2003;**160**(5):939–946.

12 Goodwin RD, Fergusson DM, Horwood LJ. Childhood abuse and familial violence and the risk of panic attacks and panic disorder in young adulthood. *Psychol Med* 2005;**35**(6):881–890.

13 Read J, van Os J, Morrison AP, Ross CA. Childhood trauma, psychosis and schizophrenia: a literature review with theoretical and clinical implications. *Acta Psychiatr Scand* 2005;**112**(5):330–350.

14 Morgan C, Fisher H. Environment and schizophrenia: environmental factors in schizophrenia: childhood trauma—a critical review. *Schizophr Bull* 2007;**33**(1):3–10.

15 Roustit C, Renahy E, Guernec G, Lesieur S, Parizot I, Chauvin P. Exposure to interparental violence and psychosocial maladjustment in the adult life course: advocacy for early prevention. *J Epidemiol Community Health* 2009;**63**(7):563–568.

16 Weich S, Patterson J, Shaw R, Stewart-Brown S. Family relationships in childhood and common psychiatric disorders in later life: systematic review of prospective studies. *Br J Psychiatry* 2009;**194**(5): 392–398.

17 Karoly LA, Kilburn MR, Cannon JS. *Early childhood interventions: proven results, future promise.* RAND Corp, Santa Monica, CA 2005. <http://www.rand.org/pubs/monographs/2005/RAND_MG341.pdf>

18 Aos S, Lieb R, Mayfield J, Miller M, Pennucci A. *Benefits and costs of prevention and early intervention programs for youth.* Olympia: Washington State Institute for Public Policy; 2004. <http://www.wsipp.wa.gov/rptfiles/04-07-3901.pdf>

19 Wise S, da Silva L, Webster E, Sanson A. *The efficacy of early childhood interventions: a report prepared for the Australian Government Department of Family and Community Services.* Melbourne: Australian Institute of Family Studies; 2005. <http://www.aifs.gov.au/institute/pubs/resreport14/aifsreport14.pdf>

20 Penn H, Burton V, Lloyd E, Potter S, Sayeed Z, Mugford M. What is known about the long-term economic impact of centre-based early childhood interventions? Technical report. In: *Research Evidence in Education Library.* London: EPPI (Policy and Practice Information and Co-ordinating) Centre, Social

Science Research Unit, Institute of Education, University of London; 2006. <http://eppi.ioe.ac.uk/cms/ LinkClick.aspx?fileticket=l5do4A7UCSo%3D&tabid=676&mid=1572>

21 **Wolfe B, Tefft N.** *Child interventions that may lead to increased economic growth* (Early Childhood Research Collaborative Discussion Paper 111). University of Wisconsin—Madison, WI; 2007. <http://www.earlychildhoodrc.org/papers/DP111.pdf>

22 **Reynolds AJ, Temple JA.** Cost-effective early childhood development programs from preschool to third grade. *Annu Rev Clin Psychol* 2008;4:109–139.

23 **Watson J, Tully L.** *Prevention and early intervention update: trends in recent research.* Centre for Parenting & Research, New South Wales Department of Community Services, Sydney 2008. <http://www.community.nsw.gov.au/docswr/_assets/main/documents/research_earlyintervention.pdf.

24 **Burr J, Grunewald R.** *Lessons learned: a review of early childhood development studies.* Minneapolis: Federal Reserve Bank of Minneapolis; 2006. <http://www.minneapolisfed.org/publications_papers/ studies/earlychild/lessonslearned.pdf>

25 **Rolnick A, Grunewald R.** Early childhood development = economic development (Editorial). *Fedgazette* (published by the Federal Reserve Bank of Minneapolis, MN, USA), March 2003. <http://www.minneapolisfed.org/publications_papers/pub_display.cfm?id=1839>

26 **Pillas D, Suhrcke M.** *Assessing the potential or actual impact on health and health inequalities of policies aiming to improve early child development in England 2009.* London: Institute of Health Equity; 2009. <http://www.instituteofhealthequity.org/Content/FileManager/pdf/economic-early-child-development-full-report.pdf>

27 **Suhrcke M, Pillas D, Selai C.** Economic aspects of mental health in children and adolescents In: *Social cohesion for mental well-being among adolescents.* WHO/HBSC Forum. Copenhagen: WHO Regional Office for Europe; 2008. <http://www.euro.who.int/__data/assets/pdf_file/0003/76485/Hbsc_ Forum_2007_economic_aspects.pdf>

28 **Scott S, Spender Q, Doolan M, Jacobs B, Aspland H.** Multicentre controlled trial of parenting groups for childhood antisocial behaviour in clinical practice. *Br Med J* 2001;**323**(7306):194–198.

29 **Hertzman C, Power C.** A life course approach to health and human development, in Heymann J, Hertzman C, Barer ML, Evans RG, editors. *Healthier societies: from analysis to action.* New York: Oxford University Press; 2006. pp. 83–106.

30 **Strohschein L.** Household income histories and child mental health trajectories. *J Health Soc Behav* 2005;**46**(4):359–375.

31 **Schreier A, Wolke D, Thomas K, et al.** Prospective study of peer victimization in childhood and psychotic symptoms in a nonclinical population at age 12 years. *Arch Gen Psychiatry* 2009;**66**(5): 527–536.

32 **Leiner M, Puertas H, Caratachea R, et al.** Children's mental health and collective violence: a binational study on the United States–Mexico border. *Rev Pan Am Salud Publica* 2012;**31**(5):411–416.

33 **Rutter M, Quinton D, Hill J.** Adult outcome of institution-reared children: males and females compared. In: Robins LN, Rutter M, editors. *Straight and devious pathways from childhood to adulthood.* Cambridge: Cambridge University Press; 1990.

34 **Rutter M.** Protective factors in children's responses to stress and disadvantage. In: Kent MW, Rolf JE, editors. *Primary prevention of psychopathology: social competence in children,* pp. 49–62. Hanover, NH: University Press of New England; 1979.

35 **Shaffer A, Yates TM.** Identifying and understanding risk factors and protective factors in clinical practice. In: Compton M, editor. *Clinical manual of prevention principles in mental health.* Arlington, VA: American Psychiatric Publishing; 2010. pp. 29–48.

36 **Elder GH, Shanahan MJ.** The life course and human development. In: Lerner R, Damon W, editors. *The handbook of child psychology,* 6th ed. New York: Wiley; 2007. pp. 665–715.

37 **Wolff J, de-Shalit A.** *Disadvantage.* Oxford: Oxford University Press; 2007. pp. 119–132.

38 **Singh-Manoux A, Ferrie JE, Chandola T, Marmot M.** Socioeconomic trajectories across the life course and health outcomes in midlife: evidence for the accumulation hypothesis? *Int J Epidemiol* 2004;**33**(5):1072–1079.

39 **Marmot Review Team.** *Fair society, healthy lives. The Marmot Review.* Strategic Review of Health Inequalities in England post-2010, London; 2010. <http://www.instituteofhealthequity.org/projects/fair-society-healthy-lives-the-marmot-review>

40 **Kuh D, Ben-Shlomo Y, Lynch J, Hallqvist J, Power C.** Life course epidemiology. *J Epidemiol Community Health* 2003;**57**(10):778–783.

41 **Moffitt TE.** Adolescence-limited and life-course-persistent antisocial behavior: a developmental taxonomy. *Psychol Rev* 1993;**100**(4):674–701.

42 **Frick PJ.** Developmental pathways to conduct disorder. *Child Adolesc Psychiatr Clin N Am* 2006;**15**(2):311–331.

43 **McCabe KM, Hough R, Wood PA, Yeh M.** Childhood and adolescent onset conduct disorder: a test of the developmental taxonomy. *J Abnorm Child Psychol* 2001;**29**(4):305–316.

44 **Brown SA, Gleghorn A, Schuckit MA, Myers MG, Mott MA.** Conduct disorder among adolescent alcohol and drug abusers. *J Stud Alcohol* 1996;**57**(3):314–324.

45 **Price RH, Choi JN, Vinokur AD.** Links in the chain of adversity following job loss: how financial strain and loss of personal control lead to depression, impaired functioning, and poor health. *J Occup Health Psychol* 2002;**7**(4):302–312.

46 **Vinokur AD, Schul Y, Vuori J, Price RH.** Two years after a job loss: long-term impact of the JOBS program on reemployment and mental health. *J Occup health Psychol* 2000;**5**(1):32–47.

47 **Allison PD, Furstenberg FF.** How marital dissolution affects children: variations by age and sex. *Dev Psychol* 1989;**25**(4):540–549.

48 **Kessler RC, McLaughlin KA, Green JG, et al.** Childhood adversities and adult psychopathology in the WHO World Mental Health Surveys. *Br J Psychiatry* 2010;**197**(5):378–385.

49 **Wolchik SA, Sandler IN, Millsap RE, et al.** Six-year follow-up of preventive interventions for children of divorce: a randomized controlled trial. *JAMA* 2002;**288**(15):1874–1881.

50 **Reiss D, Price RH.** National research agenda for prevention research: The National Institute of Mental Health Report. *Am Psychol* 1996;**51**(11):1109–1115.

51 **Levy R, The Pavie Team.** Why look at life courses in an interdisciplinary perspective? *Adv Life Course Res* 2005;**10**:3–32.

52 **Yoshikawa H.** Prevention as cumulative protection: effects of early family support and education on chronic delinquency and its risks. *Psychol Bull* 1994;**115**(1):28–54.

53 **Hegerl U, Wittenburg L; European Alliance Against Depression Consortium.** Focus on mental health care reforms in Europe: the European alliance against depression: a multilevel approach to the prevention of suicidal behavior. *Psychiatr Serv* 2009;**60**(5):596–599.

54 **Pearlin L, Schieman S, Fazio EM, Meersman SC.** Stress, health, and the life course: some conceptual perspectives. *J Health Soc Behav* 2005;**46**(2):205–219.

55 **Arseneault L, Bowes L, Shakoor S.** Bullying victimization in youths and mental health problems: 'much ado about nothing'? *Psychol Med* 2010;**40**(5):717–729.

56 **Horwitz AV, Widom CS, McLaughlin J, White HR.** The impact of childhood abuse and neglect on adult mental health: a prospective study. *J Health Soc Behav* 2001;**42**(2):184–201.

57 **Ybarra ML, Eaton WW.** Internet-based mental health interventions. *Mental Health Serv Res* 2005;**7**(2):75–87.

58 **Golkaramnay V, Bauer S, Haug S, Wolf M, Kordy H.** The exploration of the effectiveness of group therapy through an Internet chat as aftercare: a controlled naturalistic study. *Psychother Psychosom* 2007;**76**(4):219–225.

59 Pijnenborg GH, Withaar FK, Brouwer WH, Timmerman ME, van den Bosch RJ, Evans JJ. The efficacy of SMS text messages to compensate for the effects of cognitive impairments in schizophrenia. *Br J Clin Psychol* 2010;**49**(2):259–274.

60 Bauer S, Okon E, Meermann R, Kordy H. Technology-enhanced maintenance of treatment gains in eating disorders: efficacy of an intervention delivered via text messaging. *J Consult Clin Psychol* 2012;**80**(4):700–706.

61 Luthar SS, Cicchetti D, Becker B. The construct of resilience: a critical evaluation and guidelines for future work. *Child Dev* 2000;**71**(3):543–562.

62 Hawkins JD, Catalano RF, Miller JY. Risk and protective factors for alcohol and other drug problems in adolescence and early adulthood: implications for substance abuse prevention. *Psychol Bull* 1992;**112**(1):64–105.

63 Brackenreed D. Resilience and risk. *Int Educn Stud* 2010;**3**(3):111–122.

64 Boyden J, Cooper E. Questioning the power of resilience: are children up to the task of disrupting the transmission of poverty? In: Addison T, Hulme D, Kanbur R, editors. *Poverty dynamics: interdisciplinary perspectives*. New York: Oxford University Press; 2009. pp. 289–308.

65 Hatch SL, Harvey SB, Maughan B. A developmental–contextual approach to understanding mental health and well-being in early adulthood. *Soc Sci Med* 2010;**70**(2):261–268.

66 Diewald M, Mayer KU. The sociology of the life course and life span psychology: integrated paradigm or complementing pathways? *Adv Life Course Res* 2009;**14**(1–2):5–14.

67 Kawachi I, Berkman LF. Social ties and mental health. *J Urban Health* 2001;**78**(3):458–467.

68 Grote NK, Bledsoe SE, Larkin J, Lemay EP, Brown C. Stress exposure and depression in disadvantaged women: the protective effects of optimism and perceived control. *Soc Work Res* 2007;**31**(1):19–33.

69 McLaughlin KA, Costello EJ, Leblanc W, Sampson NA, Kessler RC. Socioeconomic status and adolescent mental disorders. *Am J Public Health* 2012;**102**(9):1742–1750.

70 Hales CN, Barker DJ. The thrifty phenotype hypothesis. *Br Med Bull* 2001;**60**:5–20.

71 Räikkönen K, Pesonen AK. Early life origins of psychological development and mental health. *Scand J Psychol* 2009;**50**(6):583–591.

72 Nelson F, Mann T. Opportunities in public policy to support infant and early childhood mental health: the role of psychologists and policymakers. *Am Psychol* 2011;**66**(2):129–139.

Index